The Helen Cam Bequest.

9/6

Elizabeth Garrett Anderson

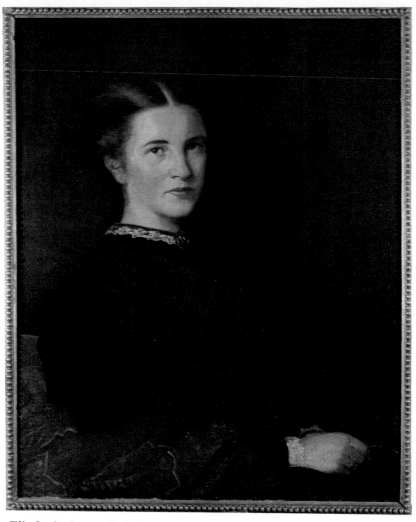

Elizabeth Garrett L.S.A. painted soon after her qualification as a doctor

Elizabeth
Garrett Anderson

by JO MANTON

METHUEN & CO LTD
11 NEW FETTER LANE · LONDON EC4

First published in 1965
© *1965 by Jo Manton*
Printed in Great Britain by
Butler and Tanner Ltd
Frome and London

To
HELEN M. CAM
C.B.E., Litt.D.

Contents

Illustrations

Illustrations

Acknowledgment for permission to reproduce illustrations is due to the following: The Misses Anderson for frontispiece, Messrs Faber & Faber for No. 1, The Radio Times Hulton Picture Post Library for Nos. 6 & 15 and the caricature on p. 222, the proprietors of *Punch* for the cartoon on p. 242, the Royal Free Hospital School of Medicine for nos. 9 & 12, Mrs M. L. Spring Rice for Nos. 4 & 5, Mr B. W. Allen for No. 2, the Elizabeth Garrett Anderson Hospital for Nos. 7 and 11*a*, and Sir Colin Anderson for the remainder.

Acknowledgments

Exactly a hundred years ago Elizabeth Garrett became a Licentiate of the Society of Apothecaries. For the first time in this country a woman had legally qualified as a doctor. She asked that no biography of her should be written and for a long time her family obeyed this command. It was not until 1939 that her daughter, Dr Louisa Garrett Anderson, published *Elizabeth Garrett Anderson*, a devoted and intimate memoir, in which she quoted, though usually in part, from many of her mother's letters. The years since then have confirmed how effectively Elizabeth Garrett Anderson changed the social history of a highly conservative profession. In her life as a wife and mother she faced problems which confront an increasing number of working wives today. Nor has her spirited charm faded with the passing of a century. For all these reasons I have ventured to attempt the life she did not want; and I am particularly grateful for the generosity and encouragement of her own descendants.

My first thanks must go to Sir Colin Anderson, who not only allowed me to use for the first time a large collection of his grandmother's unpublished papers and photographs, but has encouraged the work at every stage. Two nieces of Elizabeth Garrett Anderson, Mrs Spring Rice and Mrs Wood, and a niece and a cousin by marriage, Miss Mary Clarke and Winifreda, Countess of Portarlington, have patiently answered questions and given me much valuable first-hand information. Other nieces by marriage, the daughters of the late Dr Ford Anderson, allowed me to read their father's unpublished reminiscences, and two granddaughters, the children of Sir Alan Garrett Anderson, have given permission to reproduce the portrait which forms the frontispiece.

I should also like to thank the many institutions and individuals who have given me access to documents in their possession: the

Fawcett Society and its Librarian Miss Vera Douie for her unrivalled knowledge of the women's movement, Miss E. M. Sugden, secretary of the Elizabeth Garrett Anderson Hospital, Mrs S. C. S. Robinson, Registrar of the Royal Free Hospital School of Medicine, and Miss Woodall of the Queen Elizabeth Hospital for Children. Particulars of these documents have been given in the bibliography and references, in the hope that they may be of some use to students of the period.

For permission to reproduce unpublished documents as appendices I have to thank the following: The Dean of the Middlesex Hospital School of Medicine for Appendix I, The Worshipful Society of Apothecaries for Appendix II, The Royal College of Physicians for Appendix III and The Library of the Faculty of Medicine of the Sorbonne for Appendix IV.

Many librarians and archivists have given me skilled and generous help. I should particularly like to thank D. Charman, Esq., of the East Suffolk County Record Office, Miss Alison Reeve of the County Record Office, London, S.E.1, and Mrs Ann Saunders, archivist of the Borough of Marylebone, as well as the staffs of the Wellcome Historical Medical Library, the libraries of the Royal Colleges of Physicians and Surgeons, the Periodicals Room of the University of London Library, the Royal Free Hospital School of Medicine Library, the Guildhall Library and the Borough Libraries of Lewisham, Stepney and Marylebone. Many people have kindly answered queries on particular points, among them Professor Kathleen Tillotson, Miss Sheila Smith, Mrs Alison Aldburgham, Dr Cyril Bibby and The Rev. A. D. Browne. Any lay writer on a medical subject is dependent on the goodwill of doctors. I have been fortunate in the generosity of Dr John Sturrock, Dr Douglas Guthrie, Dr André Hahn, Dr John Bromley, Dr Norah Nicholls, Miss Louisa Martindale, F.R.C.O.G., and the late D. G. Martin, F.R.C.S. My late father-in-law, Surg-Capt F. C. B. Gittings, M.D., gave me much information about student life at the Middlesex in the nineteenth century, and it is a particular pleasure to record my debt to him.

Acknowledgments

I am grateful to E. S. Peacock, A.I.B.P., for technical assistance with old and faded photographs, to Mrs K. M. Sale and Mrs J. Findlater who typed the manuscript, and to my daughter Charlotte Johnson, who undertook the French correspondence and translation. My husband, Robert Gittings, has given invaluable advice on methods and organization of research at every stage of the work, which indeed I could not have undertaken without him. Finally, I am greatly indebted to Dr F. N. L. Poynter, Director and Chief Librarian, Wellcome Historical Medical Museum and Library, for his kindness in reading the manuscript.

Jo Manton
Chichester, 1965

PART ONE

The Medical Student

London Suffolk
1836–1841

One day in March 1841 a young man of twenty-nine named Newson Garrett brought his wife and four children by sea from London to Aldeburgh. The 200-ton Suffolk hoy had carried them a cold and comfortless journey, buffeted by the North Sea scour. Once under the high shingle bank of the River Alde, they had still to steer a nine-miles' course through brigs, wherries, drift-wood and floating sea-wrack before Aldeburgh – a sudden hill, a square embattled church tower and three windmills – appeared on the skyline. The hoy anchored off Slaughden Quay and the passengers were ferried ashore in open boats. Five-year-old Elizabeth Garrett, a Londoner born, found herself set down on a windswept jetty littered with bales and boat gear. Coastguards shouted orders which the wind snatched away. Furniture and baggage was heaved ashore and loaded into carts, the weary children following. The travellers jolted along the sandy track from the harbour, past the windmill, past the Martello tower and the fishermen's huts, past the Tudor flint and timber of Aldeburgh's Moot Hall, and up Church Hill to a new home.[1]

In coming to Aldeburgh, Elizabeth Garrett was returning to the country of her ancestors. Since the early seventeenth century the Garretts had been gunsmiths and blacksmiths in East Suffolk, hard-working, independent and strong as whipcord. There had

---

[1] White, W., *History, Gazeteer and Directory for Suffolk*, 1844, p. 173, and Clodd, E. (published anonymously), *A Guide to Aldeburgh*, 1861.

Elizabeth Garrett Anderson

always been a pioneering strain in the family. In 1636 a Puritan ancestor, Harmon Garrett, gunsmith of Wickham Market, had emigrated to New England in a party of Suffolk people led by their minister of religion. He became one of the founders of the township of Lancaster, Pennsylvania, but returned after twenty years to his native place, where he restored the church bells. His descendants worked the Wickham Market smithy until 1818, while a younger branch of the family, which passed on for seven generations the Christian name of Richard, settled at Woodbridge as makers of edge-tools. Their scythes and sickles were so renowned that blade-smiths in Sheffield had been known to forge the Garrett mark.[1]

At the end of the eighteenth century the pioneering strain reasserted itself. Richard Garrett, fourth of the name, left the old forge at Woodbridge and opened a small works at Leiston near Aldeburgh, one of the first in England to specialize in agricultural machinery. His son Richard the fifth married the daughter of a brother craftsman and inventor, John Balls.[2] This couple had three sons, Richard, Balls and Newson Garrett, the youngest, born in 1812.[3]

From the first, Newson Garrett was not the boy to be over-shadowed by elder brothers. He went to school at Grundisburgh near Woodbridge for a time, but he was a restless, impatient lad unsuited to study and he acquired remarkably little book-learning. His adult writing and spelling were a joke, in which he joined with good humour. 'What's this?' said an old schoolfellow, the mason Thomas Thurlow, thrusting back a scrawled letter into his hand. 'Well, Tom,' said Newson Garrett, after peering at it for some time, 'if you can tell me what it is about, I may be able to read it.'[4] Once he had left school Leiston offered little to young

[1] Anderson, Sir A. G., MS. draft *The Garretts of Suffolk*: Anderson family papers.
[2] He is believed to have designed the first threshing machine.
[3] Anderson, Sir A. G., op. cit.
[4] John S. Smith (Thurlow's grandson) to Dr Louisa Garrett Anderson. Thurlow made the bust of Crabbe in Aldeburgh Church.

18

Newson Garrett, since his eldest brother Richard would inherit the works and his second brother was also apprenticed as an iron-founder. So, like the youngest of three brothers in a fairy tale, and with the same boundless confidence, he set out in the world to make his fortune. Like many other ambitious young men he was drawn to London. He had already a family connection there, for in 1828 his brother Richard had married Elizabeth Dunnell, the daughter of a London innkeeper of Suffolk origin.[1]

Young Newson Garrett settled in Islington, and in the alien bustle of London made his way to his sister-in-law's parents at the Beehive Inn, Crawford Street, Marylebone.[2] He found a cheerful, prosperous house and in the landlord, John Dunnell, a man of substance. Dunnell came from a family of smallholders at Dunwich and was one of the thirty-two freemen of that famous Rotten Borough. Although he lived in London and owned at least two public houses, he still found it worth while to travel back to the crumbling village on the Suffolk coast to record his vote at elections. He was independent, even stubborn. In 1810 he went down on purpose to vote against the Barne family who controlled the Borough.[3]

The Dunnell family made Newson Garrett welcome, both as a Suffolk man and as Richard's younger brother. Newson had not come to London, however, to continue in his brother's shade. His bold schemes for the future captured the interest of the Dunnells' younger daughter, Louisa. Newson was twenty-two years old and exceptionally handsome, with fair hair, blazing blue eyes and a bright complexion; he had been, so an old Suffolk neighbour declared, the most beautiful child she had ever seen.[4] Louisa Dunnell fell deeply and lastingly in love with this impetuous young man. On his side Newson grew devoted to the

[1] St Mary, Bryanston Sq., Register of Marriages, 1828.

[2] The Beehive still exists, under the same name and on the same site.

[3] Barne Barne to Snowdon Barne, 25 March 1820. E. Suffolk County Record Office.

[4] Fawcett, M. G., *What I Remember*, pp. 29, 34.

19

young girl so slight and gentle-looking, so serious in manner. Louisa was not pretty; her natural reserve was deepened by a rigidly Evangelical piety, but she had character and brains, and John Dunnell had given her the best education he could afford. Suffolk ancestry gave the young couple a common background, and Newson's determination promised a successful future. They asked John Dunnell's consent to their marriage and, since Louisa was still under twenty-one, this he formally gave. They were married on 5 April 1834 at the handsome classical church of St Mary, Bryanston Square, just around the corner from the Beehive Inn.[1] Newson Garrett, a vigorous competitor, thus married at the same age, in the same church, and into the same family as his brother Richard. John Dunnell and Louisa's aunt were their witnesses, and the bride signed the register in her neat hand.[2]

After their wedding Newson and Louisa Garrett went to live, as their fellow-countryman the poet Crabbe had done, in Whitechapel. They settled at 1 Commercial Road, a pawnbroker's shop belonging to John Dunnell on the corner of Whitechapel High Street where the New Road, as it was called, cut through towards the docks.[3] Here, after just under a year of marriage, their first child Louisa, and sixteen months later, on 9 June 1836, their second, Elizabeth, were born. When she was three weeks old the baby was carried to Hawksmoor's great church, St George-in-the-East, whose lofty tower, crowned with a circle of columns, soared above the crowded streets of the parish. Here she was christened, after her aunt Betsy, simply Elizabeth. The parish register records: 'Born June 9th, baptized July 3rd 1836 Elizabeth dr. of Newson and Louisa Garrett, 1, Commercial Rd., Pawn-broker, by the curate.'[4]

In this parish and this house Elizabeth Garrett spent the first three years of her life. Outside the safety of home, the surround-

---

[1] St Mary, Bryanston Sq., Register of Marriages, 1834.

[2] She seems also on this occasion to have signed her husband's name, which appears in the same handwriting, with a cross beside it.

[3] Robson, *London Trade Directory*, 1835–9.

[4] L.C.C. County Record Office, p. 93/GED/16.

ings were menacing. In the 1830s London's East End was being transformed from a series of ramshackle villages strung along the river to one dense industrial slum. Relics of a country past still remained; bales of hay were stacked in the Whitechapel High Street for the open-air market, and the nearby King's Arms was a coaching inn, with open galleries, stables and a cobbled yard.[1] Yet all day along the smooth tramway of granite blocks in Commercial Road horses dragged dray-loads of sugar from the West India docks, with incessant grinding of iron-bound wheels on the stone.[2] Hogsheads of raw sugar were unloaded and boiled in the sugar bakeries, great gaunt buildings black with soot and noisome with fumes. The sulphurous smoke from their chimneys hung over the whole district; puddles underfoot were dark and scummy. The houses in Commercial Road and its side streets were long terraces of smoky brick, with a shop or two rooms opening on to the pavement and two rooms above. At the back was a close little yard, seldom larger than one of the rooms.[3] 1 Commercial Road differed from the rest only in being a corner pawnbroker's, with front door into the shop and a side door always open, as though half inviting, half repelling the visitor to the pledge office.

Louisa Garrett was a notable housekeeper, capable of creating a home even among these grim and serried rows of houses. She never feared hard work, and the first scenes which met small Elizabeth Garrett's eyes were probably homely and neat in the local fashion, with checked curtains, whitened doorstep, and bright coke fire. In the pawnshop there was scope for Newson Garrett's energy and ability, since the three brass balls, in Cockney slang the 'swinging dumplings', throve in every poor neighbourhood. Often a whole family's clothes would turn up on Monday morning to be redeemed, with any luck, for next Saturday night.

[1] L.C.C. County Record Office, Print Room, Stepney, CC 936 and CB 14721.
[2] Rose, M., *The East End of London*, p. 124.
[3] Hollingshead, John, *Ragged London*, pp. 63–7.

Petticoats, stays, gowns, shawls and bonnets, shirts, collars and even handkerchiefs lay in bundles on the shelves or hung in strings across the shop. Commercial Road was one of the districts where pawnshops were commonly used by thieves to dispose of swag stolen or smuggled from the river.[1] Newson Garrett was a licensed pawnbroker, carrying on a legitimate business, but he risked receiving stolen goods unawares, with a penalty of transportation.

It was not easy to bring up children in the Whitechapel of the 1830s. Where could two little girls run or play freely when the only open spaces were warehouse yards or derelict burial grounds? If Louisa took the children towards the river they would meet the Ratcliffe street women with their short skirts, high red morocco boots and brass heels.[2] If they played nearer home they might hear the shrill barefoot street arabs who used the name of God only as a curse. To a pious mother such thoughts were appalling. Louisa Garrett kept the children so closely by her that in after life Elizabeth seemed to remember nothing of her earliest home. Her birthplace was unknown apparently even to her children and has remained unknown until now.[3]

In November 1837, when Elizabeth Garrett was only seventeen months old and Louie still under three, their mother had another baby, this time a boy. On him the hopes of both families were fixed and he was proudly christened Dunnell Newson, as if to represent their joint ambitions. He lived through the winter, but died at six months in May 1838. The young mother's grief was terrible. She tried to pray, but the only petition her heart could frame was that God would take her too.[4] For a time even the

[1] Mayhew, H., *London Labour and the London Poor*, Vol. I, pp. 373–4.

[2] Rose, M., op. cit. p. 58.

[3] The premises were acquired in 1839 by Messrs Gardiner's, the well-known marine outfitters, and rebuilt on a much larger scale when the western end of Commerical Road was constructed in 1865. Nothing therefore remains of Elizabeth Garrett Anderson's birthplace, but it stood on the site of that East End landmark, Gardiner's Corner. *Gardiner's Centenary Catalogue*, 1939.

[4] Fawcett, M. G., op. cit. p. 9.

thought of her little girls could not comfort her, and the memory of this early sorrow was still vivid when they were grown women.

To assert his own faith in the future of their family, and perhaps to cheer his wife, Newson Garrett commissioned a family portrait, an ambitious gesture for a young man in his humble position.[1] The family is posed in an oblique line, with Louie peeping out, shy and bright-eyed, round her mother's arm. Elizabeth stands boldly on Mrs Garrett's lap in the centre of the picture. She still has the bud-like mouth and nose of babyhood, but her fluff of hair has already a russet sheen, her brows are strongly etched and her eyes have the penetrating brightness they were to keep even when she was an old woman. One small fist clutches her mother round the neck, the other waves gaily; one foot is lifted as if she were ready to walk out of the picture and advance on the spectator.

Louie and Elizabeth were not to be exposed to the dangers of another summer in Whitechapel. By the end of 1838 the family had moved from Commercial Road. Newson took over the management of a larger pawnbroker's shop at 142 Long Acre, three doors from the corner of St Martin's Lane. Here the Garretts remained for two years.[2] It was a step up in the world in every way. Newson was no longer simply a pawnbroker but a 'Pawnbroker and Silversmith'; the district was healthier than Whitechapel, and the street more cheerful for young children to look out on. Country carts passed every day on their way to Covent Garden; there were coach-houses and stables full of horses. The grass and trees of St James's were near enough for the children to play, although Trafalgar Square was not cleared until 1844 and

[1] The original canvas, by an unknown artist, was destroyed by fire, but the picture survives in a photographic copy which is said to give a good likeness of Elizabeth Garrett at two years old.

[2] The *Post Office Directory* for 1840 gives Newson Garrett's address as 142 Long *Lane*, but this number did not in fact exist and is unconfirmed from any other source. The whole corner has now been rebuilt and the Sussex public house, St Martin's Lane, occupies the site.

Lord Nelson was not yet on his column for them to admire. Close at hand Elizabeth could see the comings and goings at Northumberland House, the red coats of the Horse Guards, passing coachmen from the Royal Mews and the stage-coaches swaying down St Martin's Lane on their way to unload at Charing Cross.[1]

In June 1839, at St Martin's-in-the-Fields, a new baby was christened in the family names of Newson Dunnell.[2] Next year followed Edmund, a quiet steady child, who was devoted to his sisters. From this year, 1840, dates the one conscious memory Elizabeth retained of her London childhood. Like many childhood memories it was of night.[3] She was asleep in her cot in a dark room when her father appeared, swung her up in powerful arms and carried her to the window. Mrs Garrett hovered anxiously somewhere near, protesting that it was late and Lizzie should be asleep. 'Nonsense, dear Mother!' said Newson Garrett robustly. 'Of course the child must see it; she will remember it all her life.' The four-year-old child, still drowsy, was perched on his broad shoulder. Looking down, Elizabeth saw a fairy-tale scene of gilded coaches, the great yellow globes of the gas lamps along the street and a cheering crowd below. She remembered it so vividly that she could describe it to her own children exactly, which has made it possible to fix the date. It was the night of Saturday, 2 May 1840, when, according to the Court Circular

> The Queen and Prince Albert, accompanied by the Hereditary Prince of Saxe Coburg Gotha, honoured the Italian opera with their presence. Her Majesty's Theatre on Saturday night was attended by above eight hundred of the beau monde, and the coup d'œil was exceedingly brilliant denoting that all the world was in town and that the annual reign of fashion and gaiety had begun.[4]

[1] Boys, Thomas Shotter, engraving *Charing Cross in 1842.*
[2] St Martin's-in-the-Fields, Register of Baptisms, 1839.
[3] Anderson, L. G., *Elizabeth Garrett Anderson*, p. 26.
[4] *The Morning Herald*, 4 May 1840.

This one brilliant scene, isolated in surrounding darkness, was the first and last of Elizabeth Garrett's London memories. Before another year had passed she had moved with her family to Aldeburgh.

For some time Newson Garrett had been searching for an opportunity to return to Suffolk. He was too much of a country-man to feel at home in the city, and for complete satisfaction he wanted to achieve success under the eyes of his brother and all who had known him as a boy. His father, Richard Garrett the ironmonger of Leiston, had died in 1837, but had left little capital to his youngest son. Most of his property had been tied up in the works which naturally passed to Richard. All Newson received under his father's will was a quarter share of the 'stock, implements and interests on hand', independently valued, to be paid by instalments so that current business at the works could be carried on.[1] However, Louisa Garrett had a little money of her own, and Newson had some savings. John Dunnell, having seen his son-in-law at work, was convinced of his abilities, and gave or lent the balance of the capital. In 1841 Newson Garrett bought a corn and coal warehouse from a Mr Fennell at Snape Bridge near Aldeburgh.[2] He was still only twenty-nine, but he had years of business experience behind him, a devoted wife beside him and an iron will to succeed. Together he and Louisa packed their household goods, and prepared for the journey by sea to Aldeburgh. Thus five-year-old Elizabeth Garrett, with an almost unknown chapter of London childhood behind her, arrived at Slaughden Quay.

[1] Register of Wills, Dec. 1837, no. 835, Somerset House.
[2] Newson Garrett: Obituary notice, *East Anglian Daily Times*, 6 May 1893.

CHAPTER TWO

A Daughter at Home
1841–1854

Newson Garrett settled his family at Aldeburgh in a square white Georgian house opposite the church at the top of the town. The poet George Crabbe had served his apprenticeship as an apothecary in its panelled rooms and had known the medlar, quince and mulberry trees of the walled garden. This house, The Uplands, was the family home from 1841 to 1852. Alice, the first Garrett to be baptized at Aldeburgh, was born there in 1842. Next came two inseparable sisters, Agnes in 1845 and Millicent in 1847. Sam, Josephine and George followed in the 1850s.

Throughout these years, while his family grew, Newson Garrett's business interests expanded to keep pace with them. Bold, impulsive and impatient, he strode around the little port, or drove full-tilt across country in his dog-cart, furious if everyone else did not see at once that his plan for any project was the best, indeed the only one. Family, friends and servants were swept along on the tidal wave of his energy.

Aldeburgh appeared at first sight a backwater for a young man intending to make his fortune, but Newson Garrett knew what he was at. The warehouse he had bought lay a few miles inland where the Alde, winding in a wide, shining channel among the marshes, suddenly narrows to an arched bridge at Snape. Snape was well placed for water-borne trade; at high tide large sailing barges could tie up alongside the rambling red-brick warehouse, and the new owner could carry his goods in his own vessels. Here Newson

Garrett, short in capital but long in enterprise and courage, began to malt grain.

Malting was an expanding industry. Malt had not been made in any quantity in the near neighbourhood of London for a century or more, while the demand of the London breweries had grown outrageously. There was room to ship malt on a large scale down the coast to London or northwards to other large brewing centres such as Norwich.[1] From his central position on the Alde, near grain markets and harbours, Newson Garrett could capture both the Thames and the East Anglian trade. His small fleet plied between Aldeburgh and London, and northwards as far as Newcastle. Within three years of his arrival at Snape he was shipping 17,000 quarters of barley each year for London and other markets. To corn he added coal. At Slaughden Quay there was the sound of the shipwright's hammer and a strong smell of tar from his yard, a clatter of horses' hoofs and a rumble of coals being unloaded from Garrett's vessels into his wagons. Of twenty-four ships in the little port, other than fishing boats, twelve belonged to him.[2]

This success was Newson's answer to the triumph of Richard Garrett at Leiston. The middle brother, Balls Garrett, a mild and peaceable man, migrated to Kent, where he became proprietor of the Medway Iron Works at Maidstone.[3] Meanwhile Richard carried the Leiston works into its great days. From the first his firm specialized in agricultural machinery; the portable horse-worked threshing machine, which he manufactured, was seen all over Suffolk and further afield. By 1850 Garrett of Leiston drills and horse-hoes were the best known in England.[4] Steam engines followed traction engines for ploughing, and the steam roller, with the familiar trade-mark of a prancing horse in gleaming brass on its funnel, appeared. Machinery from the Leiston

[1] Clapham, J., *Economic History of Modern Britain*, Vol. I, p. 232.
[2] Clodd, E., *A Guide to Aldeburgh*, 1861, p. 66.
[3] *East Anglian Daily Times*, 6 May 1893.
[4] Clapham, J., op. cit. Vol. I, p. 140.

works captured the export trade and was sold all over Europe, particularly in Germany and Russia.

Newson Garrett could not bring himself to accept a position socially and economically inferior to his brother, and the two men quarrelled bitterly. Local tradition had it that the Garrett brothers did not speak to each other for thirty years,[1] though their two wives were sisters and their families were on affectionate terms. Rivalry with his brother reinforced Newson's natural ambition and drove him on like a daemon. He acquired a brick-yard and built rows of houses, of which he was the sole architect. Brudenell Terrace, Aldeburgh, towering above the old cottages of King Street and shutting out their view of the sea, was considered by the family to be his master-piece. He founded and built a gas works and became, by a natural extension of his malting interests, partner in a brewery. About 1848 he was appointed agent for Lloyds. The children, when they were allowed into their father's counting-house, spelled out the strange words on his writing paper, Agent for Lloyds and Receiver of Droits of Admiralty.[2]

Elizabeth Garrett grew up in an atmosphere of triumphant economic pioneering. In a sense she was a by-product of the industrial revolution and her precise social class was a factor in her success. Sensitive or hesitant spirits might doubt the inevitability of progress; the Garretts were not temperamentally given to doubt. If individual courage and effort could transform a backward corner of East Anglia, what might they not achieve in the world of intellect and affairs? Where Richard and Newson Garrett had succeeded in early-Victorian industry, their children were to compete successfully in the great administrative and professional class of late-Victorian England. The special achievement of Elizabeth Garrett was to see that this élite of professional ability contained women as well as men.

Belief in progress through private enterprise did not rule out

[1] Personal information: Mrs Wood, Newson Garrett's granddaughter.
[2] Fawcett, M. G., *What I Remember*, p. 11.

public spirit; Newson Garrett took, and taught his children to take, a boisterous interest in local government. Aldeburgh, like Dunwich, had remained unaffected by the Municipal Corporations Act of 1835. The Borough was still substantially the Borough of Crabbe's poem, a self-elected body capable of some extraordinary vagaries. It was not difficult for Mr Garrett to enter the Corporation; by paying the standard fee of five pounds he procured his own election as inferior and later capital burgess.[1] Newson Garrett's public life was stormy. Many of the older burgesses resented the intrusion of this self-assertive newcomer, and he had powerful enemies on the Council. On his side Mr Garrett was no peacemaker. The limitless skies of East Anglia seem to breed extreme individualists, and he was no exception to the rule. His quarrels were not restricted to his brother Richard. Those with Mr Dowler, the long-suffering Rector of Aldeburgh who was also Bailiff and Capital Burgess, were particularly scandalous because so public. If the offending clergyman were in disgrace Mr Garrett would not let his family go to Matins at the flint Parish Church of St Peter and St Paul across the lane from their front door. Instead, the children were lined up to march down the hill to the dissenting Union Chapel in the High Street. The little Garretts were very much entertained by the deference with which they were received at this humble place of worship.[2]

Such events could not be hushed up, and Mr Garrett's feuds were at once the scandal and delight of Aldeburgh. 'None of his virtues were passive,' wrote a tactful commentator. 'It may be supposed that this ... did not always in a small community make for peace, but below an occasionally stormy surface Mr Garrett had a great heart.' [3] In all Newson's storms his wife was his sheet anchor. Louisa Garrett adored her handsome husband and admired everything about him, yet devoted as she was, she took no part in his quarrels. The children were sharp enough to observe

[1] Clodd, H. P., *Aldeburgh*, p. 130.
[2] Fawcett, M. G., op. cit. p. 30.
[3] *The Aldeburgh Magazine*, May 1893.

the scenes which took place every Christmas when their parents sent gifts of poultry to neighbours in the town. Mrs Garrett would bring her list to show her husband. 'Ha!' exclaimed Newson at the sight of an offending name. 'Don't you know I've quarrelled with that fellow!' 'Oh yes, I know, Father dear,' replied Louisa, quite unruffled, 'but that don't matter.' And the chicken or turkey was sent.[1]

The truth was that the centre of gravity in the household lay with their mother rather than with their ebullient father. Tiny, deceptively frail-looking, Louisa Garrett went purposefully about her tasks. She washed, dressed and fed the children, she supervised the cooking, the baking, the laundry, the dairy, the scrubbing and polishing of the whole house. She kept minute, exquisitely neat accounts. When there was a difficult business letter to compose, 'dear Mother' would be summoned, and taking off her apron would hurry to the counting-house. There she drafted in a neat, clear hand, without mistakes of spelling or grammar, tactfully translating Newson's more forceful expressions into terms that would not give offence. For all this he respected and admired her.

Faith was the source of Mrs Garrett's strength. Her dogma, like that of her sister and ally, Aunt Richard Garrett, was of the strictest Evangelical school. Although officially a member of the Church of England, she was a subscriber to Spurgeon's printed sermons in *The Tabernacle Pulpit*, reading weekly of inner conversion versus baptismal regeneration, of the certainty of predestination, and the dangerous tendencies of biblical criticism. Each day began and ended with prayer. Mrs Garrett tried at first to put her husband in charge of family prayers as befitted his position, but praying bored Newson's restless temperament. When he read aloud from the Bible before breakfast, he took to turning over two pages at once to make the daily chapter shorter. One day, doing this, he jumped from the concluding verses of one long chapter to the beginning of another and got out of the

[1] Fawcett, M. G., op. cit. p. 34.

difficulty by closing the family Bible firmly, with the words 'For what we have *already* received may the Lord make us truly thankful.' He was never allowed to conduct prayers again.[1]

In an age when many middle-class children were confined to top-floor nurseries, Elizabeth Garrett was free to explore the lonely salt-marshes, the steep stony beach, the rope walk, the sailmaker's yard.[2] She could run without stumbling over the nets spread out to dry or knocking her head on the outriggers of the beached fishing boats; she could look into the fishermen's curing houses, or peer down the wells in the shingle where they kept their fish alive till they could be shipped to London. She knew the North Sea in all its moods, from the days in spring when waves ran softly up the shining shore to the mornings in autumn when one could hear the passing fishermen speak without seeing their ghostly boats among the mists.[3] The air of Aldeburgh is salty and biting; Elizabeth Garrett grew up with superb health and vitality, so that she could speak, at the end of her life, of having worked for seventy years without even a headache.

The children's friendships lay not among the two or three aristocratic families of the town, but among the huts along the beach, where the fishermen's wives sat at their doorways mending nets. They talked to the crew of the lifeboat that was Aldeburgh's pride, or to Bob Wilson, the old sailor in the lookout station at the top of the steps. At home there was Barham, the groom and gardener. He drove the dog-cart, looked after the pigs, killed them when the fatal moment came, turned them into bacon and was, said Millicent Garrett, the gentlest, kindest, dearest man in the world. From these early friendships Elizabeth Garrett learnt an unaffected simplicity which she kept all through her life. In an age when class-consciousness was as constricting as a strait-jacket it was a fortunate gift.

[1] ibid.
[2] The scenes of her early childhood appear in the vignettes by Charles Standfield, A.R.A., to the eight-volume edition of Crabbe, published by John Murray in 1834.
[3] Crabbe, G., *The Borough*, Book, I, ll. 42 ff.

There was no school in Aldeburgh to which the children could go, although the boys later had a tutor. Elizabeth and Louie learnt their earliest lessons in the three Rs from their mother during the time she could spare from feeding and dressing the latest baby, superintending the young maids in the kitchen and composing Newson's quarrels. By 1846 when Elizabeth was ten years old it was clear that their mother must have help, and a governess was engaged at twenty-five pounds a year.

Miss Edgeworth was a decayed gentlewoman, poor and pious. Like all governesses she had one overwhelming fear, to lose her place and fall into want.[1] Miss Edgeworth never went on holiday. She slept in the same bedroom as Louie and Elizabeth and crept fully dressed behind the curtains of her bed at night. In the morning the girls would hear faint creaking and rustling in her corner, till she appeared once more in the same genteel condition. Mornings were spent with her in the schoolroom, afternoons were devoted to a regimented walk, one mile out and one mile back along the flat straight road to Leiston. At meals the governess was careful to steer the conversation into improving channels and to agree with everything Mrs Garrett said. This was too much for Mr Garrett's bluntness. 'Bless my soul, Miss Edgeworth,' he would exclaim impatiently, 'you said just the opposite a minute ago!' Miss Edgeworth had not spent her life as a poor dependent in other people's houses for nothing. 'When last I spoke I had not the pleasure of hearing dear Mrs Garrett's opinion.' Elizabeth overheard this exchange with contempt for Miss Edgeworth's servility. She was not an imaginative child. Nothing foreshadowed a life spent in winning professional status for educated women. She despised and disliked her governess.

The boredom of the hours in the schoolroom was torture to Elizabeth's lively mind. Miss Edgeworth relied on preparing and hearing a set section of Mangnall's *Historical and Miscellaneous Questions for the Use of Young People* each day. Elizabeth found that

[1] In 1851 there were 24,770 governesses in Britain, and for one post 810 applicants were recorded.

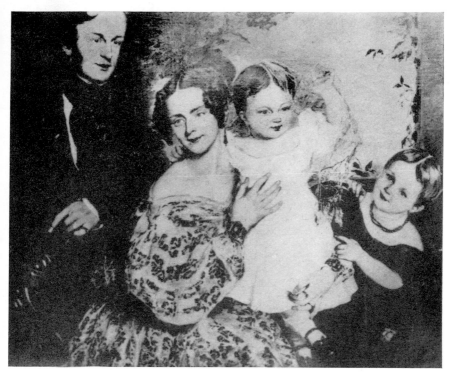

1. Newson and Louisa Garrett with Louisa and Elizabeth aged two 1838

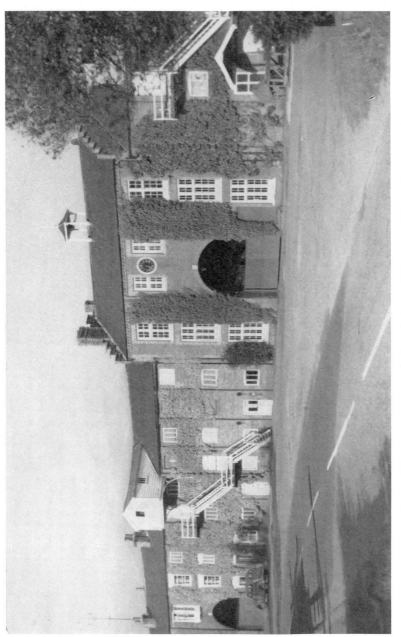

2. The maltings at Snape, the foundation of Newson Garrett's prosperity

she could confuse the governess by reversing rôles and asking questions which Miss Edgeworth had not prepared. With childish cruelty she harried her teacher and even incited the gentle Louie to do the same. The schoolroom became a battle-ground where Miss Edgeworth suffered daily defeat and humiliation. The harassed, weary teacher and the intelligent, frustrated child were both victims of the same social convention, which regarded governessing as the only female profession and amiable ignorance as the most suitable frame of mind for a lady. It was a convention into which Elizabeth Garrett would never fit.

By the time Elizabeth was thirteen and Louisa fifteen it was plain that they were too much for their governess. Reasoning, punishments and earnest prayers had no effect on them, and they were finally pronounced to be out of hand. Mr Garrett undertook to find them a school in London. He was aware of the gaps in his own book-learning, and passionately proud of his family. He intended to give his children the best education his money could buy; moreover, unlike most fathers of his time, he meant to educate the girls as thoroughly as the boys. His decision was to transform his daughters' lives. His final choice fell upon one of many private schools at Blackheath, the Boarding School for Ladies kept by the Misses Browning at 4 Dartmouth Row, S.E.[1]

Dartmouth Row lay just off the windy expanse of Blackheath, a quiet terrace sheltering behind wide sidewalks and an avenue of lime trees, each house further enclosed by its own wrought-iron railings. Many houses in the row, like number four, were small private boarding schools. The new pupils were shown into a little drawing room which seemed almost filled by a large lady, who daringly mingled scarlet, purple, green and yellow upon her ample person. She was Miss Louisa Browning, the headmistress, whose less imposing sister served as assistant. They were, they

---

[1] *The Post Office Suburban Directory 1858.* An advertisement claimed that 'the salubrity of the situation is too well known to need comment'. The fees were about £12 10s. per quarter.

never failed to explain to prospective parents or new girls, aunts of the poet Robert Browning who, it was understood, might honour the school with a visit at any moment. In fact they were step-aunts and there is no record that Browning regarded them as close connections at all.[1] However, such innocent deceptions are not unknown in academic circles, and the two ladies kept, of its kind, an excellent school.

Elizabeth, a strong-willed and demanding pupil, did not fit easily into the ladylike routine of Dartmouth Row. Later in life she used to say she remembered the stupidity of the teachers there with shudders.[2] They failed, of course, to teach her any science or mathematics but they were hardly to blame since it was impossible to find women qualified in these subjects.[3] French conversation at all times was the tedious rule. This custom, of powerful appeal to the parental pocket, was supposed to possess the advantages of a finishing school in France without the expense of the journey.[4] Intelligent conversation was confined to secret corners, while the girls dressed, ate and took their walks in crocodile to the accompaniment of heavily Anglicized French. Nor were the staff exempt. 'De l'air, toujours de l'air!' Miss Browning would cry as she swept in to open the windows.

To do them justice, the Misses Browning did not purvey accomplishments at the expense of education. Miss Browning taught English literature, French, Italian or German. They both talked well. To Elizabeth, brought up on Spurgeon's sermons, it was a revelation to hear Miss Louisa describe her two brothers, one as a devout Christian but the most selfish man she had ever met, and the other with no religion at all, but having the kindest

[1] Orr, Mrs Sutherland, *Life and Letters of Robert Browning*, p. 10.

[2] Anderson, L. G., op. cit. p. 33.

[3] In 1863 a selected group of girls from schools of good standing attempted the Cambridge Local Examinations; the examiner reported that even the senior girls showed very little knowledge of arithmetic, and it was clear to his mind that this was due to want of proper instruction. Stephen, B., *Emily Davies and Girton College*, p. 90.

[4] *The Times*, 2 July 1849. 'The Academie Française', Blackheath: advertisement.

heart in the world.[1] Their pupils probably received a better education in reading, writing and speaking English than many of their brothers in classics-dominated public schools. From them Elizabeth Garrett learnt the enjoyment of books. In poetry she read not only the fashionable Tennyson but Wordsworth, Milton and Coleridge as well. She read Gibbon and Motley for pleasure, and for relaxation Trollope, Thackeray or her favourite George Eliot. She learnt to write straightforward, vigorous English in a schoolgirl script, which developed later into a bold and springing hand. Even after the invention of the steel pen she preferred to write with the goose-quills of her schooldays. Her letters were racy and amusing.

Learning lessons came more easily to Elizabeth than learning deportment. The small boarding school of ten to twenty pupils was an extended family and Elizabeth, at home with the Aldeburgh sailors and fisherfolk, had now to mix with the daughters of professional men and gentlefolk. The criticism of adolescent girls can be crueller than any imposed discipline, but Elizabeth was intelligent enough to adapt herself. She and Louie formed friendships at school which were to affect their whole lives. Louie visited the Smith sisters at their father's country house, Suffolk Lodge, Acton, while Elizabeth found a friend older than herself in Jane Crow, a well-read and intelligent girl of about eighteen.[2]

The process of education was not all on the school's side. At the first interview, when Miss Browning listed the extras on the curriculum, Newson Garrett said his daughters would take them all, but added one more of his own, a hot bath once a week. It was a revolutionary proposal, since the reforming zeal of the Prince Consort had only just succeeded in installing the first bathroom at Windsor Castle.[3] Miss Browning might well have been a little taken aback, but reflecting that this overwhelming parent had

[1] Fawcett, M. G., op. cit. p. 39.

[2] Stephen, B., op. cit. p. 26.

[3] Possibly Mr Garrett, in whom the spirit of emulation was always strong, had been inspired by the Lord of the Manor at Aldeburgh, Leveson Vernon, whose new Marine Villa was fitted with a bathroom 'as a test'.

four more daughters still at home, she did her best. Every Saturday night the wooden washtub was placed before the kitchen range to reduce the danger of catching cold and, decently screened by a towel horse, Louie and Elizabeth sat by turns soaping and splashing in the hot water. They were known to everyone in the school as 'the bathing Garretts'.

Blackheath was still very much a village in those days. A boy at school nearby in the 1860s remembered tranquil Dartmouth Row, the wide wild stretch of the heath, the old gardens and summer-houses surrounding it, and the unpolluted Ravensbourne flowing through green fields.[1] When the daily walk took the girls to the brow of Greenwich Park, they could see the Thames winding below, and the masts of ships coming and going to the Port of London, among them their father's weekly brig from Slaughdon Quay. Two years in the mould of Dartmouth Row changed Elizabeth, outwardly at least, from a tomboy into a young lady of fifteen. She would never be pretty, for she had inherited her mother's small stature and irregular features, but she had vitality and intelligence. Her powerful, purposeful mind was as yet unformed; only a lively curiosity about the world gave any promise of what lay in the future. She was bold, yet cautious; as quick and mettlesome as her father, as reserved as her mother where the emotions were concerned. Her manners were straightforward and friendly with a note of formality when occasion demanded it; she had acquired the quiet voice and bearing of a lady. By 1851 Elizabeth and Louisa were considered to be 'finished' and left school together.

They were taken on a short tour abroad, including Paris, and an expedition through the Rhine gorge to admire the scenery. On the way home they visited the Great Exhibition in Hyde Park. The two girls were given tips by their Uncle Richard and spent some of this money on presents for their small sisters at home. Two bonnets of drawn blue velvet and lace with pink ribbons consoled Millicent and Agnes for being too young to see

[1] *The Home Counties Magazine*, Vol. VII, p. 77.

the Exhibition. The lofty roof of the Crystal Palace, and all it covered, made a deep impression on Elizabeth's mind. She sometimes talked of it, remembering herself and Louie, keen sightseers, full skirts billowing over crinolines, poke bonnets with lace behind and roses under the brims. As an old lady, honoured and famous, when she walked in Hyde Park she would say 'the Exhibition buildings came as far as this', or, looking up into the branches, 'the glass covered that elm'.[1]

After the excitement of the Great Exhibition it was time to return to Aldeburgh. For the next nine years, until she was twenty-four, Elizabeth lived the life of a daughter at home. Her brother Sam had been born in 1850, to be followed by Josephine in 1853 and George in 1854. By the time she was eighteen she had five sisters and four brothers, a healthy, noisy tribe, close-knit by a stubborn family loyalty. They were their father's children; nursery quarrels were sudden and furious, but at the first sign of opposition from the outside world the Garretts closed ranks like Grenadiers. Elizabeth's love for the young ones was almost maternal in its protectiveness.

By 1850 Newson Garrett was already a rich man. He decided to build himself a gentleman's mansion to his own design and lay out an estate at Aldeburgh, perhaps in rivalry to his brother Richard's country property.[2] Alde House was a square, handsome white building surrounded by gardens and paddocks. It stood on the crest of the hill behind Aldeburgh, then open on all sides. From the terrace the eye could see to a horizon eight miles off. On the left the old church tower showed through the trees; on the right the Alde wound among its marshes to Slaughden Quay. Green turf sloped down from the watcher's feet to the gardens behind the old houses in the High Street. Before him lay the whole stretch of the bay, studded with sailing ships from the fisher's coble to the merchantman in full sail. At night the ships dropped anchor and hung out lanterns till, said Edward Clodd, 'one might

[1] Anderson, L. G., op. cit. p. 34.
[2] Personal information: Mrs Wood.

fancy the stars had fallen from their places and were making a ring of diamond brightness round Aldeburgh Bay'. It was a scene to breed strength and inner quietness. Elizabeth Garrett loved it all her life.

By her own wish Elizabeth continued to work in the mornings at Latin and arithmetic, with help from a tutor who came to coach her brother Newson for the army. Many able girls educated themselves unofficially in this way. She was not starved of books. For a yearly subscription of a pound she could work her way through the thousand well-assorted volumes of the Aldeburgh Public Reading Room, as well as the new novels sent down from a London lending library. There is no evidence that at this time she was consciously preparing for a career, but she enjoyed using her brain and she read widely.

The afternoons were given over to country pleasures. Elizabeth learnt to ride from her father, who mounted his children on Shetland ponies as soon as they were old enough to sit in the saddle. It was a great pride to him to lead out a cavalcade, with his favourite daughter cantering by his side. Sometimes she drove with him across country to the markets where he bought corn and barley. These expeditions demanded hardihood for even in winter Newson insisted on taking the open dog-cart, and would return with hair and beard fringed by icicles. When the family went sailing in the bay he insisted that sea-sickness was an affectation. However choppy the water, the girls were not allowed to complain. Once they pointed out that the family's dog who had accompanied them was retching. Their father was immensely astonished. 'God bless my soul,' he exclaimed, 'look at that poor creature! Then it is *not* affectation after all!'[1]

They had a good many gaieties of a simple kind. In hard winters, when the marshes froze, they went skating. Elizabeth went to dances with her sisters and cousins, often riding in a farm cart with straw upon the boards to keep their satin-slippered feet warm. In summer there were croquet parties, picnics and boating on the

[1] Fawcett, M. G., op. cit. p. 14.

Alde by moonlight, a scene magically unchanged since Crabbe
had written:

> *Among those joys, 'tis one at eve to sail*
> *On the broad river with a favourite gale;*
> *When no rough waves upon the bosom ride,*
> *But the keel cuts, nor rises on the tide; . . .*
> *What time the moon, arising, shows the mud*
> *A shining border to the silver flood.*[1]

The Crimean War came no nearer to the secure world of Aldeburgh than a distant clap of thunder. Elizabeth at eighteen followed
the news through her father's papers. 'Heads up and shoulders
down!' he cried one morning in September 1855, as he strode into
the breakfast-room, newspaper in hand. 'Sebastopol is taken!'

The autumn of 1855 and the winter of terrible storms which
followed it taught her the lesson of courage close at hand.
Aldeburgh Bay was treacherous to sailing ships; in that winter
seventeen vessels were driven ashore or broken up on the shoals.
On one such day, when the coastguard's gun signalled a wreck, it
was blowing a black north-easter and even the lifeboatmen hesitated to launch their ship, Newson Garrett put them on their
mettle by climbing aboard with one of the children in his arms
and offering to go as passenger. More often he was in the water
himself, waist deep among the breakers, helping to form a human
chain along a rope and rescue the shipwrecked crew one by one.
On 22 November 1855 the rope snapped and the coxswain George
Cable was swept away and drowned before the eyes of the
watchers on the beach.[2] Instantly Newson Garrett took his place
and kept it until the rescue was complete. His wife, watching,
made no move to stop him, but prayed for his safety, as she prayed
for him every day of her life. He returned safely and received the
official thanks of the Royal National Lifeboat Institution.

[1] Crabbe, G., *The Borough*, Book IX, ll. 152–68.
[2] Clodd, op. cit. p. 142, pays tribute to the continuing courage of the
Cable family. A great-great-grandson, then aged 15, crewed with the lifeboat in 1954, although he was legally under age.

CHAPTER THREE

'I'm going to be a doctor'
1854–1859

❄

In 1854, when she was eighteen, Elizabeth Garrett and Louie went on a long visit to their school friends, Jane and Annie Crow. The girls' father was a partner in the firm of Francis Gray & Crow, alkali manufacturers, with a chemical factory at Gateshead, and the family lived at Usworth Hall, five miles out of the town.[1] The ritual of provincial visits was more or less established, drives, sightseeing and paying or receiving calls among the local gentry, 'doing company' as Florence Nightingale contemptuously called it. At one of these drawing-room gatherings Elizabeth met a young woman six years older than herself, small and rather plain, her manner conventional, her face unrevealing between smooth bands of mouse-coloured hair. She was introduced as Miss Emily Davies, daughter of the Rector of Gateshead. As they talked, and with repeated meetings they began to talk a great deal, Elizabeth found that the prim appearance was misleading. Emily Davies had a caustic wit and a clear, original mind.

'Our education answered to that of clergymen's daughters generally,' she wrote. 'They have lessons and get on as they can.' Emily Davies had learnt Latin with her brothers for her own pleasure and had written weekly English essays for criticism by her father. Yet she had been forced to stay at home, her time frittered away in a multitude of small duties, while her brothers went to public school and university. She watched her favourite brother Llewelyn bracketed fifth in the Classical Tripos at Cam-

[1] Whellan, *Northumberland Directory for 1855*, p. 396.

bridge and elected President of the Union. As she compared his life with her own she felt, slowly growing in her mind, a feeling of resentment at the subjection of woman much larger and profounder than any personal jealousy. Emily Davies spoke for many young women of her generation when she wrote of

> the weight of discouragement produced by being told that, as women, nothing much is ever to be expected of them . . . that anything like original research or profound learning is not for them to think of and that whatever they do they must not interest themselves, except in a second-hand and shallow way, in the pursuits of men, for in such pursuits they must always expect to fail. Women who have lived in the atmosphere produced by such teaching know how it stifles and chills; how hard it is to work courageously through it.[1]

These words, and others like them, stirred Elizabeth deeply. She wrote regularly to Emily Davies, and they met again in 1856 when the Garretts paid a second visit to Usworth. The friendship between Elizabeth and Louisa Garrett, the Crows and Emily Davies, lasted as long as their lives, and had an enduring influence, not only on themselves, but on their families, and on a whole generation of girls yet unborn. Millicent Garrett, a good judge, saw the Gateshead meeting as a turning point in history. There was no sudden moment of illumination, no time at which Elizabeth Garrett could say, as Florence Nightingale did, 'God spoke to me and called me to His service'. The process was slow but decisive; steadily during the five years from 1854 to 1859 she searched for some cause to give meaning to her life. At first she tried to be, as her mother wished, 'converted' in the Evangelical sense, but in spite of all her struggles it seemed fore-ordained that she should never reach the required 'converted state'. The passive acceptance it demanded was as impossible to her as it had been to Newson.

At this chrysalis stage she read Dean Stanley's *Life and Letters of Dr Arnold* and found, with all the force of a new gospel, that

---

[1] Stephen, B., *Emily Davies and Girton College*, p. 29.

it was possible to be 'at once as liberal and as Christian as Arnold was'. Everything about Arnold's life appealed to her: his golden time at Oxford with the studies and friendships she longed for herself, his sense of duty which found an echo in her own, his conception of the social responsibilities of Christian life. His biography became a sort of Bible which she read and re-read for six months. 'I suppose to everybody in the state I was then in, light in some measure comes sooner or later,' she said ten years afterwards, 'and that if Arnold had not come my way something else would have done the same for me, but still one remembers the light-bearer with unusual reverence.'[1]

Elizabeth Garrett's nature was simple and direct. Belief, for her, demanded action. She looked at her secure sheltered life and found it empty of any real purpose. Her intelligence, her native vigour, her strong will all clamoured to be put to work. There was nothing to use her powers in the life of a daughter at home, and she saw no chance of life altering. Louie had shared her pleasures and duties from the time they both left school, they loved each other intensely, forming a devoted couple within the wider circle of the family. But Louie was beautiful, according to people who knew her as a girl, gentle where Elizabeth could be brusque, tender where Elizabeth was reserved and independent. Inevitably she began to attract admirers, while Elizabeth could scarcely conceal her boredom with the stolid young merchants and farmers of Aldeburgh society. Sooner or later this beloved sister would leave her. Louie's first known offer of marriage came from her cousin Richard, son of Uncle Richard at Leiston, a clever and vigorous young man.[2] She refused him, causing another rancorous skirmish between the two fathers, but soon after, when she was twenty-three and Elizabeth twenty-one, accepted James Smith, brother of her former school friends. James and Louisa Smith were married at Aldeburgh on 10 September 1857,[3] and Louie

---

[1] Elizabeth Garrett to Emily Davies, 12 Oct. 1865. Fawcett Library.
[2] Anderson, Sir A. G., MS.
[3] Aldeburgh Parish Church, Register of Marriages, 1857.

left home to live at 7 St Agnes Villas, Bayswater. The following August their first son was born.

Elizabeth was left with the duties of eldest daughter which in such a large household were not merely ornamental. The Alde House property included, as well as the house and garden proper, stables, granaries, glasshouses, piggeries, a large kitchen garden, an ice-house, a laundry and a Turkish bath, a fantasy of Newson's known to the servants as 'Master's Sweatin' House'. Elizabeth learnt how to manage all these. There was also the annual migration to Snape to be organized. The coming of the railway had reduced the shipping trade at Aldeburgh and Newson Garrett now sent only one weekly brig to London. In spite of this he welcomed the railway with both hands and finally got, by his own exertions, a private branch line for goods to Snape,[1] his head-quarters as maltster, coal, lime and corn merchant, brick and whiting manufacturer and shipbuilder.[2] He adapted himself with energy to the new situation, building a rambling, one-storied house at Snape Bridge to be the family's home during the winter months, when malting can be carried on, and moving back to Aldeburgh for the summer.[3] Every October for many years house-hold stores, clothing, belongings, toys, had to be packed and loaded on to barges for the journey upstream, only to be re-packed and loaded once more the following May. It is not surprising that his daughter Elizabeth became an excellent household manager.

She was also leader and friend of her younger brothers and sisters. One of Elizabeth's inventions, which Millicent Garrett always remembered, was called 'Talks on Things in General'; these took place on Sunday evenings.

I can see her now on the sofa in the Alde House drawing room: George, our younger brother, on her lap, and the rest of us grouped round her while she talked on just what was upper-

---

[1] When asked to show his ticket at the Liverpool Street barrier he refused with some annoyance. Ticket collectors learned to recognize him.

[2] White, W., *History, Gazeteer and Directory for Suffolk*, 1855, p. 526.

[3] Fawcett, M. G., op. cit. p. 37.

most in her mind at the time: Garibaldi and the freeing of Italy from the Austrians, Carlyle's Cromwell, Macaulay's History of England, and modern political events and persons, such as Lord Palmerston and the chances of a Reform Bill.[1]

George, at less than five, might have been considered rather young for Macaulay and the Reform Bill, but like all the children he loved his masterful elder sister.

Mrs Garrett felt that these duties should make up a full and happy life, yet Elizabeth grew steadily more restless.

> I was a young woman living at home with nothing to do in what authors call 'comfortable circumstances' [she said later, remembering this time]. But I was wicked enough not to be comfortable. I was full of energy and vigour and of the discontent which goes with unemployed activities. 'The obscure trouble of a baffled instinct' as Coleridge finely calls it. . . . Everything seemed wrong to me.[2]

The drive and ambition which had carried Newson from Whitechapel to Alde House was strong in her. She considered herself objectively. She was not poor; she had good health, high spirits and a fair share of ability. Surely with these gifts she might do something? In this belief she was encouraged by reading a new magazine entirely devoted to women's questions.

The first appearance of *The Englishwoman's Journal* in 1858 marked the beginning of the organized woman's movement in Britain. It had grown out of a harmless and tedious magazine 'edited by ladies for ladies' which was bought by the contributions of a circle of friends and re-edited with considerable ability by Bessie Rayner Parkes, daughter of a progressive Unitarian family.[3] Its appearance was serious, not to say forbidding. No concessions were made. In the first number Coventry Patmore's *The Angel in*

[1] Fawcett, M. G., op. cit. p. 41.
[2] Elizabeth Garrett, MS. draft for a speech, Royal Free Hospital School of Medicine.
[3] She was later the mother of Mrs Belloc Lowndes and Hilaire Belloc.

the House, that idyll of married life, was praised for the charm of its style but criticized as '*unmitigatedly conventional* . . . we cannot conceive what vision Mr Coventry Patmore could in his most prolific moments embody, of a woman who could not afford to wear white kid gloves'. Close columns of small type set out the wretched conditions under which women were employed as governesses, dressmakers and factory hands, short stories were moral in tone, while strictly factual articles showed the need for educated women to work in penitentiaries, hospitals, asylums and workhouses. After a few months the editor of the journal defined its aims. 'It is work we ask, room to work, encouragement to work, an open field with a fair day's wages for a fair day's work.'

To Elizabeth Garrett and others like her, these words were a trumpet-call. At last they were not alone, for here were comrades who felt as they did. The most unexpected revolution of the century was about to begin, not in the mine or the factory but in the provincial drawing-room of the middle-class family. Where fathers had competed successfully in industry and commerce, daughters were now ready to compete in life outside the home. They were prepared to give up leisure, comfort, security and privilege for the chance to be full-grown individuals in their own right.

A regular feature of *The Englishwoman's Journal* was a series of articles on the careers of eminent women such as Florence Nightingale, Rosa Bonheur and the great Rachel. It was probably in one of these that Elizabeth Garrett first read of the American physician Dr Elizabeth Blackwell.[1] Alone, without influence or money, Elizabeth Blackwell had graduated in medicine from the small university of Geneva, New York State, in 1849 and opened her own dispensary amongst the immigrant women and children of the New York slums. Small, delicate and gentle, she had nevertheless moved unmolested among medical students, 'being able', so her sister wrote, 'by her unmoved deportment, to cause her presence to be regarded by those around her, not as that of a

[1] She was born in Bristol but emigrated with her family as a child.

45

woman among men, but of one student among five hundred, confronted only with the truth and dignity of Natural Law.'[1]

In January 1859 the newspapers announced that Elizabeth Blackwell was visiting England; she had come in fact to see her old friend Florence Nightingale and to place her name on the new Medical Register instituted by Act of Parliament the year before. Sometimes the tone of the press was friendly, if jocular, as in the neatly turned verses of a contributor to *Punch*:

> *Young ladies all of every clime*
> *Especially of Britain,*
> *Who chiefly occupy your time*
> *In novels or in knitting*
> *Whose highest skill is but to play*
> *Sing, dance, or French to clack well,*
> *Reflect on the example, pray,*
> *Of excellent Miss Blackwell.*
>
> *Think if you had a brother ill,*
> *A husband or a lover,*
> *And could prescribe the draught or pill*
> *Whereby he might recover;*
> *How much more useful this would be*
> *Oh sister, wife or daughter!*
> *Than merely handing him beef tea,*
> *Gruel or toast-and-water.*
>
> *For Doctrix Blackwell – that's the way*
> *To dub in rightful gender –*
> *In her profession, ever may*
> *Prosperity attend her!*
> *'Punch' a gold handled parasol*
> *Suggests for presentation*
> *To one so well deserving all*
> *Esteem and admiration.*

[1] Blackwell, A., *The Englishwoman's Journal*, 1858.

The original ran to four more verses, all reflecting the casual contempt which many educated men felt for the shallowness and stupidity of their female relations' lives.

Sometimes the tone of the press towards Dr Blackwell was hostile to the point of insult. 'It is impossible that a woman whose hands reek with gore can be possessed of the same nature or feelings as the generality of women,' observed a columnist.[1] This remark, or another like it, caught Newson Garrett's eye and he repeated it in the family circle at Alde House. Instantly Elizabeth Garrett sprang to the defence of the woman doctor. She could be as hasty as Newson himself but now she forced herself to speak calmly and reasonably.

'How can you judge a woman of whom you know nothing? At least find out about Dr Blackwell before you make up your mind.'[2] She suggested that her father should write to a London business acquaintance, Valentine Leigh-Smith; his cousin Barbara Bodichon, née Leigh-Smith, knew Emily Davies and was an old friend of Elizabeth Blackwell. Newson Garrett liked his daughter the better for standing up to him. He was fair-minded enough to write as she suggested and the reply came in the form of a letter of introduction from Mr Smith to Dr Blackwell herself. Meanwhile Elizabeth had heard from Emily Davies that Barbara Bodichon would like to meet her. The former Barbara Leigh-Smith was the daughter of a rich Unitarian family. Her father, a merchant grocer and Radical M.P., had educated his daughters at home and given them experience of freedom and responsibility. At twenty-one Barbara had received three hundred pounds a year and her father's blessing to do as she liked with it. She had travelled on unchaperoned holidays, painted well enough for Corot to accept her as a pupil, and built herself a country cottage in Sussex where she gathered her friends for week-end parties. She had also, in the Unitarian tradition of public service, founded an undenominational

[1] Quoted Cunnington, W., *Feminine Attitudes in the Nineteenth Century*, p. 144.
[2] Anderson, L. G., op. cit. p. 42.

school, published in 1854 a pamphlet summary of the laws relating to women, and devoted part of her capital to the founding of *The Englishwoman's Journal*. Then suddenly in 1857, Barbara Leigh-Smith had left all this to marry Eugène Bodichon, an eccentric French surgeon living in Algeria and seventeen years older than herself. 'Some people think the docteur ugly and terrific,' she wrote with satisfaction. 'I think him the handsomest man ever created.'[1] Young Millicent Garrett, when she met him, called Dr Bodichon the 'he-hag'.[2]

Barbara Bodichon lived with her husband in a villa they had built among the pines and olives of his North African estate, but she happened to be in London on a vist to her family. Emily Davies was also in town staying with her brother Llewelyn, now Rector of Christ Church, Marylebone. The letter of introduction from Valentine Smith was safely in Elizabeth's pocket, and the excuse of escorting Agnes and Milly to school at Blackheath ready to hand. Elizabeth, a born opportunist, saw a chance too good to miss. At the beginning of February 1859 she went up to London to stay with Louie. The first step was for Emily to take her to tea with Madame Bodichon. The two girls crossed quiet Blandford Square from Llewelyn Davies's rectory to No. 5, the family home of the Leigh-Smiths, where they were welcomed by their hostess. She was a tall woman, about thirty-two years old, soon to be described by George Eliot in the character of *Romola*, with 'lovely hair of a reddish gold colour, enriched by an unbroken small ripple, such as may be seen in the sunset clouds'. Barbara Bodichon took a warmhearted interest in younger women. Of course, she said, Elizabeth Garrett must present the letter of introduction, and she would arrange a meeting with Dr Blackwell in her own house. Moreover she was arranging for Dr Blackwell to give three lectures on *Medicine as a Profession for Ladies* for the purpose, she

[1] Burton, H., *Barbara Bodichon*, p. 92.
[2] He advocated large-scale euthanasia, and insisted on doing all his own laundry, both of which might have appeared unusual in conventional circles.

said, laughing, 'of opening the medical profession to women before we are all dead'.[1] Finally, in parting, she advised Elizabeth and Emily Davies to call at the offices of *The Englishwoman's Journal*. Barbara Bodichon could feel satisfied with the results of her tea-party. She had won two outstanding recruits.

Elizabeth and Emily Davies made their way to 14a Princes Street, Cavendish Square.[2] Like many new callers, they were surprised and delighted. Visitors expecting some dowdy old lady in charge found instead a group of girls who were well dressed, attractive and gay.[3] Some of them were talented and all were enterprising. A country reader, Jessie Boncherett, the daughter of a Lincolnshire squire, had joined the office to organize a Society for Promoting the Employment of Women. Adelaide Anne Proctor was a successful writer of light verse. Anna Jameson, an older woman, had dared to end an unhappy marriage and earn her own living as an author. Isa Craig, in spite of sneers in the press about 'strong-mindedness', had become assistant secretary to the recently founded Association for the Promotion of Social Science.[4] This circle of fellow-workers soon felt the need for a social centre as well as a registry office. Tentatively, on a very small scale, the *Journal* had opened a 'Ladies Institute' with a luncheon room and a reading room supplied with papers and magazines. For the first time women could taste the pleasures of being clubbable. Bonnets and muffs piled up in the hall, while crinolines whirled in and out of the crowded little rooms. The high spirits of the members brimmed over in laughter and jokes.

There was much serious work as well as laughter at the offices of the *Journal* and the Society for Promoting the Employment of Women. These pioneers had intended primarily to win a fuller, more interesting life for women of their own social class. Before

[1] Burton, H., op. cit. p. 190.
[2] *The Englishwoman's Journal* moved in Dec. 1859 to larger rooms at 19 Langham Place and its supporters became known as the 'Langham Place circle'.
[3] Stephen, B., op. cit. p. 51.
[4] Strachey, R., *The Cause*, p. 93.

long they were forced to see the desperate need of unmarried working-class women, reduced to drudgery as seamstresses or 'slaveys', for training and decent employment. Society would not help poor women; they were too exhausted and too frightened to help themselves, therefore luckier women must help them. The pioneers took up the task. It is interesting to note how many of the circle came from Unitarian, nonconformist or, like the Garretts, Evangelical homes. Even where their religious beliefs had changed, they retained the social conscience of their upbringing.

The Society for Promoting the Employment of Women achieved wonders, considering the difficulties of its work. Its officers were mostly the daughters of successful business men, hardworking, capable and conscientious. To provide employment for the crowd of pathetic, hopeless candidates they founded a printing press, a law-engrossing office and a training school which taught badly-needed arithmetic to shop assistants. They placed selected women as clerks, telegraphists and children's nurses. Yet when Elizabeth Garrett first visited its offices, the Society had still failed in one important field. The liberal professions, law, medicine, university teaching and social work were irrevocably closed to women by lack of education. Here was a new recruit, intelligent, spirited, attractive, determined above the average; perhaps she could achieve something. Elizabeth Garrett was drawn, once and for all, into the service of the women's cause. 'No one has time for everything,' she maintained, 'the passion of my life is to help women.'[1]

She joined the Society for Promoting the Employment of Women and on 2 March 1859 attended a lecture by Dr Elizabeth Blackwell. The Marylebone Hall had been hired and Barbara Bodichon had brought primroses and wreaths of greenery from her Sussex cottage to decorate the reading desk. Elizabeth Garrett studied the slight, worn figure on the platform. When Elizabeth Blackwell began to speak, her simplicity and quietness of manner

[1] Anderson, L. G., op. cit. p. 15.

strengthened the authority of her words. Dr Blackwell emphasized that it was not a theory she wished to present, but the result of eight years in practice as a physician in New York.[1] She stressed the value of women physicians to their own sex in sickness and the contribution they could make to the education of wives and mothers in healthy living, for instance in the planning of food and the rearing of young children. 'Health has its science as well as disease and everyday life should be based on its laws,' she insisted.

She went on to discuss the contribution which women ought to make to the social welfare of their own country in hospitals, workhouses, schools or prisons. She contrasted the uselessness of a mere 'lady' with the informed and well-organized work of nuns in continental countries. She spoke from her own knowledge of religious orders in French hospitals of 'active occupation, personal standing and authority, social respect and the companionship of intelligent co-workers both men and women – the feeling of belonging to the world in fact instead of a crippled and isolated life'. Elizabeth Garrett felt as if her own deepest needs were being put into words.

The lecture went on. 'We come now to the position of women in medicine itself. The fact that more than half of the ordinary medical practice lies among women and children would seem to be at first sight proof that there is a great deal women could do for themselves.' Elizabeth Blackwell rejected utterly the idea of some separate and inferior qualification for women only. They must be fully qualified, not only to serve women in every department of life, but to make their full contribution to the profession itself. 'Though they may be few in number, they will be enough to form a new element, another channel by which women in general may draw in and apply to their own needs the active life of the age.'

The lecture finished. Barbara Bodichon carried off Dr Elizabeth Blackwell to her house for a party, and Elizabeth followed. In

[1] *The Englishwoman's Journal*, May 1860, Vol. V, p. 27.

Barbara's drawing room the two women met for the first time. Elizabeth Blackwell recognized the bright-eyed girl who had listened so intently during her lecture;[1] Elizabeth Garrett looked closely at the older woman. Dr Blackwell's features were drawn, and she was disfigured by a blind eye. She had almost lost her sight from purulent ophthalmia, contracted while syringing the infected eyes of a baby at La Maternité in Paris, where she had taken her midwifery training.

Rather shyly, Elizabeth presented her letter of introduction and asked a few questions. She was dumbfounded when Dr Blackwell replied as to a future colleague. 'She assumed that I had made up my mind to follow her,' said Elizabeth. The idea both excited and alarmed her. Here was pioneering to satisfy the spirit which had carried the Garrett ancestors to the New World, a purpose in life to satisfy the conscience of the Dunnells. Yet Elizabeth hesitated. She felt she had 'no particular genius for medicine or anything else'; she had no experience of the world and she felt as if she had suddenly been thrust into something too big for her. Without committing herself, she said good night and fled home to Louie.

She might still have turned back, but for one chance. Circumstances threw her together with Emily Davies for the next few weeks. Chaperoned by their respective relations, they both stayed on in London to hear Dr Blackwell give two further lectures. Then in mid-April they both travelled to Usworth Hall to act as bridesmaids with Jane Crow at the wedding of her sister Annie. During the next weeks the three fellow bridesmaids drew up lists, wrote letters, attended dressmakers' fittings and arranged flowers. It made a pretty picture of ladylike activity and gave them opportunities for uninterrupted discussion. No one could possibly foresee that Jane Crow, Emily Davies and Elizabeth Garrett would become respectively secretary of the Society for Promoting the Employment of Women, founder of Girton College and the first woman doctor to qualify in England.[2] Their conversations con-

[1] Blackwell, E., *Pioneer Work opening the Medical Profession to Women*, p. 176.
[2] The bride herself was for a short time Mistress of Girton.

tinued undisturbed. They talked and, as Emily put it with her usual discretion, 'it came to be understood that E.G. would, if possible, enter upon the career'.[1]

The subject of women physicians was one on which Emily Davies had very decided views. As a clergy-daughter, parish visiting in the tenements of an industrial town, she had seen the realities of woman's life. She was so convinced of the need for women doctors to attend women and children that she had even considered studying medicine herself, although the subject was distasteful to her. Here, in Elizabeth Garrett, with her apparently rich father, her untapped reserves of intelligence and ambition, her unaffected manner and her magnificent health, was the ideal medical pioneer. At first Elizabeth was troubled by doubts of her own ability. She was, after all, she said, 'thoroughly ordinary'. Would she be equal to the task? And would other women follow her?

Emily Davies dismissed such fears with magnificent aplomb.

> As we look round upon medical men, we cannot help observing many physicians and surgeons who do not appear to be superior in ability to average women; and as for many years only women above the average in mental or physical strength will dare to think of entering the profession, perhaps they will not *always* go to the wall.[2]

Elizabeth Garrett was tempted by adventure; the influence of Emily Davies, whose judgment she trusted, was decisive.

Later, remembering this time, Elizabeth was careful to acknowledge her debt to her friend. 'Miss D. talked her ideas over with me' she noted in a private draft for a speech. 'It seemed to us that the duty of ministering as a physician does to the care of women and children would be work not unsuitable to a woman, and also that it was work they ought to be free to take up if they chose.' She added wryly, 'Naturally neither of us knew much of the

[1] Stephen, B., op. cit. p. 56.
[2] Davies, S. E., 'Female Physicians', *The Englishwoman's Journal*, 1861.

details of medical education, nor did we realize how long and sustained an effort would be needed before our end could be reached.'[1]

For the moment difficulties lay in the future, unconsidered and unforeseen. Elizabeth Garrett had found her vocation at last. When she went home to Aldeburgh her seventeen-year-old sister Alice was waiting to meet her at the station. Alice wanted to hear about the wedding, about London, about Louie and her baby. All this had to wait, for there was one piece of news in Elizabeth's mind which, at the moment, drove out everything else. 'I'm going to be a doctor,' she whispered to Alice, as she climbed into the pony trap.[2] She confessed afterwards that she had no idea of the difficulties which lay ahead, difficulties deep rooted in the social history of her chosen profession.

[1] Elizabeth Garrett Anderson, MS draft for a speech, Royal Free Hospital School of Medicine.
[2] Anderson, L. G., op. cit. p. 43.

CHAPTER FOUR

Wise Women and Learned Men:
a retrospect

'A doctor', observed Miss Mitford, surveying the social scene in 1824, 'is sometimes an old man, sometimes an old woman, but generally an oracle and always (with reverence be it spoken) a quack' – an unflattering opinion which reflects both on the sex and the calling. Women held a traditional, if lowly, place in British medicine. The village woman, skilled in the use of herbs, offering physic to the anxious mother as well as philtres to the love-sick girl, was a part of the rural landscape. Miss Mitford's own Dr Tubb, 'inventor and compounder of medicines, bleeder, shaver and physicker of man and beast', had inherited his practice, along with a still for drugs and a prodigious stock of impudence, 'in the female line from his great-aunt Bridget'.[1]

The ancestry of Dr Tubb's Aunt Bridget stretches into the half-light of antiquity. In prehistoric Britain, as in most primitive societies, illness and the supernatural had a common threshold. Women took a leading part in the magic ritual of medicine, which included decoction of herbs, plantain, mandragora and the sacred mistletoe, fumigation and the massage or manipulation of the patient. Among the Germanic peoples few men dared to intrude on these mysteries, as Tacitus noted: 'They take their injuries to their mothers and wives who do not fear to examine and treat their wounds.'[2]

[1] Mitford, M. R., 'Dr Tubb': *Our Village*.
[2] Castiglione, A., *A History of Medicine*, p. 290.

The primitive tradition of female medicine in Britain was re-inforced by successive invaders. Women doctors appear in Roman literature from the time of Scribonius onwards, and more frequently in funerary inscriptions under the titles of obstetrix, clinica or medica. They were often household slaves brought by their owners into Britain and other overseas provinces of the Empire.[1] Early Christian missionaries to Britain introduced the order of deaconesses who, among their religious duties, visited the sick in their homes or cared for them in hospital. The boundary between nursing and medical practice was vaguely defined, but by the tenth century the ecclesiastical law of Edgar and his adviser St Dunstan was explicit. 'Possunt et vir et foemina medici esse.'[2]

The Norman conquest brought to England an established tradition of medicine practised by women from castle to cottage. Ladies were the ordinary practitioners of domestic medicine and the skilled chatelaine could reduce fractures, probe and dress wounds or burns and prepare herbal remedies. Certain religious orders had, of course, a special vocation to tend the sick, which included diagnosis in the light of existing knowledge as well as treatment and everyday nursing. The most famous hospital in medieval Britain was probably the nunnery at Sion on the Thames, while the abbess Euphemia of the Benedictine House at Wherwell in Hampshire directed her infirmary 'in the spirit of a man rather than a woman'.

Secular practice by women was also not unknown. Male physicians were rare, since time and desire for study were almost confined to monks, Jews and others debarred from the supreme masculine occupation of fighting. Professional women doctors, trained by apprenticeship to men, by reading medical books and by continual practice in the empiric method, naturally emerged to meet the need. None in Britain attained the fame of the women professors of Salerno, but they flourished well enough to take

[1] Mozans, H. J., *Women in Science*, p. 291, note 1.
[2] Charrier, E., *Evolution intellectuelle de la Femme*, pp. 280-1.

in their turn male apprentices. At the time of the Crusades a petitioner, addressing to Edward I a plan *De recuperatione terrae Sancte*, suggested sending with the Crusaders to the Holy Land a band of women doctors to win the confidence of the local inhabitants,[1] and the tale is told of a professor at Oxford who rode forty miles to get the prescription of an old woman for jaundice. Among the surgeons, Queen Philippa, wife of Edward III, is said to have appointed as Court Surgeon Cecilia of Oxford, and by the close of the fourteenth century a few women were even recognized as surgeons by the Guild of Surgeons founded in 1389.

In the fifteenth century, however, the surgeons' guild, like other craft fraternities, grew increasingly powerful and exclusive. Before long it was strong enough to enforce the exclusion of outsiders from practice, and its few unprotected women competitors were an easy target for attack. In 1421 the surgeons' guild petitioned Parliament that no man should practise without having graduated in 'The Scoles of Fysik withynne some Universitee' and that no woman should practise under pain of long imprisonment.[2] After repeated petitions by the guild an Act of Henry V finally repealed the law of Edgar which had given medical women legal status in Britain.

The great mental leap forward of the next two centuries did not favour the woman doctor. Strong government and the growth of political order released intelligent men from fighting for a life of intellectual work. Their reading among the scientists of the classical world reawakened interest in anatomy and natural function, while the study of plant life led slowly to a more rational use of drugs. The new learning centred on the universities, where women played no part; still more important, when the practice of medicine in England passed under the control of the newly founded College of Physicians, women were excluded. In petitioning for

[1] Lipinska, M., *Histoire des Femmes Médecins*, p. 21.
[2] Power, E., 'Women Practitioners of Medicine in the Middle Ages', *Proceedings of the Royal Society of Medicine*, 1921.

the Charter of the College in 1518, Thomas Linacre pointed out the danger that

> common artificers, as smiths, weavers and women, boldly and accustomably take upon them great cures and things of great difficulty; in the which they partly practise sorcery and witchcraft, partly apply such medicines unto the disease as be very noxious and nothing meet therefor.'

The college would sometimes admit male empirics, after payment of a fine, to its examinations, but contemptuously dismissed 'an outlandish ignorant sorry woman'.[1]

Yet though the College denied them full rank women continued to practise medicine during the sixteenth and seventeenth centuries, both as amateurs and even as professionals. Following Bishop Bonner of London, the bishops issued licences to practise physic and surgery within their jurisdiction, and at least sixty-six such licences, in seven dioceses, have been traced to women. Female apothecaries were also sometimes admitted to membership after apprenticeship, usually to a relation. Bishops in the course of a visitation regularly inquired 'whether any, man or woman, within the Parish hath professed or practised Physick or Chyrurgery'. Throughout the seventeenth century St Bartholomew's Hospital employed women as official members of its medical staff, for the treatment of skin diseases. One of these women was paid as much as £125 in 1635 and another £20 in 1682 for treating 'scald heads and lepersies'. The last woman to treat skin cases was appointed as late as 1708.[2]

Descendants of the medical chatelaines played the part of military surgeon to both armies in the civil war. Lucy Hutchinson who 'dressed wounds as well as any man surgeon' was ready to face the anger of her fellow-Puritans and treat injured Royalist prisoners in the dungeons of Nottingham Castle. The Cavalier Lady Anne Halkett, who had studied medicine and surgery in

[1] Mozans, H. J., op. cit. p. 291.
[2] Moore, N., *History of St Bartholomew's Hospital*, Vol. II, p. 733.

order to help the poor, received the thanks of Charles II for her care of gunshot wounds and mangled limbs on the battlefield at Dunbar.[1] The care of the sick poor demanded not only charity but study, and domestic medicine was a serious art. Lady Falkland supplied 'antidotes against infections and other several sorts of Physick' on a hospital scale. Mrs Bedell 'Was very famous and expert in Chyrurgery which she continually practised upon multitudes', while Mrs Bury studied morbid anatomy until her skill in diagnosis was remarkable. Jane Barker read medical books with her brother at Cambridge and issued prescriptions which were filed 'with those of the regular physicians'. She was said to be particularly successful with cases of gout, and found plenty of patients under the hard-drinking early Hanoverians. The lady amateur of medicine, though excluded from official scientific education, was probably no more of a menace than the Hogarthian surgeon-apothecary of the early eighteenth century with his bleeding bowl and swingeing doses of calomel or antimony. There were however several notorious female quacks. Such were Mrs Mapp, a virago from Epsom who earned enough as a bone-setter to run her own coach-and-six, and Jane Stephens who in 1740 sold to Parliament a remedy for the stone, consisting largely of lime-water and soap.[2]

The herbalist tradition, unchecked by the Puritan zeal for witch burning, continued in country places. Many patients of the middle classes preferred to consult these village wise women, since the fee for a Fellow of the College was half a guinea, and in the words of Culpeper 'the physician is like Balaam's ass; he will not speak until he sees an angel'. William Withering, who in 1785 introduced digitalis into the London Pharmacopoeia, relates that his curiosity was roused by the secret family recipe of an old woman in Shropshire named Mother Hutton 'who sometimes made cures after more regular practitioners had failed' in heart cases, with a decoction containing foxgloves. Some people indeed in the

[1] Halkett, A., ed., Camden Society, *Autobiography*.
[2] Lipinska, M., op. cit. p. 211.

sceptical eighteenth century felt there was not much to choose between the wise woman and the learned holder of degrees. One of these was Adam Smith, the political economist. 'Do not all the old women in the country practise physic without exciting a murmur or a complaint?' he asked. 'And if here and there a graduate doctor should be as ignorant as an old woman, where can be the great harm?'[1]

Except at this humble level however the credit of the woman medical practitioner declined steeply in the second half of the eighteenth century. A combination of historical circumstances worked against her. The great wars on land and sea produced numbers of men who had served a rough-and-ready training as surgeon-apothecaries in the armed forces of the crown. It has been said that by the end of the century more than half the medical men in practice in Britain had service qualifications. They had entered the profession with no preliminary education, apart from a chance meeting with the recruiting officer or the press gang, and many of them were remarkably tough customers. Competition with them was cut-throat competition and the women could not survive it. Moreover from the 1760s onwards Britain was entering upon what Trevelyan has called 'the most potent and characteristic phase of the whole Industrial Revolution, the connection of iron and coal'. The world's money poured into British counting-houses and middle-class merchants began to aspire to the style of the gentry. The devitalizing ideal of ladylike idleness, which was to be such a bane to high-spirited Victorian girls, was born.

By the end of the eighteenth century, then, good-class medical practice had closed to women, apparently for ever. The Royal College of Physicians had established a thriving oligarchy in which royal patients, appointments at the great new voluntary hospitals of the century, university chairs and knighthoods rotated among the Fellows, to the fury of the surgeons and even of their own licentiates. There was still less room for women

[1] Turner, E. S., *Call the Doctor*, p. 118.

within that circle of privilege. At the same time social and economic changes were forcing them out of family practice. The same process was at work in France, where women were forbidden by an edict of 1758 to practise medicine or surgery except midwifery.

In Britain even the midwife was to lose her official status. Traditionally the most responsible medical work undertaken by women was midwifery. From medieval times 'a sad woman, wise and discreet and worthy to have the office of midwife' had been licensed by the bishops to attend women in labour and recognized by physicians as a reputable colleague. Peter Chamberlen the younger and his son, of the famous family of accoucheurs, attempted in 1616 and again in 1634 to incorporate the midwives into a company or college under the crown. Their proposals were carried out almost three centuries later, a record for cautious reform even in Britain. Meanwhile their successors wrote textbooks for the professional instruction of midwives. *The Female Physician* by John Mowbray, M.D., published in 1724, advertised itself as 'containing all the diseases incident to that sex in Virgins, Wives and Widows, together with their causes and symptoms, their degrees of danger and respective methods of prevention and cure'.[1] The midwife of the day, it seems, was a gynaecologist as well. When William Smellie, the father of English midwifery, began to teach in London in 1741 he hung a lantern at his front door advertising lessons for midwives at five shillings each. He taught women the use of forceps and calipers and trained them on an anatomical model constructed of real bones covered with leather.[2] In spite of this long tradition of good relations, though, the end of the eighteenth century saw women midwives, like the women physicians, fighting a rearguard action.

As the wealth of the nation increased fashionable ladies increasingly employed physicians for their confinements, and in this, as in other things, the middle-class wife followed their example. The

[1] Mead, K. H., *A History of Women in Medicine*, pp. 464–5.
[2] ibid. p. 463.

status of the midwife declined, her downfall hastened by the medical faculty which addressed its blandishments to women. 'They early persuaded them (for they love to be persuaded) that they had hitherto been very unsafe in the hands of a set of ignorant midwives and had run the greatest risk of losing their lives every time they had employed them. In consequence the midwives were dismissed.'[1] By the nineteenth century midwives had become, in the person of Mrs Gamp to whom 'a laying-out or a lying-in' were all one, a byword for ignorance and incompetence. It was said that the only essential points to observe in engaging a midwife were that she should not be either a habitual drunkard or Irish. By 1827, claimed a member of the Royal College of Surgeons, the number of midwives was so reduced that in many places pauper mothers in workhouses were delivered by boy apprentices under sixteen.

The long reign of Victoria saw a development in the character of medical practice which promised to exclude women finally and completely from the profession. In Regency England medical education and qualification had been remarkably haphazard. Some future doctors apprenticed themselves to private practitioners, some paid premiums to 'walk the wards', some attended private medical schools and some kept gentlemanly residence at ancient universities without ever attending a lecture, much less a bedside. Some, the ambitious or energetic, did all these things in turn. Once trained, some entered practice as unlicensed 'medical men', while others equipped themselves with degrees or diplomas, which were available at twenty-one different standards from twenty-one different corporations. Medical students had a reputation for brutal horse-play and a lingering association with the horrors of the body-snatching trade. When John Keats was a student at Guy's, it was so unusual as to be remarked that he was 'never inclined to pursuits of a low or vicious character'.[2] James Paget attended only two lectures in obstetrics at St Bartholomew's because he could

[1] Griffith, E. F., *Doctors by Themselves*, p. 434.
[2] Rollins, H. E., *The Keats Circle*, Vol. II, p. 210.

not endure the obscene anecdotes which formed part of them.[1]
Henry Acland described his fellow students at St George's as
'low men of low habits . . . the most bearish I have ever beheld
as a mass'.

Under this system, although the best physician might be both
learned and scrupulous, the profession as a whole could not claim
the respect given to the Church or the Law. If a doctor was called
to a large country house in early Victorian times, it was customary
to offer him refreshment in the housekeeper's room. Slowly, however, medicine began to change from a craft to a field of scientific
study.[2] The change is faithfully reflected in the novels of the
period. Dr Thorne of Barsetshire 'might constantly be seen com-
pounding medicines in the shop at the left hand of his front door'.
Dr Lydgate of Middlemarch refused to do so, and, studying 'the
higher questions which determine the starting point of a diagnosis
– the philosophy of medical evidence', proposed to found a
medical school at Middlemarch Infirmary.

The future, happily for doctor and patient, lay with the men of
science, led by the great school of French physical diagnosticians.
Specialist hospitals, of which the first in Britain was the Royal
Chest Hospital, formed new centres for study and teaching. The
passing of the first Public Health Act in 1848 and the establishment of the General Board of Health made it possible to collate
medical statistics which now took on new value. Research in the
hospitals and universities gave the physician new resources and
a new intellectual standing. At last he abandoned, with his gold-
headed cane, tricorne hat and sonorous Latin, the futile search
for a universal theoretical system of medicine, and in its place
turned to direct observation at the bedside.

Meanwhile the profession, by its own efforts, reformed its
education and code of professional conduct. The Royal College

---

[1] Paget, J., *Memoirs*, p. 39.

[2] Landmarks in this process were the invention of the stethoscope and the
improved compound microscope. Developments in histology, pathology,
physiology and clinical medicine followed.

of Surgeons, successor to the Surgeons' Company, founded in 1800 on the model of the 280-year-old College of Physicians, attempted to impose higher standards on the old-fashioned cupping and bleeding craft of the surgeon-apothecaries. In the year of the Great Reform Bill 'more than fifty medical gentlemen' met in a society 'both friendly and scientific', later to form part of the British Medical Association.[1] Two years later, in 1834, the government appointed a Select Committee on Medical Education which uncovered the tangle of conflicting claims and privileges forming the ancien régime. *The Lancet*, under its ferocious founding-editor Thomas Wakley, hounded the medical corporations to establish higher, and uniform, standards of training.

Now it was that women began to feel the full disadvantage of their exclusion from the universities and from all scientific education. Nature might have assigned to them the treatment of the sick; education, controlled by society, now gave it exclusively to men. By the mid-nineteenth century the figure of the ideal physician was clearly drawn as a scholar and a gentleman, a status to which, on both counts, no woman could aspire.

Ironically the Medical Act of 1858, excellent in its intentions, made this state of affairs absolute. The principle of this Act was that at last 'persons requiring medical aid should be enabled to distinguish qualified from unqualified medical practitioners'. This was to be achieved through the General Medical Council, which established a minimum standard of training, and a Register of qualified doctors who alone were entitled to sign death certificates or claim legal protection in their work. On paper the Medical Act of 1858 constituted no bar to the practice of medicine by women since it imposed no restrictions on candidates for registration other than having received a proper training. It had, however, failed to provide for the compulsory admission of women to universities, medical schools or qualifying examinations.

There was very little hope that universities would admit women

[1] Vaughan, P., *Doctors' Commons*, p. 8.

voluntarily, judging by the experience of Jessie Meriton White, the spirited daughter of a Liverpool shipowner. In May 1856 she wrote to the Registrar of the University of London, asking whether a woman could become a candidate for a diploma in medicine if, on presenting herself for examination, she produced all the requisite certificates of character, capacity and study from one of the institutions recognized by London University. Two months later, after taking Counsel's opinion, the Senate of London University passed a resolution that 'Miss J. M. White be informed that the Senate, acting upon the opinion of the legal advisor, does not consider itself empowered to admit females as candidates for degrees'.[1] Miss White might have done better to follow the example of Dr James Barrie, a remarkably fresh-faced subaltern who entered the army medical service in 1813, rose to the rank of Inspector General of the Army Medical Department, and was found after death to have been a woman. Jessie White gave up the idea of medicine; she found adventure instead by marrying one of Garibaldi's officers and nursing his wounded redshirts in the field. The battle of woman's entry to the medical profession remained for the moment unfought.

From 1858 onwards, in effect, the Examining Boards held the right to admit or reject aspiring woman doctors. These Boards were made up of practising members of the medical profession, representatives of an established masculine monopoly, and their judgment could hardly be perfectly unbiased. The question of the right of women to sit for medical qualifying examinations was to split the medical profession from top to bottom. Some, a minority, were warmly and sincerely in favour of women physicians. Others, though they did not like the idea personally, believed that liberal principles entitled the women to compete. One of these was the well-loved and just Sir James Paget, who wrote: 'I think them sadly mistaken in wishing for it, but I see no sufficient *grounds* on which they can justly or usefully be excluded.'[2] Others again

[1] Pratt, E. A., *Pioneer Women in Victoria's Reign*, pp. 94–5.
[2] Todd, M., *Life of Sophia Jex-Blake*, p. 444.

were prepared to go to almost any lengths in order to keep out the intruders, seizing with alacrity on the weapon of womanly purity, which lay ready to hand. One doctor remarked that no other topic roused his colleagues to such transports of righteous indignation.

> Many of the most estimable members of our profession perceive in the medical education and destination of women a horrible and vicious attempt deliberately to unsex themselves – in the acquisition of anatomical and physiological knowledge the gratification of a prurient and morbid curiosity and thirst after forbidden information – and in the performance of routine medical and surgical duties the assumption of offices which Nature intended entirely for the sterner sex.[1]

Lecturers in anatomy lamented that they would no longer be able to teach useful, indecent mnemonics; here the coming of women students was to create a revolution indeed. Prominent among the objectors were the members of the Obstetrical Society, who ran the most serious risk from feminine competition.

To sum up: since medieval times Englishwomen had been excluded from scientific study, and the great medical advances of the last three hundred years had been made by men alone. Women had been excluded successively from the medical guilds, the Royal Colleges and good professional practice, even in midwifery, so that the development of medical education and ethics alike had passed them by. By 1860 the prospects for any woman who wished to win a qualification in medicine in this country were more daunting than ever before. Vested interest, prejudice and custom, so potent in British society, all were against her.

Skill and intelligence alone would not be enough to regain the rights lost one by one over centuries. The task would call for high courage and a granite integrity of character. Nowhere in Europe was the woman who wished to study medicine so stubbornly opposed as in Britain, yet nowhere was her final victory so com-

[1] Rivington, W., *The Medical Profession*, 1st edn, pp. 135–6.

plete and resounding.[1] One has only to compare the present position of women in medicine with that in law, industrial management or banking to appreciate this. Among the reasons for victory may be found the character of Elizabeth Garrett, the first woman in this country to qualify as physician and surgeon.

[1] Lipinska, M., op. cit. p. 445, formed this opinion after an international study of the medical women's movement.

Discussions and Decisions
1859–1860

When Elizabeth Garrett returned from Gateshead hugging her new resolution, she found a threatened financial crisis at home. The enterprises of the rival Garrett brothers had grown fast during the past ten years. Early in the 1850s Richard Garrett had built the Long Shop at Leiston, a model engineering workshop of its time; by 1855 he had one of the largest agricultural machinery factories in the kingdom, covering eight acres and employing six hundred men. The plant raised its own steam power, manufactured its own gas and during 1855 constructed its own private line to the main railway.[1]

Such achievement at Leiston called for a corresponding effort at Snape. In 1859 Newson Garrett doubled the size of the maltings, marking out the foundations with his walking stick, firing the bricks at his Aldeburgh yard and ferrying them upstream under sail to raise new buildings on the Wharf at Snape Bridge. Incidentally his building lines, marked by eye alone, were slightly curved, to the confusion of subsequent architects. The new maltings formed a long rambling red-brick range with doorways, ladders and hoists of white clapboard. Under the gilded clock in the centre, an arched gateway admitted Newson's private railway like an iron horse to its stables. On a winter's day the russet glow of the buildings still lights up the bleak landscape of the estuary. It was a triumph for Newson Garrett, undertaken entirely at his

[1] White, W., *History, Gazeteer and Directory for Suffolk*, 1855, p. 526.

own risk, but to create it he had strained his self-made capital to the utmost.

Money was for the time being very short at Aldeburgh. Newson's optimism turned to gloom and expenses were cut down all round. He threw himself into preparations for an imaginary bankruptcy with the same wholehearted enthusiasm which he brought to everything else. The family sat down to their dinner of Suffolk dumpling and found its familiar accompaniment of beef had disappeared. Millicent was abruptly brought home from Miss Browning's to study as best she could in the old school-room. There was even talk of leaving Alde House.[1]

At the same time the quarrel between the Garrett brothers took a fiercer turn, probably because Newson supported one of Richard's sons in a disagreement with his father.[2] Next Newson, who had always believed himself, in spite of his innate enthusiasm for progress, to be a Conservative, wrote to Sir Fitzroy Kelly, the Conservative M.P. for East Suffolk, announcing that he would henceforward vote Liberal. Richard Garrett, searching for the worst term of condemnation in his vocabulary, called his brother a Radical. From this time onwards they hardly met and were not on speaking terms. These various stresses made Newson's temper shorter than ever. It was not the moment for his daughter to approach him with a revolutionary and expensive project.

In January 1860 Elizabeth read in *The Englishwoman's Journal* an open letter from Dr Blackwell to 'Young Ladies Desirous of Studying Medicine,[3] which described the four years of a medical course. There must be a year of medical reading, directed by 'a respectable medical practitioner', covering anatomy and physiology, chemistry and materia medica, and the close study of some ten standard medical textbooks. The second year should be divided between six months' practical work in a laboratory and six months in hospital as a nurse. 'No one who has the true spirit

---

[1] Fawcett, M. G., op. cit. p. 50.
[2] Anderson, Sir A. G., MS.
[3] Blackwell, E., *The Englishwoman's Journal*, Jan. 1860.

for this work in her, will hesitate to accept the wearisome details of the nurse's duty, for the sake of the invaluable privilege of seeing disease on a large scale.' The third year presented more difficulties, for it should be spent in a college, and the fourth should include six months' practical experience in midwifery. For these last two years Dr Blackwell could only suggest America and Paris respectively, since no British university or hospital school had ever admitted a woman. The letter ended with an estimate of the expense involved. 'I think I may safely state that £100 per annum will be necessary for four years, exclusive of travelling expenses, clothes, books and instruments. To this I must add means of support during the first years of practice, for no one should calculate on a rapid success.'

For the time being Elizabeth decided to say nothing about her plans. Meanwhile in London Louie and Emily Davies had discreetly approached the ladies' committee formed by Elizabeth Blackwell and investigated the legal position.[1] This was not encouraging. It was true that Dr Blackwell had already been inscribed as the first woman on the British Medical Register under the Act of 1858, but the Medical Council, alarmed by this, had now resolved to exclude all other holders of foreign diplomas.[2] Elizabeth Garrett and her advisers were therefore in a dilemma. She could qualify in America or in Switzerland, where medical schools were open to women, but this qualification would have no legal standing at home. To win a place on the Medical Register she must gain admission to a British medical school and a British examining body. If she succeeded, other women could follow; if she failed, the way might be closed for years.

During 1859 and 1860 Emily Davies paid several visits to Alde House. The two young women shut themselves away and talked endlessly, not of parties or dancing partners, but of matriculation, hospitals, examinations and feminism. Emily Davies was now

[1] Blackwell, E., *Pioneer Work opening the Medical Profession to Women*, p. 177.
[2] Rivington, W., *The Medical Profession*, 2nd edn, p. 97.

convinced that the only way to improve the status of women was to improve their education. It was their ignorance which encouraged men to regard them as children or dolls.

> Newspapers are scarcely supposed to be read by women at all [she wrote]. When *The Times* is offered to a lady, the sheet containing the advertisements and the Births, Deaths and Marriages is considerately selected. Almost complete mental blankness being the ordinary condition of women, it is not to be wondered at that their opinions, when they happen to have any, are not much respected.[1]

She was critical of women's lazy minds; she also had no use for their cherished ailments, which often represented an escape from responsibility.

> It is a rare thing to meet with a lady of any age who does not suffer from headaches, languor, hysteria or some ailment showing a want of stamina. . . . Dullness is not healthy and the lives of ladies are, it must be confessed, exceedingly dull. Busy people, and especially men . . . think dullness is calm. If they had ever tried what it is to be a young lady they would know better.

To all women's sufferings and failings Emily Davies found one answer, education. In private Miss Davies might refer to the opponents of the women's cause as 'the enemy', yet she was sensible enough to see that women would lose, not gain, support by shocking conventional public opinion. By sheer force of character she imposed on her lively young friend Elizabeth Garrett her own standards of propriety. 'I don't think it quite does', she wrote in a characteristic letter, 'to call the arguments on the other side foolish. They are, of course, but it does not seem quite polite to say so.'

A pair of very shrewd young eyes watched Emily Davies and Elizabeth at their discussions on these visits. Millicent Garrett, then aged thirteen, soon summed Emily Davies up.

[1] Davies, S. E., 'On Secondary Education relating to Girls', *Proceedings of the Social Science Association*, 1864.

Miss Davies had a strong and masterful character [she recalled]. She wanted women to have as good and thorough an education as men; she wanted to open the professions to them and to obtain for them the Parliamentary franchise. But she did not want any violence either of speech or action. She remained always the quiet, demure little rector's daughter.

To the younger Garretts Emily Davies was a kill-joy, but if the often-told story is true, she soon began to discern the exceptional qualities of Elizabeth's small sister. It was night in Elizabeth's room at Alde House. The two friends were talking as they brushed their hair by the bedroom fire, while the pretty, intelligent child sat nearby, listening but saying nothing. 'Well, Elizabeth,' said Emily, 'it is clear what has to be done. I must devote myself to securing higher education, while you open the medical profession for women. After these things are done we must see about getting the vote.' She turned to the little girl, still sitting quietly on her stool, and said, 'You are younger than we are, Millie, so you must attend to that.'

Elizabeth set to work to fill the daunting gaps in her education. Mr Tate, the schoolmaster at Aldeburgh, coached her in Greek and Latin and sportingly promised 'not to tell', in case her plans should come to nothing. Emily Davies, with her own incisive style, corrected English compositions by post, marking offending sentences as obscure, ungrammatical or inelegant. 'I am afraid you will find my style very dogmatic and rough. Will you make as many corrections as possible in it, please?' wrote Elizabeth. She was hard-working, objective and self-critical; gradually, with practice, her writing began to reflect these qualities. Her style was vigorous and straightforward, accurate on facts and enlivened by a youthful sense of fun. Her letters were racy and amusing; vitality overflowed from the pages. Elizabeth Garrett was happy. The change to purposeful work had brought her an almost physical relief. 'From the moment I got into steady work,' she recalled, 'and had more to do every day than I could easily undertake, the sky cleared, and it has been clear ever since.'[1] With hard work, her recreations took on meaning and pleasure. She read, rode and walked with zest, and discovered the new world of Bach and Mozart.

The years 1859 and 1860, when Elizabeth Garrett stood poised ready to begin her career, form a watershed in English thought. In 1859 William Morris's Red House at Bexley was begun; in 1860 Ruskin began to issue *Unto This Last*. The same years saw the publication of the *Origin of Species*, Mill *On Liberty*, Fitzgerald's *Omar Khayyám* and Meredith's *Richard Feverel*.[2] Elizabeth read them all steadily.

Meanwhile there were signs that Newson's financial cloud was lifting. Millicent returned to school. Sam was to go to Rugby, later to Cambridge, and there was no more talk of moving. By June 1860 Elizabeth felt she could no longer put off telling her parents about her ambitions. She waited until after her twenty-fourth birthday, and on 15 June approached her father. A letter to Emily Davies, written the same day, recounts their conversation verbatim.[3]

She began by telling him that she wished to study medicine. Newson Garrett hardly let her finish:

'The whole idea is so *disgusting*,' he burst out. 'I could not entertain it for a moment!'

Elizabeth was unshaken. 'What is there to make doctoring more disgusting than nursing, which women are always doing and which ladies have done publicly in the Crimea?' she argued. He could not tell her. Elizabeth spoke as firmly as she dared. 'I *must* have this or something else; I cannot live without some real work.' Mr Garrett shifted his ground. 'It would take seven years before you could practise.' Again his daughter was ready with an answer. 'Six, not seven; and if it were seven years, I should

---

[1] Elizabeth Garrett Anderson, MS. draft for a speech, Royal Free Hospital Medical School.

[2] Young, G. M., *Early Victorian England*, Vol. II, p. 502.

[3] Elizabeth Garrett to Emily Davies, 15 June 1860. Fawcett Library.

be little more than thirty-one years old and able to work for twenty years probably.' This was a reasonable enough point. Mr Garrett, recognizing a stubbornness to match his own, ended by saying, 'At least I cannot agree to it without more thought.'

To Elizabeth this seemed a satisfactory ending to the interview. She understood her father very well, his originality, his ambition and his intense family pride. 'I think he will probably come round in time; I mean to renew the subject pretty often. He does not like it, I think . . . but he will soon be reconciled *if I succeed*. This is an all important point.'[1]

She also realized that her father's hasty tongue might be a danger; adroitly she used the hostility between the Garrett brothers to silence him.

I told him that nothing would more certainly clinch my determination than the sneers and foolish ridicule that would be sure to come from *relations* when they knew it. If it becomes a matter of gossip, I shall never retreat, however great the wish might be. This arrow took effect well, and I feel pretty sure that he will be personally anxious to keep it quiet.[2]

Essentially, whatever their arguments, Mr Garrett and Elizabeth understood one another; but between mother and daughter an intellectual gulf began to open. However real her affection for her mother, however strong public opinion on filial obedience, it was impossible for Elizabeth to halt her own development and return to the Evangelical mould. She was infuriated to hear her mother defending Mr Dowler's 'vile' Sunday sermon, and Mrs Garrett, on her side, had to endure Elizabeth's admiration for *The Mill on the Floss* and even for its author – 'it is so impossible to believe that she has really sinned against her own conscience'. Mrs Garrett had borne eleven children, and contributed through years of hard work to the rise in the family fortunes. Now, when tranquil prosperity should have rewarded her, the news of her headstrong

[1] Elizabeth Garrett to Emily Davies, 18 June (?) 1860. Fawcett Library.
[2] ibid.

daughter's plans broke on her like a calamity. Sobbing 'The disgrace!' she shut herself into her bedroom and made herself ill with crying.[1] Elizabeth was miserable but unshaken.

A week passed, and Mrs Garrett grew calm enough for them to have a two-hour discussion. Elizabeth wanted to go to London to take advice from medical men and the president of Dr Blackwell's committee, Mrs Russell Gurney, who had sent her a kind note. Mrs Garrett countered with another proposal. Why should not Lizzie stay at home and act as governess to the younger children? Elizabeth protested, instantly and steadily, that it would be completely impossible for her to live at home all her life, an argument which met with total incomprehension.[2] In this uneasy state the family had to welcome a party of visitors, including some cousins, John and Sarah Freeman. Elizabeth insisted that nothing must look odd to the guests, but Mr Garrett could not resist bringing up the subject of women physicians as the party sat round the dinner table.

He asked Sarah Freeman her opinion and she opposed women in medicine, not in an intelligent way, thought Elizabeth, but evidently only from prejudice. Newson was roused to say 'I should prefer a woman attending my wife and daughter, if I could be thoroughly well satisfied that she was qualified.' Sarah objected that Miss Blackwell was not so strictly examined as men were. Opposition at once put Newson on his mettle. 'I should have expected the examiner to be *more* strict with her than they are usually', he maintained. Elizabeth's brother Edmund, a natural conservative, joined in. 'If I had been an examiner, I would have refused to examine any woman,' he said. Alice and Mr Garrett both opened their mouths to speak at once. Newson won. 'That would have been very mean and cowardly of you,' he said. Elizabeth, sitting quietly in her place, heard her father with satisfaction.[3]

[1] Anderson, L. G., op. cit. p. 47.
[2] Elizabeth Garrett to Emily Davies, 26 June 1860. Fawcett Library.
[3] Elizabeth Garrett to Emily Davies, 28 June 1860. Fawcett Library.

By the end of the month he did as she wished. Feeling, in a typical family phrase, that 'he could not let Elizabeth fight the first round without an ally', he came with her to London and arm-in-arm they walked down Harley Street, calling on the leading consultants. They made a striking pair, the handsome vigorous father with the tang of Suffolk in his speech, and the daughter slender and self-possessed. Clearly they were people of substance, accustomed to having their own way, but no one would offer them any encouragement. 'My dear young lady', said one eminent consultant, 'why not be a nurse?' For a moment Elizabeth Garrett allowed a flash of spirit to show through her demure disguise. 'Because,' she said in her soft, ladylike voice, 'I prefer to earn a thousand rather than twenty pounds a year.'[1] It was her one indiscretion; otherwise she kept her temper and replied courteously to distasteful advice. Everywhere they got the same answer. Miss Garrett might waste her father's money on lectures, but no medical school would admit her to practical work and no corporation would allow her to sit for its qualifying examinations. Without these she could not hope to get her name on the Medical Register and practise legally. Some of the physicians laughed at her, some were barely civil; no one offered help.

Elizabeth was anxious about the effect of so much discouragement on her father. In particular the suggestion that she should nurse was dangerous to her plans, for 'lady nurses' were much in the public mind at that moment. In a few days' time, on 9 July, the training school for nurses, endowed with the proceeds of the Nightingale Fund, was to open at St Thomas's Hospital. During the next decade it became an accepted convention for 'lady pupils', on payment of a premium, to undergo a shortened period of hospital training. They were carefully segregated from ordinary nurses, with private rooms to sleep in, reserved seats in chapel and special uniforms.[2] Society at large was now favourably in-

[1] Anderson, L. G., op. cit. p. 50.
[2] At Guy's they wore 'stately black alpaca gowns', at the Middlesex they 'were attired in a dress of violet hue with a small train three inches in length,

clined to nurses. 'Here is an opportunity for showing how a woman's work may complement man's in the true course of nature' ran an enthusiastic magazine article. 'Where does the character of the "helpmeet" come out so strikingly as in the sick room, where the quick eye, the soft hand, the light step and the ready ear, second the wisdom of the physician, and execute his behests better than he himself could have imagined?'[1]

It was precisely this tone of sentimental, rather patronizing, approval which made Elizabeth reject nursing. The trained nurse, by her very training, must carry out the doctor's orders. The woman physician or surgeon by contrast asserts her right to independent professional judgment. This Elizabeth Garrett, whatever the cost, was determined to do.

Newson Garrett was recalled on business to Aldeburgh, leaving Elizabeth, anxious but determined, to stay on with Louie in London. In fact she need not have worried. The frustrating excursion to Harley Street had done her cause more good with her father than any number of reasoned arguments. Mr Garrett was a living example of Blake's axiom that 'Damn braces, bless relaxes'. Opposition always put him on his mettle. Once at home, surrounded by the brick and mortar evidence of Garrett enterprise and success, fatherly pride and sheer East Anglian obstinacy kindled in him. He had never failed in his ventures and Elizabeth must not fail in hers. It took him less than a week to decide, and, once resolved, not even Mrs Garrett's renewed tears and threats that the disgrace would kill her could make him change his mind. It was the most remarkable thing he ever did in a remarkable life, to set his individual sense of justice against the established social order; Mr Garrett's decision was of historic importance, not only for his own family. On 8 July he wrote Elizabeth a generous letter. 'I have resolved in my own mind after deep and painful

which swept the floor behind them', and concealed their ankles from the prying eyes of students. Abel-Smith, B., *A History of the Nursing Profession*, p. 31.

[1] Abel-Smith, B., op. cit. p. 18.

consideration not to oppose your wishes and as far as expense is concerned I will do all I can in justice to my other children to assist you in your study.'[1] By the time Elizabeth read these words her plans were already far advanced, for she had spent the intervening week in ceaseless activity.

The first step was to meet Dr Blackwell's representative; Llewelyn Davies arranged an introduction and his sister at once took Elizabeth to call at Mrs Russell Gurney's house. Emelia Gurney, wife of the Recorder of London, was in her late thirties, an intelligent, well-read woman of great warmth and charm. Her welcome was balm to Elizabeth, still smarting from the friction with her own mother, and an affectionate relationship grew up between them. On Wednesday, 4 July, Mrs Gurney took Elizabeth for a carriage drive, and next day invited her to breakfast. One by one they discussed eminent men who could be relied upon to give Mr Garrett a favourable impression of the situation. Among these Mrs Gurney mentioned William Hawes. This name struck Elizabeth as familiar, and she soon learnt that Mr Hawes, a former business acquaintance of her father's, was a governor of the Middlesex Hospital. 'I am pretty sure his opinion will have weight,' she said.[2] Mrs Gurney arranged another breakfast party on Saturday morning, 7 July, for Elizabeth to meet him.

Mr Hawes proved an excellent adviser, friendly and realistic. He approved in principle of women studying medicine, but stressed that the difficulties to be overcome would need strong determination, and great individual fitness in the first candidate. He questioned Elizabeth searchingly.

'Have you any idea of the nature of the difficulties?' he asked. She admitted that she had not. 'It is because I feel so ignorant about them that I dare not speak or think confidently of the strength of my determination.' 'Then I suggest some test should be found to prove your powers of endurance before any time is spent on direct medical studies.' Mrs Gurney and her husband

[1] Anderson, L. G., op. cit. p. 56.
[2] Elizabeth Garrett to Emily Davies, 4 and 5 July 1860. Fawcett Library.

78

agreed, and Elizabeth, considering these 'great unknown difficulties', was honest enough to see the idea was reasonable. Although fixed in her determination not to limit herself to nursing,
she was quite willing to nurse for a time, as means to an end.
'I suggest that I should spend six months as a hospital nurse at
once,' she said.

Mr Hawes agreed to go at once to the Middlesex Hospital to
arrange it with the treasurer and the matron, on condition that
Elizabeth would face the full ordeal of a surgical ward. The
Gurneys, thinking how lonely she would be, wanted to advertise
for another lady pupil, but Elizabeth, who was anxious to start
now, next day if possible, would not wait. She must, she wrote,
'go through the test and assure myself and my friends of the
stability of my resolve; and if I am to fail, the sooner the question
is settled the better for me in every way'.[1] The arrival of Mr
Garrett's letter promising financial support clinched the Middlesex
plan. Louie, although she now had a second baby to occupy her,
supported her sister on a round of family calls to break the news.
The Dunnell relations were startled by Elizabeth's plans, but her
enthusiasm and Louie's gentleness won them round at least to
verbal agreement. Through it all, Elizabeth managed to keep an
appearance of calm, but she was so strung up that when she went
to say goodbye to Mrs Gurney the older woman's kindness brought
her dangerously near to tears.[2]

She returned to Aldeburgh to make final arrangements on
12 July, and next day wrote a formal letter to Aunt Richard
Garrett, setting out her plans in terms which made it plain she
would accept no interference.[3]

For some time I have been gradually making up my mind to an
important step. . . . During the last two or three years I have
felt an increasing longing for some definite occupation which

[1] Elizabeth Garrett to Emily Davies, 8 July 1860. Fawcett Library.
[2] Elizabeth Garrett to Emily Davies, 11 July 1860. Fawcett Library.
[3] Elizabeth Garrett attached importance to this letter, for she made a
careful copy of it. Quoted Anderson, L.G., op. cit. p. 57.

should also bring me in time a position and a moderate income. I think you will not be surprised that I should feel this longing, for it is indeed far more wonderful that a healthy woman should spend a long life in comparative idleness, than that she should wish for some suitable work, upon which she could spend the energy that now only causes painful restlessness and weariness. I have decided that the study of medicine offers more attraction to me than any other kind of work and I have decided to enter upon it.

She added pointedly, 'I need scarcely say that I should not make this attempt without my dear parents' sanction.

This plain speaking did not prevent Aunt Richard Garrett and the Freeman cousins from offering a liberal dose of advice, which Elizabeth ignored. Their morbid prophecies of a breakdown and early death did not alarm her at all. She already had the common-sense approach to health which were to mark her work as a physician.

I am determined by God's help to keep in good health if care can do it. I shall ride as often as my funds will permit of the outlay and I think with an occasional gallop, frequent bathing and daily walking, I shall be able to prove that it is not necessary to break down under the physical and nervous difficulties.[1]

She did not want any old friends to learn of her decision at second hand, so she took the trouble to go round Aldeburgh seeing them each in turn and telling them herself. Criticism she must learn to meet with calm, civil obstinacy.

When visiting was done and the last letters written, all that remained was to do her packing. Clothes were a problem. To emphasize her student status, Elizabeth declined to wear nurse's uniform, but ordinary clothes were hardly suitable for hospital use. A typical frock of the season had a flounced crinoline, a tight bodice heavily worked with bead or braid, long, pointed sleeves

[1] Elizabeth Garrett to Emily Davies, 19 July 1860. Fawcett Library.

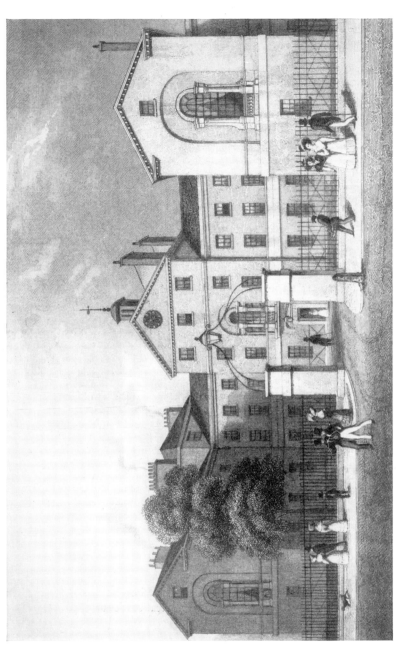

3. The Old Middlesex Hospital showing the fore-court by which Elizabeth Garrett entered the building

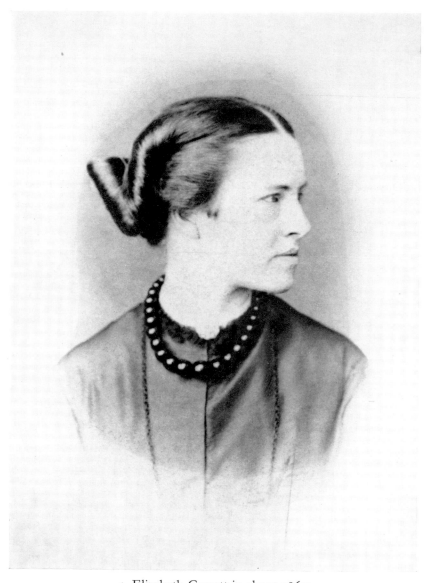

4. Elizabeth Garrett in about 1860:
the Suffolk girl who became a medical student

of Gothic inspiration, and full under-sleeves of snowy lawn. In the end Elizabeth provided herself with linen aprons and a note-book and decided to keep an open mind about dress. The end of the month approached. In spite of Mrs Garrett's occasional tears and protestations, Elizabeth left for London at the end of July 1860.

CHAPTER SIX

The Surgical Nurse
August 1860 –January 1861

On 1 August 1860, at eight o'clock in the morning, Elizabeth Garrett passed for the first time through the gateway of the Middlesex Hospital. The entrance from the street was through wrought-iron railings and a paved forecourt. Before her was a wide façade of red brick with pediment, cupola and gold clock face. On either side were wings, added as the number of beds grew, and lit by tall Palladian windows.[1] It was a handsome building, fitting the dignity of the charity founded in 1745, and removed in 1757 to a site in the open fields north of Oxford Street noted for good snipe shooting. A hundred years had seen the hospital gain size and reputation, while the city closed around it; by 1860 it stood among the crowded streets of Soho. From the first, apprentices and pupils had walked the hospital with individual physicians and surgeons. In 1835, on the initiative of the great Sir Charles Bell, the hospital had opened its own Medical School, so that in his words 'the experience afforded by upwards of two hundred beds; by the observation of 1,600 in-patients and 5,000 out-patients in the course of every year should not run to waste'.[2] After some early difficulties the Middlesex Hospital Medical School had prospered; in 1853 it had enlarged its museum and library, and by the time Elizabeth entered the hospital it was in the first rank.

[1] Sanders, H. St G., *The Middlesex Hospital*, p. 25.
[2] Thomson, H. C., *The Story of the Middlesex Hospital Medical School*, p. 27.

The Medical School was, of course, the goal of her ambition, and privately she did not shift an inch, but she judged it wise to say nothing of this for the present. The fiction that she was a nurse satisfied the conventions and must be maintained. Inwardly trembling with excitement, but schooled to decorum, she unpacked her apron and notebook and presented herself at her first ward. She had been warned to expect horrors and was determined to outface them. 'Everyone seemed to fear that my health and nerves will break down'; she wrote, 'therefore I am determined by God's help to come through.'[1] The bare boards, the long whitewashed room and the rows of curtained beds were orderly enough, but the smell in any hospital ward was such that visitors had been known to vomit at their first entrance.

In 1860 the Listerian revolution still lay five years in the future. The surgeons at the Middlesex, as everywhere, wore their old frock-coats in the dissecting rooms. Eventually the coat, stiffened with blood and pus until it stood upright, found its way to the operating theatre. An operation was a dirty job, and an irretrievable coat the most suitable wear for it. Occasionally the operator turned up his cuffs, but his assistants never; to do so would have been an affectation of importance on their part. They gathered round the wooden table, stained rusty brown and sprinkled round with sawdust like a butcher's block. The house surgeon stood ready with a bevy of threaded needles for suturing, the long silken threads trailing to the floor from his coat lapel, where he had fastened them. Behind him the throng of students pushed and jostled.

The most common operation was amputation, for malignant growths, tuberculous joints and almost all compound fractures. Irons were kept aglow in a brazier to sear growths or septic wounds. One case of sepsis was enough to infect every wound in a ward. Gangrene, carried from patient to patient on the dressers' hands, attacked the stumps, which lay upon zinc trays, where drops of pus slowly collected into pools. None of this appeared to disturb

[1] Elizabeth Garrett to Emily Davies, 29 Sept. 1860. Fawcett Library.

Elizabeth Garrett. She approached nursing objectively, with detachment. Within a few days she established her own routine.

At eight o'clock every morning, having walked from Bayswater whatever the weather, she appeared in one of the two surgical wards. She went at once to a side table and began to prepare for the day's dressings, spreading ointment, cutting lint, rolling bandages and making poultices without supervision. Next, polite and composed, she accompanied the ward sister on a dressing round. The simpler cases she could soon dress herself, the more difficult ones, such as cancer, were dressed by the sister while she watched closely, with interest. There was plenty in the ward for her to observe. A table at the end of the room bearing test tubes and one or two standard chemical reagents served for a laboratory; there the clerks or dressers under the supervision of the house physician or surgeon made the few routine clinical investigations.[1]

Indiscriminate bleeding was on the wane, but the process of cupping still survived. Every morning an active old gentleman, Mr Briggs, cupper to the hospital, called at the ward door and asked, 'Any orders for me today, Sister?' He wore a dress-coat and white neckcloth and had the urbanity of a bygone age. His deftness in cupping was phenomenal to watch and the younger members of the medical staff regarded him as the last of the Barber Surgeons.[2] Elizabeth finished the dressings in time to go upstairs and visit two medical wards with the house physician, Dr Willis, before returning for the visit of the surgeon, Mr Worthington, at eleven. After this she gave out medicines all round her ward and went to the museum to read for an hour. She swallowed a quick lunch and was back in the ward for the consultants' visits between one o'clock and three. She walked back to St Agnes Villas in time for tea with Louie or a game with her small nephews, changed for dinner, and later studied alone in her room until bedtime.

On 7 August, when Elizabeth was going about her usual duties,

[1] Thomson, H. C., op. cit., p. 71.
[2] Anderson, J. F., 'Memories of a Medical Life', broadcast on 12 Oct. 1931, when the speaker was ninety-one years old.

there was a small operation in the ward. The staff surgeon performing it, T. W. Nunn, observing this young woman who did not flinch at the sight of blood, explained the case to her and made her see exactly what he was going to do. She responded so intelligently that he offered to take her to his out-patient clinics, and Elizabeth, elated with this first success, resolved to get as skilful as she could in the meantime so that she should not annoy him by awkwardness.[1] The house surgeon and physician, taking their cue from their senior, did all they could to be helpful during the next few weeks. Mr Worthington, the surgeon, was courteous in giving information, and Dr Willis allowed her to watch for an hour and a half as he examined new cases for admission and taught her to listen to chest and heart sounds through his stethoscope. He paid her the compliment of not trying to spare her modesty in any conventional manner. Elizabeth was grateful that he seemed to think it 'quite natural for me to see and hear everything professionally'.[2] To curb her rising elation she had to remind herself that these junior medical officers would have no say in her acceptance by the Medical School.

After the first weeks of mastering routine work, Elizabeth found time to notice the students who followed their various professors on the teaching rounds in the ward. The idleness and rowdiness of the Middlesex students had led only four years before to the appointment of a Dean to control 'pupils disorderly in their conduct'. The current Dean by a fortunate chance was Mr T. W. Nunn, the surgeon who had volunteered to show Elizabeth his out-patients. He was a Pickwickian figure with bald head, mutton-chop whiskers and an engaging sense of humour; when colleagues rebuked him for allowing the whole hospital to call him 'Tommy', as detrimental to the dignity of his office, he maintained that he preferred that to some of the nicknames by which they were secretly known. He had struggled for two years as Dean with students who showed a natural tendency to attend bars rather than

[1] Elizabeth Garrett to Emily Davies, 7 Aug. 1860. Fawcett Library.
[2] Elizabeth Garrett to Emily Davies, 17 Aug. 1860. Fawcett Library.

lectures and to use the dissecting rooms as a boxing arena or ratting pit, but by the time Elizabeth entered the hospital his authority was established and at least half of the students were hard-working young men. They were poor but cheerful, lived in lodgings off the Tottenham Court Road and conducted their social life in the pubs which stayed open until after midnight. Sometimes there was a mild scuffle, sometimes they rang the night bells of distinguished consultants and ran away. Every morning they collected their racing tips from John the hospital hall porter, and hurried out of their nine o'clock lectures to place the day's bets. Another way of supplementing their allowances was by poaching in the surrounding country and in times of financial stress they returned with sackfuls of rabbits, which they sold to the various landladies from whom they rented rooms. The more sporting hunted at Edgware or Hendon, the dashing frequented music halls, and card players could generally join an all-night poker game kept up by the midwifery clerks. The unfortunate turned up at Vine Street where five shillings was the usual sum to pay for a bad headache.[1]

All in all, they resembled most medical students before and since. Some of them, taking their cue from the Dean, were courteous and helpful, and Elizabeth pleaded for friendly relations with them.

> The pupils seem inclined to treat me as a student [she wrote to Emily Davies]; several of them have volunteered scraps of information and as long as they merely speak to me of the matter in hand, I think it is wiser not to appear too frigid or stiff with them. If they *will* forget my sex and treat me as a fellow student, it is just the right kind of feeling. It does seem to be wrong in theory to treat them all as one's natural enemies.[2]

Emily Davies continued to take a guarded view of medical students as a class.

[1] Thomson, H. C., op. cit. pp. 66–9.
[2] Elizabeth Garrett to Emily Davies, 17 Aug. 1860. Fawcett Library.

Elizabeth remained unselfconscious even though many curious eyes watched her all the time. She was self-confident intellectually, but convinced from her Aldeburgh experiences that she must be completely plain and lacking in charm for men. She looked her critics squarely in the face with level brows and mouth obstinately set. Her colouring refused to conform to convention; her hair, smoothly brushed back from a wide forehead, was an as yet unfashionable auburn, her skin was smooth and clear but pale, her dark hazel eyes were uncomfortably intelligent. Her hands were small and supple with square-tipped capable fingers, the 'lady's hand' of the good surgeon. She wore well-fitting dresses in dark silk or velvet, with immaculate lace collars and cuffs. She spoke and moved quietly, yet with a subdued, gay zest for life. Observing her slender figure and light step, the Dean found it hard to believe Miss Garrett was more than eighteen years old.

Elizabeth found she was not squeamish, and after five weeks at the hospital stood among the students in the theatre watching her first operation, 'a stiffish one', with an excitement that quickened all her vitality and left her afterwards tired but happy.[1] Even more remarkably, she was without prudery at a time when even the enlightened paid lip-service to a false refinement.[2] Elizabeth Garrett had a country upbringing; she found herself unembarrassed by the body and its workings. Moreover she discovered a delight in impersonal thought for its own sake, which outweighed conventional modesty.

> I don't find it makes any difference whether the doctors are young or old, married or single, as far as being taught by them goes [she wrote]. Dr Willis takes everything so calmly that I do not feel half as much awkwardness with what he says to me

[1] Elizabeth Garrett to Emily Davies, 6 Sept. 1860. Fawcett Library.

[2] A correspondent in *The Englishwoman's Journal* wrote that it would be difficult to teach women physiology because of 'the extreme repugnance, amounting to disgust, felt by many girls to this class of knowledge'. *The Englishwoman's Journal*, April 1862.

Elizabeth Garrett Anderson

and shows me as I do with the hesitation and would-be modesty of some of the old physicians.[1]

As she found her feet and gained confidence it became clear that pioneering in a new profession was not enough for her; she would attempt, and with success, to create a new working relationship between the sexes, friendly, equal and detached.

Elizabeth Garrett's character was developing fast under the stimulus of independence and responsible work. She wished more women would try getting away from home and making a start as she had done. What women needed, she felt, was 'a great deal more stirring up'.[2] In September she was left for a time without a home. Louie and James gave up their Bayswater house and went away for a family holiday until their new house in Manchester Square should be ready. Elizabeth moved into lodgings at 58 South Audley Street, where she consented to have James's sister, Sarah Smith, with her as chaperone, but insisted on living independently and having the evenings to herself for study. Fortunately Sarah, a keen church-worker, went out often visiting the poor or to missionary meetings, which was as well, since Elizabeth could be ruthless in defence of her new-found freedom. When Mrs Garrett, alarmed by this new move, wrote once again of the life-long pain she would feel at her daughter's chosen career, Elizabeth dismissed the letter coolly as 'morbid throughout and coming at a time when many women suffer from nervous weakness',[3] an explanation presumably congenial to her medical mind. In spite of letters of remonstrance from numerous relations, Elizabeth did not go home and Mrs Garrett recovered. For a daughter to defy a parent in 1860 was to defy society itself, and this, from a sense of reasoned conviction, Elizabeth was prepared to do. To her family and the world she insisted on maintaining a confident front. 'It is rather provoking', she complained, 'that

[1] Elizabeth Garrett to Emily Davies, 6 Sept. 1860. Fawcett Library.
[2] Elizabeth Garrett to Emily Davies, 9 Sept. 1860. Fawcett Library.
[3] Elizabeth Garrett to Emily Davies, 17 Aug. 1860. Fawcett Library.

people will think so much of the difficulties, in spite of my assurances that so far from being appalling I am enjoying the work more than I have ever done any other study or pursuit.'

Elizabeth Garrett's anxieties, which she kept to herself, were real enough; they concerned the theoretical side of her work. Empirical observation, at which she excelled, still formed an important part of medicine, but by the second half of the nineteenth century a physician needed a preliminary training in the principles of physics, chemistry, anatomy and physiology. Elizabeth, having made her way into the wards without proper pre-clinical training, found much of what the medical staff said incomprehensible and was mortified when Mr Nunn, by a quick glance, showed his surprise at her ignorance. She acquired a prospectus of the Medical School course and attempted to read the syllabus by herself in the museum, but was hindered by the continual need to look up unfamiliar scientific terms. Finally she realized she must get help to draw up some orderly scheme of reading.[1]

She was further troubled by the fact of being in a false position at the hospital, nominally a nurse but without any duties or regular scene of action. 'I may go into any ward and learn anything and do anything', she wrote, with a mixture of pride and chagrin. 'Dr Willis treats me as a pupil and the house surgeons do the same, and I am in the surgery every morning getting the teaching and practice gratis for which the students pay a fee.' As a merchant's daughter her code of fair dealing would not allow this to continue. In October, her third month at the hospital, determined to regularize her position, she demanded an interview with the treasurer of the Medical School. Campbell de Morgan, F.R.S., the treasurer and lecturer in surgery, was an impressive figure, distinguished as a surgeon, with a fine presence and a grave, dark-bearded face.[2] Elizabeth, after some secret tremors, faced him bravely and asked to be allowed to pay the usual student's fees, hoping to bring him

[1] Elizabeth Garrett to Emily Davies, 9 Sept. 1860. Fawcett Library.

[2] Thomson, H. C., op. cit., group photograph of Medical Staff facing p. 60.

round by personal influence, which she was beginning to find she could often do. This time she was less successful than usual.

'I could not allow you to pay any fees, as that would be recognizing you partially as a student,' said the treasurer. 'However, you may make a donation to the hospital and stay through the winter learning all that you can as an amateur.' It was not the moment to quibble at this unpleasing term. 'I may continue in the surgery, and attend the house doctors in their rounds and go to operations and have the run of the house as at present?' asked Elizabeth. The treasurer agreed. He also offered, on behalf of the Board, a room in which she could read and keep her belongings, and permission to arrange private tuition with the hospital's apothecary. When Elizabeth asked about the ultimate chances of getting into the college he shook his head and said it was impossible. When she pressed him for reasons, he was inclined to treat the whole subject with amused contempt. 'A lady's presence at lectures would distract the other students' attention,' he said. 'All the London colleges will refuse to admit you and you might as well go to America at once.'[1]

Elizabeth refused to be discouraged. She at once approached the hospital's apothecary about coaching, thinking privately that this would suit her very well instead of nursing work as an excuse for coming constantly into the hospital. Mr Joshua Plaskitt agreed to accept her as a pupil in Latin, Greek and materia medica, for three or four hours daily in the dispensary at the hospital, for six months, as soon as her nursing probation was finished. He proved to be intelligent and liberal and, as she hastened to assure Miss Davies, 'though young, so very quiet and unflighty that no one would *say anything* in connection with him'.[2]

On 9 October Elizabeth moved into her room at the hospital, a small cottage-like apartment with many shelves containing an oppressive amount of crockery, perhaps a disused pantry. The nurses were kind; one offered to cook for her and all were willing

[1] Elizabeth Garrett to Jane Crow, 9 Oct. 1860. Fawcett Library.
[2] Elizabeth Garrett to Emily Davies, 23 Oct. 1860. Fawcett Library.

to help, but Elizabeth preferred an independent mutton-chop and ale. She felt the luxury of studying by her own fireside and invited an acquaintance of the Langham Place circle, Miss Ellen Drewry, to come in and read chemistry with her. To her dismay Miss Drewry appeared in short skirts and a hat like a saucepan.

> I wish the D.s dressed better [she lamented to Emily]. After the arrangements were made for her to come, I was almost afraid it was unwise on my part. She looks awfully strong-minded in walking dress; short petticoats and a close, round hat and several other dreadfully ugly arrangements, but as my room is out of the way, I hope she will not be supposed to belong to me by the students.[1]

It would be fatal to start the legend that a medical woman must be a she-dragon. Elizabeth herself, calm and well groomed, took pains to dress well and felt helped rather than hindered by looking as attractive as lay within her powers.

In the middle of October, after less than three months' training, she was put on night duty alone. She had difficulty in persuading the sister to let her undertake it, but insisted on being allowed because 'having the sole care teaches one so much. When the nurses are present they will not allow me to do anything at all difficult!' The eight hours on duty seemed to pass fast. She worked methodically, careful to make no noise, and went regularly round the darkened rows of beds. Between rounds she sat by the fire with screens around her and a gas lamp burning low on her desk, studying. She had never felt more alert or more watchful.[2]

In the morning she rejoiced in the curiously fresh sense of life it gave to be awake while others still slept.

> I am so fresh and hungry by six o'clock and have generally had a walk and gone through all sorts of business by eight. . . . As the maid who is supposed to wait upon me and the officers who live in the adjoining rooms does not come till eight, I am glad

[1] Elizabeth Garrett to Emily Davies, 12 Oct. 1860. Fawcett Library.
[2] Elizabeth Garrett to Jane Crow, 9 Oct. 1860. Fawcett Library.

to put my room neat at once and get breakfast. Dusting and polishing was always a favourite amusement of mine and I like the manual work after the night's duty. When I sit down to breakfast it feels uncommonly like college life, and if one had but 'fellows' with whom one could be friendly it would be very jolly.

Sleeping by day caused her no trouble; when tired she slept ten hours without a break and woke fresh and tranquil.[1]

At about midnight each night, as she sat alone in the ward, Dr Willis the house physician appeared on his last round. Often when it was over, he seemed in no hurry to go, but sat with her for half an hour, talking quietly in the darkened ward. The strangeness of the hour, the sense that for once she was not being watched by curious eyes, lowered the barriers of Elizabeth's reserve; she found herself telling the young doctor how hard it was to read alone, or to learn at the bedside without planned reading. He advised a tutor to direct her reading and supervise her work regularly.

'How would it be', wrote Elizabeth persuasively to Emily Davies, 'to ask Dr Willis to come to Manchester Square one evening (or two if he could) and act as tutor? I should not think he would be annoyed at my asking.' Emily Davies did not think it would be at all wise, and said so, but her letter arrived too late to have any effect. On the last of Elizabeth's nights on duty Dr Willis offered himself as tutor in anatomy and physiology for three evenings weekly at the modest cost of a guinea a week. Elizabeth accepted without waiting, as she would have done a few months earlier, for Emily's advice. Mr Garrett, when asked, generously agreed to meet the cost of any private tuition she might need. Elizabeth was becoming confident that she could mix with men on her own terms and set an easy, natural tone to their relationship 'as between men', whatever vulgar gossip might say.

[1] Elizabeth Garrett to Emily Davies, 12 and 14 Oct. 1860. Fawcett Library.

For the first time in their friendship she set Emily Davies's opinion on one side. Three months of independence, of hard study and responsibility, had changed her from the eager disciple of Aldeburgh days. Now she meant to use her own judgment. 'Your advice will make me more than ever cautious,' she wrote, 'though I cannot *act* positively upon it.'[1] Tactfully she asked the older woman still to criticize her manner, speech and writing, a criticism which she was prepared to take, and in an objective spirit.[2]

By the end of October 1860 Elizabeth's three months of probation at the Middlesex were over. Throughout it she had been happy and well. She had learnt her way around the stone staircases, corridors and courtyards of the hospital, and could go up and down twenty times in a day to fetch notes from the out-patients, drugs from the dispensary, clean linen from the laundry or stores from the matron's room, without complaining of feeling tired. The sisters found her reliable, the nurses liked her and there had been no gossip about her and the medical staff. Against all expectations but her own, she had come through the test. By November all pretence of her being a nurse had been dropped; somehow, without fuss or argument, by sheer tenacity, she had become an unofficial medical student. She made independent rounds in the wards, and followed the teaching rounds until it was time to start her daily two hours' work in the dispensary with Mr Plaskitt. From there she might be called to the casualty department to see a newly admitted patient, and she was amused to see the incredulity with which new patients stared at the young woman in working apron and sleeves. Evidently they thought that their symptoms and treatment were for some reason being explained to the cook, so unthinkable was the idea of professional training for a woman.

Elizabeth's two teachers made a good team. Personally, she preferred Joshua Plaskitt, who was thoughtful and widely read,

[1] Elizabeth Garrett to Emily Davies, 23 Oct. 1860. Fawcett Library.
[2] Elizabeth Garrett to Emily Davies, 30 Oct. 1860. Fawcett Library.

but he worried her somewhat by refusing to allow medicine the status of an exact science and she criticized him for leaning on the old calomel and bleeding of empirical practice. Dr Willis, an Edinburgh graduate, was the medical man of the future, believing that medicine was an exact science, and that it was disgraceful to act on the empirical plan when it could possibly be avoided. He told Elizabeth he thought the science and practice of medicine the finest pursuit possible.[1] Her own mind being above all orderly and systematic, Elizabeth sided with Dr Willis. All through the early days of grinding away at minute, unrelated facts, she struggled to arrange her information and to see natural connections. She had not, as she herself recognized, a mind of the highest calibre. If one compares her with the first generation of university women, she lacked the profound originality of Jane Harrison, or the creative flow of Constance Garnett. She had entered upon medicine almost by chance and might have done equally well at law, business or administration. Her strength lay in her power of work, and in the peasant obstinacy of her ancestors, refined into an impersonal determination, an intense will to succeed. Hospital visits, private tuition and hard study filled her entire day during the winter of 1860–1. She was often very dissatisfied with her own progress, regarding herself merely as a painstaking plodder. On the other hand her two teachers, who set her examination papers in December on the work of the last five months, were struck by the thoroughness of her reading. Her first textbooks, Barrett's *Outline of Physiology*, and 'Quain',[2] she learnt almost by heart.

Before Christmas the Garrett parents came to stay and to inspect James and Louie's new house, 22 Manchester Square. Elizabeth was pleased to see them and relieved to find her mother cheerful and affectionate, fussing over her daughter's broken chilblains as though Elizabeth had never left home. Yet she would not put

---

[1] Elizabeth Garrett to Emily Davies, 18 Nov. 1860. Fawcett Library.
[2] Presumably *The Elements of Anatomy* by Jones Quain (1796–1865), since the better-known *Dictionary of Medicine* by Sir Richard Quain (1816–1898) was not published until 1882.

away her books, even for the week of the family visit. Sometimes she felt a longing for friends, for society, for music or even for some reading that was not medicine, yet for the present, until she made some headway against ignorance, she would not allow herself to relax.[1] She went home to Aldeburgh for a brief Christmas holiday with the family, happy to see again the familiar things and places of her childhood. Yet these days at home, she saw, could only be an interim in her life. At the New Year she looked back on the past months and forward into the enthralling future, summing up her thoughts next day in a long letter to Dr Blackwell in New York. She recalled her early doubts, how far away they seemed, her offer to serve as a nurse, her early desultory reading and her final determination to cover the groundwork in anatomy, chemistry and materia medica. She related her dealings with Mr de Morgan, Mr Plaskitt and Dr Willis and described her daily routine. She stressed her enjoyment of the work, her happiness in hospital life and her hopes for the future. 'The general feeling seems to be', she wrote, 'that each doctor is willing to help me privately and singly, but they are afraid to countenance the movement by helping me in their collective capacity. This will, however, come in time, I trust.'[2]

[1] Elizabeth Garrett to Emily Davies, 12 Dec. 1860. Fawcett Library.
[2] Elizabeth Garrett to Elizabeth Blackwell, 2 Jan. 1861, reprinted in Blackwell, E., *Pioneer Work opening the Medical Profession to Women*, pp. 184–5.

CHAPTER SEVEN

A Medical Student Dismissed
January–July 1861

Early in January 1861 Elizabeth returned to Manchester Square to be present at the birth of the niece and god-daughter who became another link in the chain binding her to Louisa. The child Dorothea never forgot the devotion she witnessed between her mother and her aunt. At the end of her own long life she recorded how their lives were inspired by their great love for each other.[1] Louisa Smith, an unassuming housewife, possessed a grace and radiance of character from which her sisters, and especially Elizabeth, drew spiritual life. To her Elizabeth returned after each day's work at the hospital with a sense of coming home. Millicent, a schoolgirl on leave from Miss Browning's at Blackheath, remembered visits to Louie as the joy of her life. The three sisters walked in Kensington Gardens, or listened at home while Louie read aloud from Wordsworth, the *Ode on the Intimations of Immortality* or *The Happy Warrior*. His character

> *Whom neither shape of danger can dismay,*
> *Nor thought of tender happiness betray;*
> *Who, not content that former worth stand fast,*
> *Looks forward, persevering to the last,*
> *From well to better, daily self-surpast*

came near to expressing Elizabeth's ideal.[2] On Sundays the sisters

[1] Dorothea Lady Gibb to Sir Colin Anderson, 11 Dec. 1943: Anderson family papers.
[2] Fawcett, M. G., op. cit. pp. 42–3.

and James Smith walked to St Peter's, Vere Street, where, in spite of protests to the Bishop of London signed by large numbers of the Anglican clergy, the Christian Socialist, Frederick Denison Maurice had been instituted as Rector the year before.

Maurice's preaching, however incomprehensible to the literal-minded, gathered around him a band of disciples of whom Elizabeth became one. She was in quest of a faith, having rejected the teaching of her girlhood, and at Vere Street she found what she sought. Maurice captured her imagination by the fineness of his character and the beauty of his wonderful eyes with their look of seeing the invisible. Sometimes when he soared away, as he was liable to do, from the subject in hand, his listeners had to follow as best they could or await his return, but usually Elizabeth Garrett managed to make full notes of his sermons which she submitted to Emily Davies in the form of English exercises. She was never converted to Maurice's Christian Socialism, since the Garrett bias towards successful free enterprise was so strong, but she did believe his teaching that the Fatherhood of God must imply the brotherhood of man. Its effect was to strengthen her inherent sense of social responsibility. Inherited wealth, social position, privilege did not trouble her conscience, since she was determined to use them for the good of other women. In fighting for her medical education she could quote Maurice's words, spoken at the inauguration of Queen's College for Women, 'We look upon all studies as religious, all as concerned with the life and acts of a spiritual creature.'[1]

To Elizabeth Garrett's surprise and regret, however, Maurice strongly disapproved of women in the medical profession. She found it hard to see what his reasons were, since he had always taught that the Christian doctrine of the equal spiritual status of men and women must lead to their equality in society. One of the first public questions he had tackled was the sweated labour of women dressmakers and milliners. To supply women teachers with some professional training he had opened Queen's College

[1] Maurice, F. D., 'Inaugural lecture for Queen's College', 1848.

in 1848. Later he supported public day schools for girls and the admission of women to the degrees of London University, but his conception of 'female knowledge' did not extend to biology lessons, still less to medicine. His college, he claimed, would

> remove the slightest craving for such a state of things, by giving a more healthful direction to minds which might entertain it. The more pains we take to call forth and employ the faculties which belong characteristically to each sex, the less it will be intruding upon the province which, not the conventions of the world, but the will of God, has assigned to the other.[1]

Elizabeth Garrett honoured Maurice, whom she called the Prophet, but did not let the Prophet's disapproval deflect her from her work.

For practical advice Elizabeth Garrett could always turn to Emily Davies's brother, the Rector of Christ Church, Marylebone. Llewelyn Davies was one of the few people whose judgments she trusted without question. He combined the idealism of Maurice with the clarity of mind which was his own family's special gift. After a brilliant career at Cambridge he had served as curate in two East End parishes, St Anne's, Limehouse, and St Mark's, Whitechapel, a time of struggle against poverty and suffering which led him to Christian Socialism. Since coming as Rector to Christ Church, Cosway Street, in 1856 he had undertaken social work in the slums around Lisson Grove, which would now be divided between half a dozen welfare agencies. Llewelyn Davies believed firmly that a Christian society could not be built until women played a responsible part in it. As a wise and experienced parish priest he was a valued friend to the women's cause in general and to Elizabeth Garrett in particular.

On 16 January 1861, when Louie's baby was a week old, Elizabeth returned to the Middlesex Hospital and was delighted to find herself welcomed back as an old friend. At first she attempted to avoid Dr Willis, since she was too busy at home to begin even-

[1] Maurice, F. D., *Lectures to Ladies on Practical Subjects*, 1855.

ing tutorials yet, but he traced her to the men's accident ward where she was helping, and soon study was in full swing again. For the next two months Elizabeth would not even allow herself to go to Denison Maurice's Bible class, but spent all her spare time between ward rounds in the museum reading room, working through Tacitus with a dictionary to improve her shaky Latin.[1] She was doubtful about using a crib; the method saved so much time and worry and she progressed so fast that she suspected there must be something wrong with it.

In March, with nearly six months' intensive study behind her, and an encouraging letter from Dr Blackwell, Elizabeth Garrett felt ready to take the next step towards establishing herself as an official medical student. She was disappointed to learn that she must lose Joshua Plaskitt, who was leaving the hospital for private practice, but this only confirmed the need for her to follow the normal course of instruction. She applied to the Dean for admission to the dissecting room and to the chemistry lectures, which she confidently regarded as the thin end of the wedge for the lectures generally.[2] She pointed out that many of the doctors who had been most sure she would meet with unheard-of insults from the students, now admitted the experiment might safely be tried, and she promised to 'grind away at anatomy to be ready for the D.R.'

The Dean was sympathetic. He himself controlled the dissecting room and undertook to admit her for the next session beginning in May; further, he approached the chemists on her behalf, telling them roundly that there could not be any more awkwardness in men and women working together than in their going to church together.[3] Heisch and Redwood Taylor, the chemistry lecturers, did not need persuading; they were delighted to invite Miss Garrett to the remaining lectures of the present session. On Wednesday, 20 March, Elizabeth attended her first

---

[1] Elizabeth Garrett to Mrs Garrett, 9 Jan. 1861. Anderson family papers.
[2] Elizabeth Garrett to Emily Davies, 6 March 1861. Fawcett Library.
[3] Elizabeth Garrett to Emily Davies, 19 March 1861. Fawcett Library.

chemistry class. Expecting a boisterous reception from the students, she went early to the lecture theatre and took her seat before they came in. They were too astonished by the sight of a girl waiting with notebook and pencil to allow themselves more than an occasional grin, and the lecture went off quietly. Thanks to her private preparation she followed it well and found it interesting.[1]

Every Saturday the lecturer questioned the class on the week's work, allowing the quickest-witted to answer first. On her first Saturday Elizabeth Garrett tried to speak but could not bring herself to utter a word. Plaskitt told her she must overcome her shyness and show she felt like an ordinary student, so next week she answered the first question and many more. She even allowed herself to join in the general laughter at the replies of the chronic dunces in the class. The lecturer, V. R. Heisch, struck by her intelligence, kept her in the laboratory afterwards, showing her microscopic slides and lending her an excellent French textbook, since she read the language fluently.[2]

In the dissecting room also things went well. Mr Nunn was cautious; he would not allow her to work there unless he or one of the demonstrators were present. 'The work itself is not the objection,' he explained. 'Men and women could do that together as well as anything else; it is the general larkiness of the idle students.'[3] Accordingly he took her on her first visit, perhaps curious to see how she would react. Elizabeth Garrett found none of the horrors which had been painted for her by ghoulish acquaintances, no bodies hanging over chairs or by their feet from the ceiling, simply a number of small tables, those not in use neatly covered with calico sheets. The subjects, in fact, did not look like human beings at all.[4] Elizabeth chose a table facing the window with her back to the rest of the room and set quietly to work. As

---

[1] Elizabeth Garrett to Emily Davies, 20 March 1861. Fawcett Library.
[2] Elizabeth Garrett to Emily Davies, 23 March 1861. Fawcett Library.
[3] Elizabeth Garrett to Emily Davies, 25 April 1861. Fawcett Library.
[4] Elizabeth Garrett to Emily Davies, 23 March 1861. Fawcett Library.

well as doing theoretical work with Willis all the winter she had practised the manipulations with Plaskitt and worked on 'bits and pieces' which she carried off to study alone in her room. Now she found the work not too difficult and extremely interesting. Watching her, the Dean was impressed.

With these achievements Elizabeth's hopes soared. She knew well enough the dangers of her father's sanguine temperament in her and she had seen all her life the conflicts it provoked. She ought to have been cautious; but she was young and inexperienced, the friendship of the Dean gave her confidence and the pleasure of stretching her intellectual wings was dizzying. As March went by in apparent triumph she grew dangerously bold. She could not stop herself from glorying in 'my *widening* hospital work. There is constantly some small advance being made, either in friendliness towards some one, or new openings for study. I have felt very much set up this week as to the enjoyment I shall have in student life when it really begins.'[1] For the first time she allowed herself a note of confidence over the amazing ignorance of some fellow-students: the physician's clerk who regarded the chief good of lectures as getting one's attendance 'signed up', the chemistry students who had neglected their previous reading and could not follow the mathematical formulae on the blackboard, the second-year man who could not even distinguish the healthy heart sounds. Such an attitude of mind can betray itself in a word or a look, and from this time Elizabeth Garrett began to make enemies among the students. She was quite unaware of her danger and the letter she wrote during a spring holiday at Aldeburgh to *The Englishwoman's Journal* has a confident tone which suggests that she did not know how precarious her position was. To encourage other women to follow her example, she dwells on the friendliness of the doctors, the respectful courtesy of the students, the freedom of wards, theatres and dispensary and the privilege of a private room which had been accorded her, and concludes: 'I was soon delighted to find that both personal and social difficulties

[1] ibid.

had been overstated.'[1] The truth was that her youthful enthusiasm had not yet perceived what the difficulties were nor where they lay. The open letter produced no volunteers to join her, and she continued in her rôle, essentially more congenial, of a solitary independent pioneer.

In the summer session Elizabeth began, as she said, 'making up to the physicians', and proved extremely adroit in approaching them for permission to work in their wards. Her first choice fell upon Dr Thompson, lecturer in materia medica, a tall man to whom fluffy white whiskers and an air of mild surprise gave a look of Don Quixote, and who spoke in an inaudible mumble. This manner, however, was misleading; he was a distinguished physician and she wished to be taught by him since she knew he was a Fellow of St John's College, Cambridge, and an examiner to the Royal College. She approached him on the first day of the session, just as he was leaving the ward followed by an unusually large train of pupils, reasoning correctly that in front of them he could hardly put her off with excuses about the unpleasantness of studying with young men. Firmly, so that they could all hear, she asked to be admitted to his lectures. Dr Thompson looked astounded; he stammered that he had no personal objections and should be glad to see her. She went away triumphant, carefully avoiding him all next day in case he should have repented and changed his mind.[2] Sometimes she felt ashamed of her tactics: 'I feel so mean trying to come it over the doctors with little feminine dodges,' she confessed.[3] Mrs Gurney, however, when consulted, replied firmly that it did not matter, and that feminine arts were lawful in a good cause.

Some members of the staff offered help unasked. Dr A. P. Stewart, the distinguished physician who demonstrated the difference between typhus and typhoid, invited her to accompany his ward rounds, and though she found him 'a horribly unpunctual

[1] *The Englishwoman's Journal*, June 1861.
[2] Elizabeth Garrett to Emily Davies, 6 May 1861. Fawcett Library.
[3] Elizabeth Garrett to Mrs Garrett, 4 May 1861. Anderson family papers.

man' – he was notorious for working by night and sleeping by day – she was grateful to accept. Stewart thought highly of her and later used his influence to forward her career. The lecturer and demonstrator in practical chemistry, the thoughtful, idealistic V. R. Heisch, also showed himself a friend. At demonstrations this quiet dark man in the shabby frock-coat settled Elizabeth beside him at the bench, her feet swinging from the high stool on which she was perched. He showed her how to manipulate gas-tube and burner, blow-pipe and box of testing materials. Under his influence the men behaved perfectly, and Elizabeth found the work an amusing change from the solitary grind of the Reading Room.

She was particularly anxious to win round Mr de Morgan, and sought another interview with him on the excuse of paying fees for her chemistry lectures. As usual she reported their conversation in detail to Emily Davies.[1] The treasurer took the money and entered her name in the book without comment, which made her bold to say 'I want to be admitted fully in October, but I have no intention of asking this formally until you and a decided majority of the committee show themselves really willing to receive me.' Mr de Morgan avoided a direct reply and asked, 'Are you going in for prizes, Miss Garrett?' She reminded him that prizes were only open to those who attended the full session, to which he replied, 'But at least you may get a certificate of honour for each separate course of lectures.' Finally he produced a book in which, to her delight, Elizabeth had to sign her name in token that she would not smoke in the garden or hospital, but comport herself in every way as a gentleman. She felt this made her a real medical student at last. The days were now filled with dissecting, lectures and laboratory work, the evenings with revision and test papers set by Dr Willis. When her father visited her, she confidently introduced him to the Dean and the chemistry lecturer as the two members of staff who would encourage him most heartily about her progress. She moved through the wards, laboratories and lecture rooms with the assurance of one who felt herself at home.

[1] Elizabeth Garrett to Emily Davies, 6 May 1861. Fawcett Library.

Elizabeth Garrett Anderson

When questions were asked Elizabeth Garrett answered them calmly and clearly. In June 1861 she obtained a certificate of honour in each class examination; indeed she did so well that the examiner who gave her the list added, 'May I entreat you to use every precaution in keeping this a secret from the students?'[1] This was a warning. So, if she had heeded it, was a certain coolness among the physicians and a decline in friendliness in the out-patient department. Opposition to her presence was growing. Many of the students had been willing to tolerate her presence as 'a lark', assuming that she would soon find the work too disagreeable or too difficult and give up. It was disturbing to find her an able and ambitious student, a future rival in practice, who was all too likely to succeed. From making jokes at her expense, the Middlesex students found themselves the butt of rival hospitals for allowing a girl to share their masculine privileges. Always, infuriatingly, Elizabeth Garrett was there, a small, composed, red-headed figure at lectures, clinics or operations, behaving as though she had some natural right to a place in a man's world.

Her cool composure was more irritating than any provocative behaviour. On 5 June a visiting physician was conducting his class around the ward with Elizabeth, as usual, moving quietly among them. Pausing beside a patient's bed, he asked a question about the case. None of the men could think of a reply; the silence was broken by the low, clear voice of Miss Garrett giving the correct answer. A crisis must have come sooner or later, but that moment of confidence ended her chances of ever being accepted at the Middlesex Hospital Medical School as a recognized student.

The round finished, the class dispersed and a party of some forty students met in the theatre to discuss what should be done to dislodge the intruder. A large class of students had the potential strength of a mob. The hospital buzzed with rumours of their intentions. Joshua Plaskitt hurried to warn Elizabeth of the meeting, but she was inclined to treat it contemptuously as the work of a handful of mischief-makers.

[1] Anderson, L. G., op. cit. p. 80.

Next day, however, 6 June, she accompanied one of James Smith's sisters, who was not well, on a private visit to a senior physician at the Middlesex, Dr Priestley. When the consultation was over he asked Elizabeth what she thought of the memorial the students were drawing up against her admittance.[1] Elizabeth said she had heard something from Mr Plaskitt, but hoped he was mistaken. Dr Priestley quickly disabused her. The student meeting had decided to memorialize the lecturers against her presence in the hospital. They had been very civil about it, he said, and nothing had passed about her personally at the meeting that she would have disliked, but the memorialists declared their intention of leaving the hospital if women were admitted. 'And if any lecturer opposes them', concluded Dr Priestley, 'he would probably have a most unpleasant class in consequence of his unpopularity. The lecturers are disposed not to make any opposition to you, but the memorial could force them to do so.'[2] Elizabeth excused herself somehow and walked from his consulting-rooms to the Middlesex, giddy with shock. 'I felt all afloat and not able to think of anything but *memorial*.' Mercifully she found the person she most longed to see, Louisa, sitting in her room at the hospital. Elizabeth told the whole tale and while they were talking an idea struck her. Why not write directly to the students and try to stop the memorial? She took pen and paper at once, while Louie left her to the task.

Elizabeth Garrett made her appeal to the students friendly in tone.[3] She offered to memorialize the lecturers herself 'not to make the slightest change or omission in their lectures in consequence of the admission of women' and she appealed to the chivalry of the men by pointing out how completely she was in their power. 'I *may*, unwillingly, make you lose some teaching,' she concluded. 'You can certainly shut me out from all.' Somewhat comforted, as she always was by action, Elizabeth went to bed.

[1] Elizabeth Garrett to Mrs Garrett, 7 June 1861. Anderson family papers.
[2] ibid.
[3] Appendix I.

Next morning, 7 June, she went to lectures as though nothing had happened, and watched some of the students reading her letter in the garden. Her friends made loyal attempts to cheer her. 'The memorial has been got up by a minority, and not by the best men,' declared Mr Plaskitt. 'The signatures are mostly of the idlest set and many of the good ones stood up for you like bricks.'[1] One of the medical assistants, whom Elizabeth hardly knew, was seen pitching into the memorialists with a flushed face and an air of great annoyance. The hospital on this question formed a microcosm of the medical profession as a whole: on the one hand Elizabeth's opponents, inspired by a mixture of vested interest and real disapproval; on the other her friends, whose freedom from prejudice and personal generosity was finally to admit medical women as colleagues. Elizabeth still refused to admit that the memorial was serious. 'On the whole,' she wrote to Emily Davies with determined hopefulness, 'it perhaps may do as much good as harm.'[2]

When she got back to Manchester Square on the evening of 7 June, she found a reply from the students which had been delivered by hand in her absence. Its contents were discouraging; they refused to withdraw or delay their memorial and justified their decision by 'the impropriety of males and females mingling in one class while studying subjects which hitherto have been considered of a delicate nature'. They embellished their refusal with an expression of 'respect for the purity of your motives and high admiration for the self-sacrifice to which you submit under the influence of your enthusiasm' – using the word by implication in its eighteenth-century sense of fanaticism. Elizabeth laughed at this condescending tribute, but none the less she was now seriously alarmed. After tea she took the letter and hurried round with it to Mr Nunn's house in Stratford Place, Oxford Street. The Dean, as always, was delightfully kind. He read the students' letter, ejaculating comically, 'Well! This is a spree – this is a spree!'

[1] Elizabeth Garrett to Mrs Garrett, 7 June 1861. Anderson family papers.
[2] Elizabeth Garrett to Emily Davies, 7 June 1861. Fawcett Library.

until Elizabeth almost found herself believing the whole thing was a practical joke. He tried to reassure her, as Joshua Plaskitt had done, by pointing out that the signatures were not those of the better students, and was distressed to see her anxiety. 'Now, come, tell me all about it,' he said coaxingly. 'You weren't vexed, I hope? Not "*hurt*" I mean, as the ladies say?' Elizabeth was so grateful for his kindness that she felt almost like kissing the stout little man,[1] and went home amazingly set up.

The week-end followed and on Sunday, 9 June, Elizabeth celebrated her twenty-fifth birthday. 'Twenty-five seems to be getting *old*, doesn't it?' she wrote, thinking of all she still meant to achieve. 'I feel as if it must be the prime of life.' On Monday she went back to the hospital, determined to behave as though nothing were wrong. On Tuesday she learnt that the memorial had been presented and that the Medical School Committee was to hold a special meeting in two days time to consider it. On Wednesday morning, 12 June, the chemical class was due to be examined. Heisch, the chemistry lecturer, now her devoted friend, advised her not to sit the examination as she would be left alone with the students for the papers and the practicals, and might meet with insults from them. 'As I mentioned the examinations expressly at the time I paid the fees, I will not be frightened out of them,' said Elizabeth coolly. 'The students dare not be rude and if they were, I should survive it.'[2]

She sat for the papers and returned to spend Wednesday afternoon drafting a long businesslike letter to her parents, asking them to endow a medical scholarship for women at the Middlesex, since the financial risk to the school of her continued presence was one of the strongest points against her. Hard-headed in money matters, she felt cash might speak louder than words. She also submitted the draft endowment scheme to the Treasurer and called personally on all the members of the committee who might vote in her favour. Such fighting spirit did not pass unnoticed. Five of

[1] ibid. This passage is heavily crossed out in another ink.
[2] Elizabeth Garrett to Emily Davies, 11 June 1861. Fawcett Library.

Elizabeth Garrett's friends among the students wrote warmly assuring her that the forty-four memorialists did not represent the whole of the school.[1] Elizabeth was so touched that she found herself almost unable to reply. Another comfort was the companionship of Emily Davies, in London on a visit to her brother in Blandford Square. She promised to come to see Elizabeth at the hospital after the meeting, and go with her to hear a performance of Bach's *Christmas Oratorio*. 'As my fate will then be sealed,' wrote Elizabeth, 'I shall be able to listen.'

Thursday, 13 June, awaited with such apprehension, came and went, but Elizabeth did not hear a word. She tried to persuade herself that the meeting had been adjourned and that further consideration might be hopeful to her case. On Friday, 14 June, she began to feel that her friends at the hospital were avoiding her. The Dean, Mr Heisch and Dr Willis were not to be found in their usual places. Students and nurses looked at her but said nothing. By the end of the morning Elizabeth could bear the uncertainty no longer, and on her way into an examination she button-holed Dr Thompson to ask him what had been decided. The physician answered nervously and in painful embarrassment: the School Committee would not consider the endowment scheme, nor would they admit Miss Garrett to any more lectures when the ones she at present attended were over. He withdrew hastily before she could expose him to the fit of hysterics he expected. Elizabeth went mechanically into the examination room, took up her paper and thought about the questions as best she could. She passed third out of the class, with 66 per cent, the top mark being 73 per cent.[2] It was only later that she learnt in more detail what had happened at the committee meeting the previous day.[3]

Mr Shaw had taken the chair, with Dr Thompson, Mr Nunn and Mr Heisch, all of whom Elizabeth counted as friends, Dr

[1] Appendix I.
[2] Elizabeth Garrett to Mr and Mrs Garrett, 15 June 1861. Anderson family papers.
[3] See Appendix I.

108

Murchison and Mr de Morgan, who had shown themselves doubtful, as well as seven other lecturers on the staff. The committee read and considered a formal memorandum from the students asserting that the mingling of the sexes in the same class was 'a dangerous innovation likely to lead to results of an unpleasant character'. As Elizabeth had foreseen, the memorialists complained that the presence of a woman prevented the lecturers from speaking freely of essential medical facts, and that the appearance of 'young females as passive spectators in the operating theatre is an outrage on our natural instincts and feelings and calculated to destroy those sentiments of respect and admiration with which the opposite sex is regarded by all right minded men'. They also complained that the presence of Miss Garrett exposed them to ridicule, so that 'the Middlesex School has become a byword and a reproach among similar institutions in the metropolis and that its members are subject to taunts of a nature calculated to undermine those feelings of pride and satisfaction which ought to possess every Student in reference to the School with which he is connected'. Forty-three students signed the memorial in the hope that 'a knowledge of the feelings which exist among their Students may be of some service in guiding them in their future deliberations on this important matter'.

This document made disquieting reading for the committee. Individually they might be friendly to Miss Garrett and liberal-minded on the subject of medical women, but collectively they had to consider the implied threat to their school of a mass withdrawal of students or noisy, disorderly classes. Newson Garrett's offer, now formally submitted in a letter from Elizabeth, to invest two thousand pounds in the funds as an endowment for a woman's scholarship at the school would hardly offset the financial loss they might expect from his daughter's continued presence at the hospital. After discussion the Committee resolved that 'although the Lecturers are unable to agree with much of the reasoning in the Memorial they have come to the conclusion that for several reasons it will be inexpedient to admit Ladies to the Lectures in future sessions'. This motion was carried by a majority of seven to one, with five other members apparently abstaining.[1]

It is easy to blame the committee's timidity, but hard to see how, as servants of an institution dependent on students' fees and voluntary charity, they could have acted otherwise. They lived in an age of social conformity; members of the women's movement were equally discreet, for instance, in avoiding official association with George Eliot, however much individually they might admire her. Evidently, however, the lecturers felt they had treated Elizabeth shabbily, for they directed that a letter should be sent to her, regretting the necessity of their decision 'in the case immediately of a lady whose conduct had during her entire stay at the hospital been marked by a union of judgment and delicacy which had commanded their entire esteem'.[2] Elizabeth must take what comfort she could from that.

All she could feel at first was a determination to remain decently composed, so that the memorialists should not have the satisfaction of seeing how completely they had wrecked her hopes. 'I suppose one will outlive it somehow,'[3] she wrote wearily. Next morning, after a night's sleep, her stubborn courage reasserted itself. The thought of giving up did not cross her mind, and it must not be allowed to cross anyone else's. 'You must not think', she wrote firmly to her parents on Saturday, 15 June, at the end of an exhausting week, 'that I do take this disappointment as a sign the attempt is wrong or mistaken.'[4] Any woman, having received such a public affront, might have wanted to escape as soon as possible from the scene of her humiliation. Elizabeth Garrett would not allow personal feelings to deflect her from a course she had chosen on principle. She would not let her friends protest or write to the newspapers on her behalf, seeing that this

[1] See Appendix 1.

[2] Elizabeth Garrett, MS. draft for an article in *The Hampstead Express*, 29 Oct. 1870. Fawcett Library.

[3] Elizabeth Garrett to Emily Davies, 14 June 1861. Fawcett Library.

[4] Elizabeth Garrett to Mr and Mrs Garrett, 18 June 1861. Anderson family papers.

could only damage her chances elsewhere. She suffered, but she would not give up. For another six weeks, with complete self-command, she went daily to the Middlesex, finishing the course of lectures and demonstrations to which she was entitled, sitting her exams and qualifying for her certificates, while all the time, calmly, she re-made her plans for the future

CHAPTER EIGHT

The Siege of London University
July 1861–June 1862

❋

Elizabeth Garrett was determined to stay near the centre of the medical world, and not be recalled to Aldeburgh. Skilfully suiting the argument to the person, she dealt with the reactions of her parents to the setback she had suffered. Mrs Garrett canvassed unfavourable opinions and interpreted it as a sign from heaven to give up medicine. This her daughter would by no means allow.

> I need not say [she wrote firmly] that since the late difficulties have arisen, I have been going over the question afresh, and I am more than ever convinced that it is a good thing to work for. If I had taken it up hastily, or as a freak, I might naturally give it up now, but having a clear and deliberate conviction it is right, it would be mean and despicable in the extreme to give it up at the first breath of difficulty. If I am mistaken, God will show it to me through something more reliable than the bigotry and low tone of men of Dr Basham's[1] type. Much of what he said was not true and the whole view of the subject was taken from an essentially impure point of view. It is not true that there is anything disgusting in the study of the human body: if it were so, how could we look upon God as its Maker and Designer?[2]

[1] Dr Basham was a local practitioner whose opinion Mrs Garrett had sought.
[2] Elizabeth Garrett to Mrs Garrett, 4 July 1861. Anderson family papers.

Patiently, Elizabeth explained once again her love and need for work.

> I don't believe these tastes are wrong, they are simply the result of a healthy, active energy coming into the play of adult life. And recognizing these activities and not thinking they were given to be crushed down, I do not see that it is wrong to turn them into what I believe to be a very legitimate direction. You would not think it wrong or undutiful in a son to want some defined work and position, and why should it be so in a daughter?

She employed her best feminine arts upon her mother. She was affectionate, dutiful: she confessed to overstrain and proposed a little holiday for them together.

> It is a cool thing for me to propose you will say, but you are all so unselfish, and a little selfishness will be a pleasant variety. Anyone else would say 'take Alice' or anyone but me, but I say 'take me dear Mother', I should like to go very much and it would be good for me. Ever yours lovingly, E. G.[1]

To win over Mrs Garrett her daughter was willing to do anything except give up her own plans. Newson Garrett, by contrast, needed restraining rather than cajoling. Incensed with the Middlesex Hospital authorities and smarting from the blow to his family pride, he proposed to fight for Elizabeth's lecture certificates, which had somehow been delayed. Tactfully his daughter persuaded him that to do so would only make enemies for her, and by the end of July had secured certificates of honour in chemistry and materia medica, through the friendly assistance of V. R. Heisch.[2]

As well as managing her family, Elizabeth Garrett had to face the world at large. She was already the subject of considerable gossip in the medical world and *The Lancet*, under the title

[1] Elizabeth Garrett to Mrs Garrett, 29 July 1861. Anderson family papers.
[2] Elizabeth Garrett to Mr Garrett, 21 and 30 July 1861. Anderson family papers.

A Lady among the Students,[1] publicized her recent misfortunes with heavy-handed jocularity.

> The apple of discord is to be cast into our hospitals. A lady – Femina causa belli – has penetrated to the core of our hospital system, and is determined to effect a permanent lodgment. . . . How should the fair intruder be received? Is she to be welcomed as on all other occasions we should welcome a lady and desire to aid a woman aiming to benefit her sex not less than herself? Or should we resist the charge of parasols, and run the risk of 'taking our quietus with a bare bodkin'?

Under the pretence of complimenting Elizabeth Garrett on scientific earnestness, the editorial marvelled that 'this lady is able calmly to go through the manipulations of sounding for stone in the male bladder . . . insensible to the unpleasant feelings which her presence must arouse'. The writer congratulated the Middlesex students on their determination to be rid of her and prophesied that all other schools would follow their example. Elizabeth, though extremely annoyed, followed Joshua Plaskitt's advice and ignored the article. She was soon defended by a correspondent signing as an eye-witness[2] who pointed out that the male bladder in question belonged to a child of about two years old,[3] and that the article had therefore given a maliciously false impression. It was more difficult to answer an editorial in *The Lancet* of the following week, which maintained the uselessness of educating women in medicine when they could not obtain a valid diploma of qualification, and dismissed all Elizabeth Garrett's efforts as a restless, morbid agitation in which no worthwhile principle was involved. This seemed to be the general attitude of the profession; the Grosvenor Street and Westminster Hospital Schools rejected her application to study by a few votes and the London Hospital by the unanimous resolution of the

[1] *The Lancet*, 6 July 1861.
[2] It is likely though not certain that this was Plaskitt himself.
[3] *The Lancet*, 27 July 1861.

lecturers.[1] The reason given by the schools was always the same, that no medical examining body would admit women candidates for degrees and the schools would therefore be educating illegal practitioners.[2]

Elizabeth Garrett did not despair, and as she said, what was more remarkable her friends did not either, but she was learning in a hard school the need for caution. Although for reasons of pride she would not show it publicly, the débacle at the Middlesex had affected her profoundly. She never again made the mistake of underestimating difficulties, or of refusing to see warning signs of trouble ahead. Henceforward she proceeded with her old determination, but with a more cautious judgment. It was clear that at present the most urgent need was to find an examining body willing to admit her as a candidate. She sent off letter after letter to different universities, hoping that the discipline of thinking, writing and waiting patiently would be good for her natural impetuosity. The Gurneys canvassed influential friends on her behalf, but all in vain. During the summer of 1861 Elizabeth wrote to the examining bodies of Oxford, Cambridge, Glasgow and Edinburgh. All refused her application to be examined. The most uncompromising refusal came from the Royal College of Surgeons, which, when she applied to take its diploma in midwifery, replied that it would in no way countenance the entry of women into the medical profession.[3] Elizabeth considered writing to *The Times* on the injustice of this attitude, but was warned that she would only provoke a hostile editorial; with her new-found prudence she remained silent.

One sole examining body remained to be tried. The Society of Apothecaries had separated in 1617 from its parent 'Mystery of Grocers in the City of London', a company importing spices and drugs from the Levant. In spite of its mercantile origin the Society

[1] *The Lancet*, 3 Aug. 1861.
[2] Elizabeth Garrett to Elizabeth Blackwell, 8 May 1862, reprinted in Blackwell, E., op. cit. pp. 186–9.
[3] Stephen, B., *Emily Davies and Girton College*, p. 66.

obtained by royal charter in 1815 the right to examine and license candidates in medicine who had completed five years' apprenticeship, six courses of lectures and six months' attendance on the practice of a public hospital or dispensary. By the terms of the charter the Society was constituted a legal examining body independent of the Royal Colleges, and one which could provide a long-needed minimum qualification for the family doctor. Time had improved the curriculum for the Apothecaries' Licence; physiology was added the year after this act, midwifery in 1827 and additional hospital practice in 1830. By 1850 there were three compulsory years of lectures, demonstrations and hospital attendance. The previous examination proved 'more respectable' than Elizabeth had thought, requiring Latin, Greek and mathematics. Five out of every six students in London were working for the Apothecaries' qualification. Moreover, the Apothecaries Act of 1815 referred to 'all persons', desirous of practising medicine, without specifying the sex of the candidate. It was worth considering this humblest of medical qualifications.

As a preliminary Elizabeth wrote at once in June 1861 to Mr Plaskitt, asking if he would accept her as apprentice in the merely nominal way the Apothecaries' Hall demanded. He replied with his usual courtesy that, provided his partners did not object, he would regard it as an honour.[1] Thus duly apprenticed, Elizabeth Garrett applied through an acquaintance, Dr King, to be registered as a student by the Apothecaries' Council. After some strong opposition to the whole idea of women candidates, the Council decided to take Counsel's opinion on the terms of its charter. Once again Elizabeth had to wait as hopefully as she could. 'I am inclined to think it well to know the legality of the question, for if they legally can examine women, they cannot legally refuse to do so,'[2] she wrote, trying to put the question in the most favourable light to her parents.

[1] Anderson, L. G., *Elizabeth Garrett Anderson*, p. 85.
[2] Elizabeth Garrett to Mr and Mrs Garrett, (?), July 1861. Anderson family papers.

The summer session at the Middlesex ended, and at the end of July she left regretfully but in no unfriendly spirit. Once home at Aldeburgh, it was a comfort to get a kind and serious letter from V. R. Heisch; gratefully she sat down the same day to write him a reply. The summer holiday of 1861 at Alde House was not an easy time. Newson Garrett was restless and despondent about the uncertainty of her plans and Mrs Garrett and Alice preoccupied with housekeeping. There were thirteen visitors staying in the house beside the family, imposing a routine of picnics, garden parties, watching cricket matches and continual polite conversation. Elizabeth had the good sense to see that she must disarm prejudice, and under the critical eye of her relations was carefully feminine, doing drawn-thread work and playing croquet. Yet secretly, when she could escape to the attic to read or think for a while, she felt a sense of isolation from her family,[1] a separation more complete after one year of independent work than Louie's after four years of marriage. She had been so profoundly interested in medicine that even the sunshine and the delicious air were 'half spoiled by being obliged to pretend to enjoy stupid nonentities'.

It was difficult to appear calm under so many eyes when on 20 August at a crowded dining table she had to open a letter from the Apothecaries' Hall. To her great surprise, for she had become hardened to refusal, the Society was willing to examine her if she could fulfil its regulations. One, the indenture to Mr Plaskitt, she had already achieved. The second, spending three years in a medical school in the United Kingdom, would be more difficult, but for the moment optimism ignored these technicalities. The letter was welcomed with a 'hurray' from the young people and congratulations all round the table.[2] What Mrs Garrett said is not recorded.

This need to admit Elizabeth Garrett came as a surprise, and an unpleasant one, to many members of the Society of Apothecaries themselves. They had, however, submitted their charter for

[1] Elizabeth Garrett to Emily Davies, 21 Aug. 1861. Fawcett Library.
[2] ibid.

117

interpretation to Mr Hannen, Q.C., and his opinion was unequivocal: the purpose of the charter was to enable them to regulate the selling of drugs, and as there was no legal ground for refusing to allow a woman to sell drugs, they could not refuse to admit a woman to the examination imposed on candidates for their licence.[1] The Council of the Society was forced to recognize the indentures of Elizabeth Garrett to Mr Joshua Plaskitt and to accept his testimonial of moral character on her behalf. In return, Elizabeth received what she hoped would be her passport to the medical profession, a folded double sheet of foolscap, showing the courses of lectures she must complete and have 'signed up' before she could qualify.[2]

Elizabeth could already ask Dr Thompson and Heisch to sign a declaration that she had followed the statutory courses in materia medica, chemistry and the first session of clinical medical practice. An intimidating number of blanks remained, but Elizabeth refused to be intimidated by them. Somewhere and somehow she would find teaching in physiology, anatomy and dissection, morbid anatomy, principles and practice of medicine, midwifery and diseases of women, and forensic medicine, as well as the two further required sessions of clinical practice. Armed with the Apothecaries' schedule she redoubled her efforts to get into a medical school.

On 30 September 1862, after a struggle with Newson, who thought she could as well study at home, she returned to London. Her insistence at being at the centre of things was soon justified. Bessie Rayner Parkes, editor of *The Englishwoman's Journal*, introduced her to Dr John Chapman, proprietor of *The Westminster Review*, whose office receptions in the Strand were a meeting ground for advanced social reformers. Chapman's sympathies were roused by the struggles of the woman medical student, and since he had taken a St Andrews M.D. four years before, and

[1] Anderson, E. G., 'History of a Movement', *Fortnightly Review*, March 1893.
[2] See Appendix II.

practised as a physician,[1] he was able to give Elizabeth an introductory letter to the Regius Professor of Medicine at his old university. Elizabeth wrote at once to St Andrews and Professor Day's reply, though cautious, was helpful. During the winter of 1861-2, on his advice, she worked at Latin, Greek, history, geography, logic and mathematics, with the aim of matriculating as a university student.

To lighten a winter of solitary work Dr Chapman proposed some courses of lectures, followed by scientific reading with a private tutor. The first course required for the Apothecaries Hall certificate was in botany, which Elizabeth took at the Pharmaceutical Society, and rather to her surprise enjoyed. It included demonstrations at the Physic Garden in Chelsea. The second course in physics was that given at the Royal Institution by the Professor of Natural Philosophy, John Tyndall, who in company with Darwin and Huxley used the full range and depth of his learning in the mid-century struggle to give science a place in the accepted philosophy of living. At the time of delivering these lectures Tyndall was writing the classic *Heat as a Mode of Motion*, which he published two years later. The third series of lectures, to which she went by Chapman's personal introduction, was the course in natural history and physiology given for teachers by T. H. Huxley at the South Kensington Museum. 'The modern world is full of artillery,' said Huxley, opening the course, 'and we turn out our children to do battle in it equipped with the shield and sword of an ancient gladiator.'[2] This was precisely Elizabeth's judgment on her own early education. Huxley had doubts about admitting women to scientific meetings, since five-sixths of them were 'in the doll stage of evolution', but he admitted that most of their disabilities came from their mode of life. He refused to have his own daughters 'got up as mantraps for the matrimonial market', and his educational ideal was to educate

[1] His remedies were Spartan; he advocated the application of an ice-pack to the spine in cases of sea-sickness or stomach-ache.
[2] Bibby, C., *T. H. Huxley*, p. 22.

women as comrades, fellows and equals of men. 'Let us have "sweet girl graduates" by all means,' he wrote. 'They will be none the less sweet for a little wisdom; and the "golden hair" will not curl less gracefully outside the head by reason of there being brains within.'[1]

Elizabeth Garrett found, like all his students, that Huxley was a prince among class lecturers, 'embroidering his blackboard', as one student remembered, 'with different coloured chalks while he talked like a book'. The first lecture dealt in detail with the physiological differences of sex, from which Elizabeth's private tutors had shied away, and she felt the full advantage 'of learning clearly and well on that very point', in the calm atmosphere of a scientific exposition. Huxley was clear, deliberate, logical and inspiring. He was also at this time an extremely controversial figure, conspicuous in the arguments surrounding the publication of Darwin's *Origin of Species* two years before. It was a bold step to attend Huxley's lectures publicly, and one which marked Elizabeth Garrett's final breach with the Evangelical orthodoxy of her girlhood.

Mrs Garrett continued to regard Sunday travel as a sin, to subscribe to societies for converting the Jews, or sending, as her daughters said, moral pocket handkerchiefs to Andaman Islanders. Elizabeth Garrett, like many able young men and women all over England who had been brought up in the atmosphere of Evangelicalism, was repelled by something in its code and searched for a wider Christianity.[2] There was nothing in her religious beliefs to conflict with scientific study. She saw knowledge as God's gift to man, to be used wisely for man's and especially woman's benefit. She was aware of the lack of science in her own education, and seized this chance to repair it. Although she lacked opportunity for independent scientific work, it was of incalculable value to have followed Tyndall and Huxley's lectures. No medical student of her time could have had a better introduction to the

[1] Bibby, C., *T. H. Huxley*, pp. 35–6.
[2] Brown, G. K., *Fathers of the Victorians*, p. 518.

whole concept of a scientific culture, and she was prepared by this to receive the great advances in medicine during her career in a rational spirit, by no means universal in the medical profession. For the present, however, she felt conspicuous as the solitary woman in the large lecture-theatre, so Dr Chapman, with great kindness, brought his young daughter to hear the lectures also, and introduced the girls to Huxley, who took trouble to show and to explain to them the specimens in the Museum. It was a triumph when he officially recognized their presence by beginning his lecture 'Ladies and Gentlemen'.

On the same evening, 19 October 1861, two sisters of Octavia Hill appeared at the lecture; they were accompanied by a large, heavily built young woman with a masterful stride and flashing black eyes. This was Sophia Jex-Blake, who after a stormy childhood in which elderly, pious parents wept and prayed over her in vain, had won the right to live in London and work as mathematics tutor at Queen's College, even, to her father's horror, drawing the salary for the post. When the lecture was over the young women walked back together from Kensington to spend an hour at Manchester Square.[1]

It was an uncomfortable evening. Sophia Jex-Blake, speaking with some violent half-expressed feeling, went out of her way to shock the others. Elizabeth saw that Louie neither liked nor understood what the newcomer was saying, and that the Hills were distressed by her 'Westminster-Review-like' arguments. She herself disliked Sophia's slighting references to Maurice's conventional views on female propriety. She could not know that Sophia Jex-Blake was in the torments of an emotional crisis. For the past year she had lived in passionate friendship with Octavia Hill. 'She sunk her head on my lap silently,' she wrote of one of their long conversations, 'raised it in tears, and then – such a kiss!'[2] Octavia Hill's mother had come to resent Sophia's

[1] Elizabeth Garrett to Emily Davies, 19 Oct. 1861. Fawcett Library.
[2] Elizabeth Garrett to Mrs Garrett, 27 April 1862. Anderson family papers.

domineering presence in the house. This very week Mrs Hill had issued an ultimatum and within a few days the greatest grief of Sophia's life was to befall her, the breaking of their friendship by Octavia's own flint-worded command. Till the close of her life she grieved over it; in pathetic wills she left the whole of her little property to her friend. No wonder that to those who met her this autumn she seemed brooding and intense, as unpredictable as a gathering storm. To Elizabeth, shrewd and experienced beyond her years, Sophia was a jarring personality, with a judgment and temper she could not bring herself to trust. Years of enforced work together could not efface this disastrous first impression.

Sophia soon left London to continue mathematical training in Edinburgh, while Elizabeth stayed for a hard-working winter at Manchester Square. In spite of rebuffs and disappointments, it was a happy time. Her mouth may have become firmer, her lower lip more prominent, but she remained hopeful and serene.[1] Now that she no longer went to hospital each day Elizabeth could join with Louisa in the activities of the Langham Place circle. The 1860s were the heroic age of the Women's Movement in many spheres of life. In 1861 a pioneer party of educated women, conducted by Marie Rye, emigrated to New South Wales, where most of them found situations as governesses. Emigration of women and orphan children continued through the decade in spite of the outcry that Miss Rye was sending all the good domestic servants to Canada and Australia. In the same year Louisa Twining undertook a campaign for the humane care of pauper incurables, and after a few years saw the first bedridden patients moved from the steamy, rancid halls of old workhouses to infirmaries where trained nursing could gradually be built up. In 1861 Mary Carpenter, so busy with work for her voluntary reformatory schools that she always ate 'with her loins girt and her umbrella close at hand', persuaded public authorities of the need for schools to shelter children found begging, abandoned or exposed to criminal influences. Frances Power Cobbe, having traced in 1862

[1] Todd, M., *Life of Sophia Jex-Blake*, p. 86.

the careers of eighty girls brought up in a single London work-house, discovered that every one of them was on the streets; she founded a system of volunteer visitors to befriend and mother lonely young servants. The Langham Place offices, with Jane Crow as secretary, were pioneering employment for women. To their original book-keeping and law-copying, they added classes in plan-tracing, with shorthand and typing for 'lady typewriters'. Their funds were not large enough to establish a technical school, as they would have liked, but they could and did pay apprentice-ship premiums. This aspect of the work interested Louisa Smith. 'Surely now,' she remarked to her hairdresser, 'hairdressing would be a very suitable work for women?' 'Great heavens, no, madam,' exclaimed the man in horror, 'Why, it took *me* a fort-night to learn it!' Nevertheless the Society did help apprentices to train in hairdressing, telegraphy, pharmacy and commercial art.

All this Elizabeth Garrett followed with a generous enthusiasm, not complaining that other women's careers seemed to advance while her own stood still. The reason now is clear, for the work opened by the Society for Promoting the Employment of Women was either of minor status and modestly paid, or in new fields such as the social services, where there were no vested interests to resist competition. Elizabeth, almost alone, proposed to challenge an entrenched and profitable monopoly of the male sex.

Life in London was not without its lighter side. Elizabeth could still revisit the Middlesex Hospital in a friendly spirit; she loved concerts, garden parties in strawberry time, picture galleries, dining out. To her surprise she found herself in demand for her lively mind and intelligent, amusing conversation. The Garrett bluntness had a brusque charm of its own, and people who met Elizabeth Garrett did not forget her. She made friends among women and, which surprised her more, among men of distinc-tion. All this should have prepared her, though it apparently did not, for the shock when in the New Year of 1862 Heisch made her a declaration of love. She refused him, and Louie reasoned with

123

him when he still spoke of 'going on beyond friendship', but the whole affair imposed an unwelcome stiffness and caution on her behaviour. It was not so easy as she had hoped to maintain relationships with men on her own terms. 'I suppose I was a goose', she wrote ruefully to her mother, 'to believe in the possibility of friendship'.[1]

There was little time in the spring of 1862 for affairs of the heart, since Elizabeth had decided to apply in April to matriculate at the University of London. The first step was to obtain leave to sit the matriculation examination. Elizabeth turned once again to Emily Davies, whose father had died the previous autumn, and who now brought her mother to live at 17 Cunningham Place, St John's Wood. 'It will be very nice to have you so near,' wrote Elizabeth. 'I keep imagining all manner of ways of getting help out of your presence.'

There are clear signs of Emily Davies's generalship in the campaign which followed. She had the force of character to prevent Newson Garrett from precipitate action and the tact to circumvent well-meaning friends who proposed 'separate examinations on subjects adapted to the female mind'. Once Elizabeth's application was sent in, the two young women wrote, with Llewelyn Davies's help, to every member of the Senate, pointing out that London University had been founded to provide education for all classes and denominations without any distinction whatsoever. Elizabeth sent a statement to the *Star*, *Telegraph*, *Daily News*, *Globe* and *Atheneum*, as well as *The Medical Times*. She regretted that she could not enlist the support of Florence Nightingale, after Queen Victoria the most influential woman in the country, but Elizabeth, unconfused by the glamour of the Scutari legend, recognized that Miss Nightingale was immersed in her own concerns, and 'would probably make a public statement of her indifference or dislike to the scheme'.[2]

By contrast Elizabeth hoped for the support of Lord Granville,

[1] Elizabeth Garrett to Mrs Garrett, 2 March 1862. Anderson family papers.
[2] Elizabeth Garrett to Mr Garrett, 13 March 1862. Anderson family papers.

Chancellor of the University. In pursuit of legal arguments she went alone to take Counsel's opinion from Mr Hannen, the Q.C. who had given advice on the Apothecaries' charter. He was struck by the intelligence of his young client, who had come with the facts of Miss Jessie White's case in 1856 at her finger-tips, and both he and his wife were kind and friendly. With his approval, she followed up her letters by calling in person on several members of the Senate, including Mr Grote the Vice-Chancellor and his wife, the towering 'Grotesque' in white muslin of Sydney Smith's *bon mot*. After all this effort to win support, once more Elizabeth had to discipline herself to wait patiently. On 29 April 1862 the Senate considered Miss Garrett's application and decided by one vote 'that it saw no reason to doubt the validity of Counsel's opinion given in the case of Miss Jessie Meriton White in 1856'. Newson Garrett, resentful of this further defeat, saw the Attorney General in person, but legal opinion was clear: the Senate had no power under the present charter to admit women, and therefore there was no alternative but to demand the insertion of a new clause authorizing them to do so. 'Lizzie is certainly a wonder', wrote Louie, breaking the news to their mother; 'she is bearing her disappointment beautifully. Poor old lady, if practice makes perfect she will grow very accomplished in meeting and overcoming one drawback after another.'[1]

Elizabeth Garrett and Emily Davies were determined not to lose the goodwill they had built up. Since the University of London was about to receive a new charter, a 'crafty document' was drafted in the shape of a memorial to be submitted by Newson Garrett to the University Senate for debate. The memorial proposed that, under the new incorporation, the University and its examinations should be opened to women. It was clear that the only chance of winning admission to the degrees was to avoid the controversial question of medicine or other new professions for women, so the petition approached the question on the most general grounds that 'it appears very desirable to raise the stan-

[1] Louisa Smith to Mrs Garrett, 29 April 1862. Anderson family papers.

dard of female education, especially in the more solid branches of learning'.[1] To gain support for this memorial Elizabeth Garrett and Emily Davies sent out 1,500 copies of a circular to distinguished public men and women. The favourable opinions, when they came in, included those of Gladstone, Cobden and Monckton Milnes, and the list of supporters sent to the Senate of London University was impressive. The heavy expenses were met as far as possible by Elizabeth out of her own allowance, and beyond that by Newson's generosity.

On 7 May 1862 Mr Grote moved in the Senate that by the new charter women should be admitted to London University degrees, though not to Convocation. The discussion was long and anxious; it continued until half-past seven in the evening, when the Senate divided. Of twenty-one members present, ten were for, ten against and one neutral. The Chancellor, Lord Granville, whom Elizabeth had looked on as a friend, then had the casting vote, which he gave against the motion, destroying her hopes.

The narrowness of the division was in itself an achievement. However, that did not alter the fact that for practical purposes Elizabeth must give up hope of an English M.D. 'I am trying to go on working', she wrote, 'as much as if the exam., were still in view, but you can imagine how much harder it is to do so than when the work *must* be done and every moment used.'[2] The day after the meeting of the Senate she sat down to write a detailed, calm analysis of her various defeats for Dr Elizabeth Blackwell, accepting them quite impersonally, but regretting the loss of encouragement to parents generally to give their girls a better education.[3] Her own plan, since London University and the London hospitals were closed to her, was to try the Scottish universities, first Edinburgh and failing that St Andrews. Time was getting late if she hoped to enter in the Michaelmas term. By mid-day she had written to Sophia Jex-Blake in Edinburgh, and Sophia,

[1] *The Englishwoman's Journal*, Oct. 1862.
[2] Elizabeth Garrett to Mrs Garrett, 10 May 1862. Anderson family papers.
[3] Elizabeth Garrett to Elizabeth Blackwell, 8 May 1862.

who never could refuse a demand for help, wrote asking her to come and see what could be done there.

Elizabeth Garrett waited only long enough to attend the summer meeting of the Social Science Association, which she felt bound to support. The National Association for the Promotion of Social Science had been founded in 1857, on the model of the British Association, for the purpose of social studies, and Emily Davies had been quick to see its possibilities as a platform for the Women's Movement. From the first, women seized the chance to contribute papers on questions affecting their fellow-women, Mary Carpenter on Reformatories, Louisa Twining on Workhouses and Emily Davies on Medicine as a Profession for Women. All this, modest as it was, was enough to excite the British press to paroxysms of mirth, concerning 'the Universal Palaver Association' and 'the problem of female loquacity'.[1] Elizabeth was indignant at these cheap sneers and loyally continued to support the Association, though she herself admitted that her practical mind doubted the value of so much theoretical discussion.

> I don't feel sufficiently alive, [she wrote to her mother from this 1862 meeting] to the good likely to result from such a universal pow-wow about everything, to go out of my way to hear it . . . but it would look churlish not to go, so I shall get a ticket and diligently attend the week's meetings. It presents an opportunity for doing some knitting, if I were great in that line. I believe the meetings go on incessantly, with relays of fresh subjects and speakers (and audiences too it may be hoped) for nine days.[2]

On 30 May, as soon as the meeting was over, she set off to try her fortune in Scotland.

[1] Strachey, R., *The Cause*, p. 93. *The Illustrated London News* attended a soirée given by the Association on 21 June 1862, and reported with amazement: 'On gazing at the unwonted scene one might almost imagine that "women's rights" had been ceded and that the feminine portion of creation had been admitted to full participation in the blessings of the representative system.'

[2] Elizabeth Garrett to Mrs Garrett, 19 May 1862. Anderson family papers.

CHAPTER NINE

A Year in Scotland
June 1862–July 1863

'Miss Garrett and her strength!' Sophia Jex-Blake had written in her diary on 19 May 1862, 'making me break the Tenth Commandment. She doing Trigonometry, Optics etc. Running where I crawl!' Nevertheless, with habitual generosity she bustled round Edinburgh, making appointments for Elizabeth Garrett to see influential people, and on the 29th sent off a telegram to make sure she would really come the next day. Elizabeth stayed with her for a fortnight at 3 Maitland Street to canvass Edinburgh University for admission. She could not altogether overcome her unease at Sophia's intensely emotional temperament. 'She has some peculiarities which do not quite harmonize with my own and which I felt a good deal at first,' Elizabeth admitted to her mother. Sophia on her side seemed quite unaware of any cloud between them. Though four years younger than Elizabeth she looked older and was quite equal to managing anything; it was impossible not to respond to her kindness and enthusiasm. Elizabeth suppressed her instinctive hesitation and gratefully accepted help. The two young women went about interviewing important citizens, many of whom were surprised to learn that Sophia Jex-Blake was not the pioneer. She was so tall and high-spirited, with flashing dark eyes, while the real heroine was small and, so people noted in surprise, almost pretty. Influenced by Elizabeth's appearance, a well-wisher, discussing the difficulties in the way of practical anatomy, fatuously hoped that Miss Garrett could obtain 'nice *little* subjects'. The two girls, united by high spirits and a common sense of the ridiculous, could hardly keep straight faces.[1]

To celebrate Elizabeth's twenty-sixth birthday on 9 June they made an expedition into the Trossachs, using third-class carriages and temperance hotels to save money. Sophia Jex-Blake took command and Elizabeth was content to leave the master-rôle to her friend, entranced as she was by the beauty of the countryside. The rush of the waterfall near her bedroom window entered her dreams, and pelting showers could not spoil her pleasure in the fern-covered crags. They went rock-climbing together, each in characteristic fashion, Sophia choosing always the steepest and most dangerous places, and Elizabeth, though determined not to show her fear before her bold companion, prudently choosing a route where trees and bushes gave a foothold. Their energy was overflowing. On Sunday morning before breakfast they climbed Craig More; when they were fairly at the peak they indulged in a shout of triumph and then sat down and read the Collect for the day.[2]

After three days they returned to Edinburgh, where Newson Garrett joined them for a further round of interviews at the University. A letter came from Dr Blackwell urging them to persevere, but the immediate results were disappointing. A meeting of the physicians to consider the question of admitting Miss Garrett rejected her by 18 votes to 16.[3] Calming Newson's impatience, his daughter persuaded him to come with her to St Andrews where her friendship with George Day, Regius Professor of Medicine, was now well cemented by letter. Dr Day received them warmly in the room on the ground floor of his house where he passed his life. This highly intelligent Welshman, still under fifty, had been a Wrangler at Cambridge and, after qualifying in medicine, a lecturer in materia medica at the Middlesex Hospital School, which he left to take up his chair at St

[1] Todd, M., *Life of Sophia Jex-Blake*, p. 118.
[2] Elizabeth Garrett to Mrs Garrett, 8 June 1862. Anderson family papers.
[3] Todd, M., op. cit. p. 119.

Andrews. There, with vigour and tact, he persuaded his colleagues in the faculty to reform the notorious St Andrews M.D., of which it was said that the candidate could be sure of an interesting journey and excellent golf with the minimum of disturbance from the examiners. Day's election as a Fellow of the Royal Society had crowned his career when suddenly, climbing upon Helvellyn during his vacation in 1857, he fell and suffered appalling injuries. Shock and the crippling disabilities which followed reduced him to a life of invalidism, though he struggled with persistent courage and continued to publish medical articles in periodicals. The arrival of Elizabeth Garrett, young, intelligent, vital and determined, was a pleasure to Dr Day and his wife. They introduced father and daughter to Principal Tulloch of the University who received them with civility. Day himself was hopeful. He offered to tutor Elizabeth in any subjects she might need, though the lack of any hospital at St Andrews made clinical work impossible and, as he was careful to point out, admission to the faculty did not lie in his hands alone.

Newson Garrett by now was impatient with this long-drawn-out cautious exploration. Let Elizabeth go to America, where she was sure of a degree, and he would foot the bill! Patiently, she persuaded him that she would rather return to St Andrews for the winter session and try to gain admittance there. This wish to stay in Britain was not blind obstinacy; her reasons were fully thought out and clear enough to be set out convincingly on paper. Her father had returned to Aldeburgh, so she wrote to him on 18 June 1862:

> Believing as I do that women physicians of the highest order would be a great boon to many suffering women and that in order to have them the legal recognition must be given here or in England, I think my work is tolerably clear and plain, viz. to go on acting as pioneer towards this end, even though by doing so I spend the best years of my life in sowing that of which other students will reap the benefit. I feel very much that

probably there is a divine and beautiful fitness in my being the
one appointed to do the work. If I had a more decided genius
for medicine or anything else, it would be wasted now for want
of room and fair play, while with my good health and spirits
and a certain talent for pushing the question in a creditable
manner (which I fancy I have) I can stand the wear and tear
better than most people and with more chance of ultimate
success than many. It is a great thing for anyone in my position
to be alive to the necessity for exercising tact and showing
womanliness of manner and externals, and I fear that if I at all
gave up the post, some one less fitted for it . . . might take it
and disgrace the cause.[1]

This shows a remarkably sound, objective judgment of her own
talents and limitations, revealing how much Elizabeth had learnt
from her experience of the past year. Also, in spite of their attempts at friendship, the disciple of Emily Davies had evidently
winced at the personality and conversation of the overpowering
Sophia Jex-Blake. The two women parted soon after, Sophia to
teach at a girls' school in Germany and Elizabeth Garrett to go
south with her father for a summer holiday before returning to
Scotland for the winter. In September 1862 Elizabeth took up her
old place with Louie, keeping house at the birth of her sister's
fourth baby, Alice. On 27 September Elizabeth went to the
Apothecaries' Hall to take the arts examination, a general pre-
clinical test which she found 'more respectable than I had thought'.
Her candidature presented less difficulty for herself than for the
clerk, who was obliged to strike out 'Mr' and 'Son of' on the
printed form and to substitute in manuscript 'Miss Elizabeth
Garrett, Daughter of Newson and Louisa Garrett'. Her testimonial of moral character was provided by Joshua Plaskitt, as
was her indenture of apprenticeship, back-dated to 1 October
1860, when she first began to receive coaching from him.[2]

[1] Elizabeth Garrett to Mr Garrett, 18 June 1862. Anderson family papers.
[2] See Appendix II.

At the end of October 1862 Elizabeth Garrett arrived in St Andrews again, ready to seek admission to the winter session at the University. She took lodgings at 10 Bell Street with a Mrs Pringle who seemed astonished at her requirements in the way of hot water. Elizabeth, however, thought it would be as well to let her landlady see she was fastidious. The mattress was very hard and the nights already freezing, so that Elizabeth, usually spartan in her habits, was forced to allow herself a flannel night-gown and a hot-water bottle in order to get to sleep. She made up for it by a cold bath in the morning and two hours' astronomy before she walked out through the keen morning of 29 October 1862, under the clear grey-blue sky of a Scottish winter, to call on Dr Day.

His advice was to try for matriculation as soon as possible. Elizabeth expected an examination, but to her surprise he said, 'No, it is merely a fee of one pound for which a student receives a ticket as a member of the University, on the strength of which he is allowed to take tickets for the several classes'. Accordingly that afternoon Elizabeth called at the office of Mr McBean, Secretary of the University, and put her request. 'I am going to attend Dr Day's class and he has informed me I must first receive a matriculation ticket.' To her joy, Elizabeth told Louisa,

> the dear old buffer quietly said 'Oh, very well', and pulled down the University ledger, told me to write my name, which I did gleefully, received the coin – such small change I thought it was for that precious card – and gave me instead a card bearing the magic words 'civis universitatis sanctis Andrewsensis' beneath my name.[1]

Dr Day was delighted by this easy victory and sent her off next day, armed with her matriculation card, to take a class ticket for Dr Meddie's chemistry lectures. On 31 October, by the same means, she took a ticket for the anatomy lectures, both courses

[1] Elizabeth Garrett to Louisa Smith, undated but probably 30 Oct. 1862. Fawcett Library.

being due to start on 17 November.[1] Elizabeth could hardly believe it; in this medieval university of wintry towers and scarlet gowns she had found the home so long denied her.

On 1 November, in the afternoon, she returned from a walk with Mrs Day and heard that the university secretary was waiting to see her. 'Will ye see him?' asked the landlady with an alarmed look; 'he's a very nice gentleman.' Elizabeth, thinking he had called out of politeness, said she would be very glad to see him. The secretary was shown into her room looking very uncomfortable and almost ready to cry. This respectable elderly gentleman found himself in disgrace. The Senatus Academicus had met that day and resolved that he had given the matriculation and class tickets without due authority and that a committee be appointed to consider this novel point. 'Indeed,' said poor Mr McBean, 'I *never* have had anything to do which I hated so much!' With these words he deposited a little wrapped packet on the table. Elizabeth looked at it, mystified. 'Oh, ma'am, I can't help it!' he exclaimed. 'It's the fee!' 'I know you have no more to do with this than I have,' said Elizabeth to comfort the old man, 'but you must pick it up again, for receive it I will not.' She pushed the wrapped sovereign over to the secretary and when he refused, sent it back in an envelope to the Senate, with a letter saying that until the question was legally decided against her, she would not consent to have the matriculation fee returned.[2]

If the St Andrews Senate had expected to be rid of Elizabeth Garrett so easily they were destined to be disappointed. Her acute mind saw the possibility of a point of law and she at once sat down to draft a long and clear memorial of her case which she sent to Edinburgh for Counsel's opinion. In particular she asked, 'Did the payment of the matriculation fee and the class fees for chemistry and anatomy complete a contract binding on the Professors of the College?' Meanwhile Newson Garrett, warned by tele-

[1] *The Englishwoman's Journal*, Dec. 1862.
[2] Elizabeth Garrett to Louisa Smith, undated but probably 2 Nov. 1862. Fawcett Library.

gram, sought advice in London from Mr Hannen, Q.C., and Sir Fitzroy Kelly, the Attorney General, on the same question.[1] Elizabeth's friends rallied round her in the battle. The University Senate attempted to evade Dr Day by holding its meetings in a room up some stairs which he could not climb. He retorted by telling the members that 'Newson Garrett would not think 100 guineas too much' to spend on legal proceedings. The Vice-Chancellor was reported to look very thoughtful on hearing this. As an editorial in *The Spectator* of that week remarked: 'The chance to secure all wealthy female medical students is worth something to a small university.' On the other hand, dons fear nothing more than the ridicule of rival dons. Hot words were said to have passed between medical professors, who favoured the innovation, and theologians, who opposed it. 'You ought to be very grateful to me,' said Day to Elizabeth; 'I have been telling a dreadful number of crams for you!' The students, almost to a man, were on her side, feeling that the Senate had treated her very unjustly, and the mere mention of 'female education' in a lecture was enough to bring a storm of applause.

Elizabeth, who felt that the ladies of St Andrews regarded her as 'a social evil', would have been glad to have the company of a sister in this crisis, but Alde House was fully occupied with the departure of Alice to marry a young barrister at the Indian bar[2] and in persuading Newson not to send back a tea-set offered by the Richard Garretts as a wedding present. Elizabeth was not to be left alone, however, for Emily Davies, unasked, took the long cold journey to Scotland to stand by her friend at this time. Her unruffled presence was a blessing in the rather strained social life of the little town. She even dealt with the daughter of crusty Christopher North, a woman whose tongue was the scourge of university dinner parties, but who, after one encounter with Miss

[1] *The Englishwoman's Journal*, Dec. 1862.
[2] Newson Garrett, who disapproved of the match, insisted on giving her the return fare to India 'because you are sure to want to come back when you see him'.

Davies, became very civil all the rest of the evening.[1] Elizabeth tried to put on a confident air at these gatherings of professorial families. She wore her best light silk dress with all her rings and tried to appear as rich as she could in order to frighten the University off litigation. 'This is such an education for low cunning', she wrote to Louie, with a certain enjoyment in a battle well fought.

Nevertheless it was anxious work, even with the support of friends, to wait a fortnight from 1 November to 15 November for the Senate's decision, with the attention of town and gown alike focused upon her. Dr Day was too busy to teach her, for examinations were in progress. They were the last but one under the old St Andrews system which had made 'Scotch doctor', in many minds, a term of just reproach.[2] Unlicensed practitioners could present themselves for the M.D. without having attended lectures or kept residence at the University. Mrs Pringle's lodging-house filled with candidates. The fellow-lodger above Elizabeth was an old man, as deaf as a post, so that she could hear through the ceiling every sympathetic word the landlady shouted at him. He had eight children, had been an unqualified assistant for years and was approaching the examination with considerable dread. 'Poor old fellow,' said Mrs Pringle, 'I wonder anyone so old and deaf should care to be an M.D.!' Yet he and scores of similar medical hacks were eligible to qualify. Only Elizabeth Garrett, young, intelligent and ambitious, was excluded.[3]

Elizabeth tried not to let her spirits rise and fall with each day's news. Her Edinburgh Counsel, J. C. Smith, was of opinion that she might have a case against individual professors. Sir Fitzroy Kelly thought the opposite, but she hid his letter in her deepest petticoat pocket and said nothing about it to anyone. She tried to occupy herself with long walks in the bare, windswept country, with reading *Orley Farm* and with doing her own housekeeping,

[1] Elizabeth Garrett to Mrs Garrett, 12 Nov. 1862. Anderson family papers.
[2] Paget, S., *Memoirs of Sir James Paget*, p. 39.
[3] Elizabeth Garrett to Mrs Garrett, 12 Nov. 1862. Anderson family papers.

carefully comparing the value of cold beef, neck of mutton hash and ham at a shilling a pound, which she felt was rather dear. Her health under the strain remained buoyantly good; so did her appetite. 'I think serenity of digestion is a great thing to be thankful for,' she wrote to her mother; 'all through the worry of this week I have never quarrelled with my food.' The one thing she was afraid of was looking afraid. Dr Day laughed at her for imagining the Senate could think this. 'I assure you whatever they think,' he told his pupil, 'they do not imagine you will let them bully you without risk. You have a grand character for wide-awakeness.'[1]

On 15 November the Senatus Academicus met and by a majority ruled 'the alleged matriculation of Miss Garrett to be null and of no effect'. They therefore returned her lecture fees.[2] The decision reached Elizabeth by messenger late that night and she hurried with it to Dr Day's house, where she found him indignant on her account. He was startled by the next move she proposed. She was going to Edinburgh alone by the first train next morning to see the Lord Advocate himself. If he believed her cause was just, she was willing to force her way into the lecture rooms, with the help of her solicitor and friendly students, even though the college porters attempted to turn her back at the gates. At six next morning, 16 November, while it was still dark, Elizabeth was in the train. The ferry-boat was crowded, noisy with drunken sailors and bitterly cold. At Edinburgh she went to the Advocates' Library to find her counsel, Mr J. C. Smith, and with him at her side demanded an audience. Boldness repaid her; before long they were admitted to the Lord Advocate's room. Elizabeth told the whole story of her treatment at St Andrews very carefully and clearly to the Rt Hon. James Moncrieff. The distinguished lawyer, famous for learning and probity, heard this unexpected and unknown woman quietly to the end.

'You have been very badly used by the Senatus, Miss Garrett,'

[1] Elizabeth Garrett to Mrs. Garrett, 12 Nov. 1862. Anderson family papers.
[2] *The Englishwoman's Journal*, Dec. 1862.

he said, 'and I doubt not but that you could get damages for expenses incurred. Also I am of opinion that they could admit you to classes if they would do so. I suppose the classes are what you want, not the right to graduate?' 'No, certainly not,' Elizabeth told him. 'Classes I can get with comparative ease. The *graduation* is the most important. Could I be legally admitted to the examinations and degrees of the university?' At this, the crux of her case, the Lord Advocate hesitated. 'That is a much more difficult thing than the question about classes. I think as the Charter is now, with all the common usage of all universities against you, no woman could be admitted to university degrees.' As she heard the Lord Advocate's sentence, agreeing so closely with the independent opinion of the English Solicitor General, Elizabeth Garrett feared her eyes might fill with tears. The two men were very gentle, seeming to feel as much for her distress as she did herself. Saying to herself, 'What a mercy it is to have self-control when one wants it most,' she managed to keep her voice steady as she asked, 'Does the matriculation ticket constitute a contract in the legal sense?' 'No,' said the Lord Advocate definitely. 'A body like the Senatus could not be contracted with by an act of their secretary, unless he were formally authorized by them.' She was determined to have the whole matter thrashed out at last. 'Do you consider there would be any chance of proving our point in a court of law, on the ground of their knowledge of my intention, prior to my matriculation?' But the Lord Advocate gave her no hope. 'I fear there is none. You might get damages if you cared to sue for them; but you cannot compel the Senatus to do what their Charter does not give them the power of doing.'

There was no more to be said, and it was half-past twelve; Elizabeth Garrett thanked him and took her leave. There was just time for luncheon and a brief rest before she went, still with the devoted Mr Smith in attendance, to the office of the proprietor of *The Scotsman*, where she told her own story in her own words to the Editor. The effort to overcome natural reticence and plead her own cause was exhausting; she judged it necessary, however, for she was already looking to the future when patients might need convincing that the lack of an M.D. after her name was no fault of hers. For the moment all her will-power was concentrated on remaining calm and civil. The rest of the day was spent in similar calls and in copying papers for publication in the press. It was late at night before she was in the train again, writing in hasty pencil to her parents a long, detailed account of the day and its outcome.[1]

As the train swayed and rattled through the darkened countryside, she had time at last to face the facts. Nothing less than a special Act of Parliament would be needed to admit women to university degrees. She had been spared the public humiliation of an unsuccessful lawsuit, but her dream of being a Doctor of Medicine would remain a dream. All she had left was the belief in her own fitness for the work she had chosen. For the first time Elizabeth Garrett broke down under the strain of continuous effort, loneliness and monotonous disappointment. She had given up so much: friendships, pleasures, any immediate prospect of marriage, even the right to be her spontaneous, lively self. She had learnt, with much self-discipline, to be discreet, tactful, self-effacing. Was all this effort to be useless after all? Emily Davies had been recalled by family duties to London; all that night Elizabeth wept secretly and alone.

It was bitter to her fighting spirit to read the contemptuous verdict of the *British Medical Journal*. 'The female doctor question has received a blow instead of a lift at St Andrews University. It is indeed high time that this preposterous attempt on the part of one or two highly strong-minded women to establish a race of feminine doctors should be exploded.'[2] Elizabeth could no longer bear to remain in St Andrews where everyone knew of her humiliation. She left the town for a three-hour walk along the coast, scrambling over the rocks and watching the wintry sunset glow

[1] Elizabeth Garrett to Mr and Mrs Garrett, 16 Nov. 1862, headed 'Train from Edinburgh. Sat. night'. Anderson family papers.
[2] *British Medical Journal*, 22 Nov. 1862.

on the cliffs and the water. It was what she needed. 'I came back into town feeling disreputably dirty but very happy. I have now shaken hands with the dear M.D. and have recovered my spirits with my usual speed,' she wrote to reassure the sympathetic and anxious Louisa.[1]

The case had won her fame, not only in her own country. On 3 December 1862 the Paris journal *Le Temps* published with sympathetic comment an open letter to Miss Garrett, which ended with the encouraging words, 'Quelle que soit l'issue de ces débats, votre cause est gagnée devant l'opinion publique . . . L'Europe vous regarde, la France vous applaudit.'[2]

Russell Gurney, the Recorder, wrote from London about the effect of the St Andrews affair upon legal men of his own standing, neither young nor quite middle-aged. He reported that most lawyers had been greatly interested in the case, and were in favour of the general principle of admitting women to universities. In her disappointment, Elizabeth felt it heart-warming to receive such encouragement. Encouraging, too, was the attitude of Dr Day. He laughed at her openly for thinking so much about an M.D. 'Except when had from London University, it is no proof of anything particular,' he said. 'Its absence or presence makes no difference at all to my estimation of a person; everything depends on character, very little on legal recognition.' Elizabeth was forced to smile at her own obsession with the magic initials. 'I think I must have a great deal of the child in me yet.'[3]

Dr Day left her no time to brood. She came to his house every evening to be taken through a complete course of anatomy and physiology, for which he demanded thorough preparation. He had spent much time since his accident in writing the medical articles for *Chambers's Encyclopaedia*, and this practice in clear exposition, as well as an unusually wide scientific culture, made

[1] Elizabeth Garrett to Louisa Smith, undated (Dec.) 1862. Fawcett Library.
[2] Reprinted in *The Englishwoman's Journal*, Jan. 1863.
[3] Elizabeth Garrett to Mr and Mrs Garrett, 19 Nov. 1862. Anderson family papers.

him an excellent teacher. He arranged for a fisherman to bring Elizabeth a supply of 'all the sea beasts to be found here' for dissection and microscopic work. There was no hospital near for clinical practice, but in daily contact with a physician of such calibre she did not feel the lack of it. Soon she was as busy and happy as she had ever been. The days felt too short for all she wanted to do.

One important point, however, had to be settled. Would the Apothecaries' Hall examiners accept this private course of lectures? Elizabeth Garrett wrote to the Court of Examiners, asking if they would accept a certificate of private lectures 'if equal to the course usually given in public'. By now she had learnt to put her case well; perhaps also the distinguished name of George Day had its effect. At its next meeting the Apothecaries' Court resolved 'that Miss Garrett be informed that the Court of Examiners only demand that the certificates on the various subjects required by the Court be obtained from recognized lecturers of acknowledged schools of medicine'.[1]

So, undramatically, the problem of qualification was solved. Elizabeth was now independent of any institution, if she could find private tuition in all her subjects. The letter announcing the Apothecaries' decision was cordial; they would not only accept Dr Day's certificate in anatomy and physiology, but her Middlesex Hospital certificates of honour in chemistry and materia medica and the Pharmaceutical Society's botany course as well. Looking back in later life, she saw this as a turning point. 'From this time the road was open.'[2] Elizabeth Garrett stayed at St Andrews working steadily through the winter of 1862–3 and living alone in lodgings. She had become a celebrity in the town, and wits among the students proposed 'Miss Garrett for Lord Rector'.

In May 1863 Elizabeth, having completed her theoretical anatomy and physiology, said a grateful goodbye to Dr Day and

[1] Anderson, L. G., *Elizabeth Garrett Anderson*, pp. 107–8.
[2] Elizabeth Garrett Anderson, MS. draft for a speech, Royal Free Hospital School of Medicine.

moved on to Edinburgh. It was stimulating to her lively mind to be in a capital city again. 'I was quite amused', she wrote to Louie, 'with the happy feeling which came over me in the crowd of a Saturday afternoon in Princes Street. It was a reminder of London to see people close together, cabs and carriages.' She received an encouraging welcome from Dr Stevenson Macadam who acted as secretary to the Medical and Surgical School at Surgeons' Hall, where courses qualified for examination by the Royal Colleges of Physicians and Surgeons of Edinburgh. He opened his class to her, inviting her to his ten o'clock lectures at the School of Art in Adam Square, and his practicals at Surgeons' Hall itself. Given this firm lead by their tutor, his students apparently raised no objection. Unfortunately Dr Macadam's subject was practical and analytical chemistry, in which Elizabeth had already made a very good start. He tried to persuade his colleagues in anatomy and physiology to follow his example, which would have been an immense help to her, but they were too nervous of their students, or possibly of their seniors in the Faculty.[1] Apart from this, Elizabeth did not renew the hopeless struggle with the College of Physicians for admission to university courses, but presented herself to the best-known living doctor in the world, Professor James Young Simpson.[2] Simpson, now at the height of his fame, kept open house at 52 Queen Street for as many as fifty lunch-time guests. His house was crowded with visitors and the patients of his enormous practice, waiting for the Professor's arrival. 'When I called for him', wrote a colleague, 'his two reception rooms were as usual full of patients, more were seated in the lobby, female faces stared from all the windows in vacant expectancy and a lady was ringing at the front doorbell.' Equally crowded was the company in the dining room where noblemen, statesmen, antiquaries, scientists and artists sat down together. At the centre of the hubbub was the Professor himself, short,

[1] Report of a speech by Dr Macadam, *The Scotsman*, 16 Feb. 1891.
[2] It seems likely, though not certain, that Dr Day gave her an introduction to him. Many of Simpson's private papers remain unsorted and uncatalogued.

stout, with small feet and a step so quick that companions had almost to run to keep up with him. He had a large head, dishevelled hair and a keen eye; nothing escaped him. To young people he was kind and generous, admitting them to his conversation and even to his study, where a photograph of the first child he had delivered under chloroform – a doctor's daughter unfortunately christened Anaesthesia – hung above his desk.

Elizabeth Garrett later said she had spent some months 'in Edinburgh, working under Professor Simpson', but there is no record that she attended Simpson's lectures at the University, or his bedside teaching in the wards of the Infirmary. His prestige was vast, and to have been his pupil, even in a nominal way, would be a great help to her career. For teaching he referred her to his neighbour, Alexander Keiller of 21 Queen Street, Lecturer and Examiner in Midwifery at Surgeons' Hall and Physician to the Edinburgh Maternity Hospital. The two men had been friends since their boyhood, when Keiller, learning medicine the old-fashioned way as a chemist's assistant at a shop in Dundas Street, first noticed 'a little fellow with a big head' who took down every drug from the shelves and looked it up in the Pharmacopoeia. Keiller was now in his late forties, a diffident, kindly man, with an almost childlike simplicity, content to remain in the shadow of his famous friend, though with a little more push, said a colleague, he might have won a place in the obstetrical textbooks. Keiller's lectures were painstaking, his papers rich in clinical experience, and in his women's ward at the Royal Infirmary he had instituted for the first time systematic clinical teaching in gynaecology. 'It is quite magnificent,' wrote Simpson of his work.[1] Elizabeth Garrett was fortunate to be accepted as Keiller's pupil. He not only taught well; he was able to provide what she badly needed, clinical experience in midwifery at the Edinburgh Maternity Hospital.

This hospital, which bore the title 'Royal' apparently from its earliest days, had been founded in 1844. It formed the subject of an interesting report presented in 1848 by Simpson to the Edin-

[1] *Edinburgh Medical Journal*, Jan. 1893.

burgh Obstetrical Society, of which he was president.[1] The hospital was probably the first to experiment in the use of anaesthesia in labour. Simpson himself was aware of the dangers of this crammed house in the poorest quarter of the city where tall stone tenements were scarcely separated by narrow wynds; he noted the convalescence of the mothers was often interrupted by 'febrile and inflammatory attacks'. When Elizabeth Garrett came as an extra-mural pupil in 1863 the hospital occupied Chapel House, formerly the home of Andrew Melrose, the famous tea and coffee merchant, who had lived there in patriarchal style with his family and thirty apprentices. It was a handsome city mansion of dark granite, with a broad flight of steps leading up to the front door and room for twenty-six to thirty-six beds. The impressive building however was quite unsuited for use as a maternity hospital, where the death rate from sepsis was even higher than in general hospitals. 'The wards were filthy in the extreme,' wrote a physician who joined the staff in 1867, 'the beds were not fit for human beings to occupy, the food of the patients was so bad and so ill-cooked that they frequently could not eat it. It was not remarkable, therefore, that the mortality should have been comparatively high.' Elizabeth Garrett had the misfortune to study midwifery, as she had first seen surgery, at the very end of the pre-Listerian era, but she refused to let its horrors dismay her. She saw, too, poverty at the grimmest and most squalid, but accepted it with the same matter-of-fact interest she brought to all new experience.

In the year she was at the Royal Maternity, a house surgeon, Dr David Murray, reported twenty-five cases of successful vaccination of the new-born, a subject in which Elizabeth retained a life-long interest. Midwifery itself she found deeply satisfying. Reserved as she was, it was only to Louie that she could reveal how much she was moved by her first delivery.

> My dear little first born has just entered the world. You cannot imagine how fond I feel of him. . . . I wonder if one will

[1] Sturrock, J., 'Early Maternity Hospitals in Edinburgh', *Journal of Obstetrics and Gynaecology*, Feb. 1958.

143

go on feeling an immediate affection for the little creatures that come first into your hands! It was my turn to be assistant, so of course I was up the whole time, the others except the principal in charge go to bed until they are called. The poor little baby was stillborn and all Dr Thornton's efforts to restore it were useless. We kept up artificial respiration for more than 20 mins. but it was no use. It is very sad to see a dear little healthy looking child lost in that way. This was the consequence of the mother's folly. She had been out dancing during the evening and had brought on haemorrhage wh. no doubt killed the child. Well when we went to bed about 5½ feeling sure I was hoping to have at least the rest of the night in peace. However, about 6.20 I was called with 'Miss Garrett here's a case and it's yours'. I being chief for the first time. Of course I was up and dressed in a twinkling considerably excited with the prospect of a case 'all to myself'. However, as I did not like risking relying on my very immature judgement I sent for the doctor and he called and I had his confirmation of all I had diagnosed. He was very kind and encouraging and I was glad he stayed that I might be sure my ignorance would not do mischief. We went steadily till ten when a very nice boy came into the world. He weighs 8 lb and is 22 ins. long, so you see he is a good size. I did everything a doctor does usually, and found it very easy.[1]

Between May and the end of July 1863 she herself attended twelve cases of labour and 'witnessed upward of a hundred'.[2] She also attended Keiller's lectures on the diseases of women and secured his signature on her lecture schedule.

Legally, the nine months in Scotland had been barren. Practically, they had been of the greatest value. Elizabeth had secured distinguished teaching and gained experience in midwifery and diseases of women. Moreover she had shed the last of her illusions; she knew now that however intelligent, hard-working and well behaved she might be, no medical school or university

[1] Elizabeth Garrett to Louisa Smith, undated. Fawcett Library.
[2] See Appendix II.

would admit her on equal terms with men. The dream of opening
a training to other women students was ended; that remained for
others to do. Meanwhile, since she was paying for private tuition,
she intended, with Garrett hard-headedness, to get the best
training money could buy. Her aim now was as simple as it was
daring: to become a great physician by her own efforts and in her
own right.

CHAPTER TEN

In the Fortress
July 1863–September 1865

The most urgent need for Elizabeth Garrett in the summer of 1863 was to work at practical anatomy; she had done no dissecting since leaving the Middlesex two summers before. She spent July at Manchester Square with Louie, writing to medical men all over England and Scotland, and offering a fee of twenty-five guineas for the anatomy certificate required by the Apothecaries' Hall.[1] Newson Garrett, who was now utterly committed to her success, would have been willing to spend a large sum upon the endowment of a separate 'Female Medical College' if Elizabeth had not discouraged him. 'Something "just as good" is not good enough,' she said roundly. 'People get sick of hearing the same thing said over and over again and nothing done.' Doubting her father's discretion and knowing his fiery temper, she persuaded him not to attend public meetings on feminist questions except under the restraining escort of Emily Davies.[2]

Meanwhile the answers from the anatomists began to arrive, each one like a slap in the face, till Elizabeth grew to dread the postman's knock.

> I must decline to give you instruction in Anatomy [wrote a surgeon from Aberdeen]. I have so strong a conviction that the entrance of ladies into dissecting rooms and anatomical theatres

[1] Elizabeth Garrett to Dr Canton, 25 July 1863, Royal Free Hospital School of Medicine.
[2] Elizabeth Garrett to Mr Garrett, 7 Jan. 1863. Anderson family papers.

is undesirable in every respect and highly unbecoming that I could not do anything to promote your end. . . . It is indeed necessary for the purpose of surgery and medicine that these matters should be studied, but fortunately it is not necessary that fair ladies should be brought into contact with such foul scenes—nor would it be for their good any more than for that of their patients if they could succeed in leaving the many spheres of usefulness which God has pointed out to them in order to force themselves into competition with the lower walks of the medical profession.[1]

Elizabeth's natural steel had been tempered by her experiences of the last three years in London and Scotland. She was far beyond the stage when a snub of this kind could deflect her from her purpose. Mastering her resentment, she continued to write her letters of polite request. She was rewarded when L. S. Little, demonstrator at the London Hospital Medical School, agreed to take her for the full course of anatomical demonstrations and dissections and later for the morbid anatomy required by the Apothecaries' Hall. This young man of twenty-three, son of the great W. J. Little, was already an orthopaedic surgeon of brilliant promise. He had been elected assistant surgeon at the London Hospital at the age of twenty-one, in the year in which he qualified.[2] As curator of the hospital museum he was sure of a supply of clinical material, and like his father, he was an excellent practical teacher. Elizabeth Garrett worked on dissection under his guidance from October 1863 to 30 March 1864.

At the same time as dissecting with Little she followed a course of lectures in descriptive anatomy by John Adams, F.R.C.S., a member of the Council of the Royal College of Surgeons and lecturer on surgery at the London Hospital School, as well as

[1] Reprinted in Anderson, L. G., *Elizabeth Garrett Anderson*, p. 109.
[2] *Lives of the Fellows of the Royal College of Surgeons*, Vol. I, pp. 720–1. In the spring of 1864 Little volunteered as surgeon to the troops during the Schleswig-Holstein campaign and had charge of 2,000 wounded Danes, Austrians and Russians.

surgeon to the hospital itself. Everyone liked 'honest Jack' Adams. On his side, he found the diminutive, apparently demure Elizabeth Garrett a change from the large and rowdy class which he habitually subdued by banging his fist on the table and shouting, 'If you don't stop this bloody row I will close the lecture!' Nor did his lady pupil receive his attempts at anatomical illustration with noisy and ironical applause, even when he confessed, 'I never could draw anything but corks!'[1] Adams had an enthusiasm for his subject, and Elizabeth Garrett found herself with some surprise enjoying surgery more than medicine. She worked under Adams for a full six months and by the end of March 1864 had completed the required course, although she did not, at this time, intend to practise as a surgeon.

At the same time Elizabeth Garrett had to make up the required clinical practice for the L.S.A. No hospital seemed willing to take her and rather than stir up opposition by applying once more to teaching hospitals she decided to attend clinics at the London Dispensary. This institution, founded in 1777 at 21 Church Street, Spitalfields, treated some two thousand outpatients a year[2] from the network of narrow streets east of Liverpool Street station. Once it had been a city merchant's house. Now patients sat in rows upon benches filling the entrance hall, waiting for the porter to shout their names through a hatch hacked out of the panelling. There they returned after seeing the doctor on duty and waited again for the dispenser to hand out the old beer or stout bottles containing their free medicine. It was charity at its bleakest.[3] Spitalfields was a tragic district of old houses divided into one-room tenements where the poorest families in London sheltered. The 'profitable strangers', the Huguenot silk weavers, with their arts of mulberry growing and flower-gardening, had declined with the coming of the power loom. In their place had come families of poor Jews from Russia

[1] *London Hospital Gazette*, Vol. LX, no. 3, p. 82.
[2] Scott, J. H., *A Short History of Spitalfields*, p. 43.
[3] Sims, G. R., ed. *Living London*, Vol. III, p. 34, illustration.

and Poland, living six and eight to a room and working for a 'sweater' in the shoddy clothing trade. It was, said the Rector of the Parish, 'seventy-three acres which is one dead level of poverty and of almost hopeless misery'.

Although the dispensary was useful Elizabeth felt increasingly the lack of hospital teaching. She was convinced that 'there is nothing like bedside practice when you know the theory and want the skill and tact of experience'. At some time during the autumn of 1863 she applied to the London Hospital authorities to be admitted as a student, and received the inevitable refusal.[1] They had already rejected her in 1861 and were not likely to change their views now. In the New Year of 1864 Elizabeth Garrett decided, with the greatest reluctance, to resort to the tactics which had gained her entrance to the Middlesex Hospital, and applied to attend the London for nursing experience. There was every hope that she would be admitted, since for the last twenty years the hospital had been admitting Protestant Sisters of Charity as pupils. On 9 February the London Hospital House Committee met and noted

> Read a letter from Miss Elizabeth Garrett requesting permission to attend in the Wards of the Hospital to gain experience in Medical and Surgical nursing. Resolved that the required permission be granted and that Miss Garrett be referred to the Matron for information as to the conditions to be annexed to the permission in question.[2]

When the House Committee met, Elizabeth had already been lodging for a week at 8 Philpot Street, Commercial Road, five minutes' walk from the hospital. Philpot Street, joining Whitechapel High Street and the Commercial Road, was a cutting between grimy, stock-brick houses, narrow, fog-shrouded in winter, haunted by wizened, half-wild children. It was a gesture of extraordinary daring for a girl in her twenties to live alone in

---

[1] Elizabeth Garrett to Emily Davies, 18 Feb. 1864. Fawcett Library.
[2] *London Hospital House Committee Minutes*, 9 Feb. 1864.

the East End, then a region of superstitious horror to the middle classes. The wide boulevard of Whitechapel High Street was like a foreign city, flanked by shop fronts with incomprehensible signs, noisy with the speech of foreign immigrants. Tenements and workshops were supplied with crude gin in two-gallon wickered stone jars for mass consumption. The homeless huddled against the workhouse wall as a shelter from wind or rain, waiting for the casual ward to open. Coroners' inquests, reported in *The Times* from July to December 1866, record five verdicts of 'Starved to Death'. A boy growing up in the district at this exact time recalled 'women, swearing, fighting, clawing, *ritu ferarum*, with lacerated bloody faces and breasts'.[1] Elizabeth Garrett was protected in Whitechapel, as she had been in Spitalfields and in the slums of Edinburgh, by a cast of mind that was realistic rather than imaginative. Later, when it lay within her power to do something practical, she would make immense efforts to help the poorest women of London. Until then, she would not let the spectacle of their sufferings distract her from her immediate aim, which was to qualify. What might have been a defect proved a strength and she settled into Philpot Street with the most matter-of-fact calm. She was, in fact, within half a mile of the house where she was born, and must have passed 1 Commercial Road on every journey to the West End. It is impossible to say if she remembered her birthplace. On this point she remained utterly silent; either she did not know about the pawnshop, or she had her reasons for concealment. If so, these were not idle snobbery. Elizabeth Garrett already carried heavy professional disadvantages without the additional handicap of a self-made father and an East End birth.

On 18 February 1864 Elizabeth attended the London Hospital for the first time, going in the early morning and staying in the wards until the patients' dinner time. Since the St Andrews controversy she was a celebrity, and the medical school was in an uproar at her coming. Toughened as she was, Elizabeth suffered under the ordeal of 'standing about with nothing definite to do,

[1] Okey, T., *A Basketful of Memories*, p. 56.

In the Fortress 1863–1865

and the consciousness of being under a fire of criticizing eyes, nurses, patients and students!'[1] She forced herself to hope they would watch her less closely when the novelty wore off, and endured her distress for the sake of clinical experience. There were at that time four hundred in-patient beds at the London, as well as the evil-smelling underground hall, where the dressers applied splints to crooked bones, Scott's dressing to enlarged joints and strapping to ulcerated legs. The old receiving room, a bare hall painted stone colour and bearing an aspect of callous unconcern, was never closed. To its deal benches and stained leather sofa came street accidents, a man 'with the red bone-ends of his broken legs sticking through his trousers', a woman dripping foul mud who had been dragged out of the river, a scalded and dying baby. It was no place for the squeamish, but there was no finer clinical experience to be had. In-patients were the responsibility of the 'residents', students on duty for the week with a standard provision of bread, cheese and beer. The first regular training scheme for London Hospital nurses did not come into force until 1874, yet some of the old nurses, stout, coarse and without education, were possessed of enough skill to train any student. Elizabeth soon found out which of the senior students were 'on my side' and was able to learn a good deal by observing their work and asking them questions. Otherwise instruction was mainly by 'following the box', a box of instruments carried behind the surgeon as he made his ward rounds. Used instruments were put back into the box for use on other patients.[2]

Elizabeth Garrett's main purpose in attending the hospital was to follow the course in practical midwifery[3] and vaccination. Obstetrics at the London were dominated by Dr F. Ramsbotham, a florid, rotund gentleman with the perpetual smile of the fashionable ladies' doctor. The only subject which could rouse him was

[1] Elizabeth Garrett to Emily Davies, 15 Feb. 1864. Fawcett Library.
[2] Morris, E. W., *The London Hospital*, p. 174.
[3] This was a different course from that of midwifery and diseases of women, which she had completed in Edinburgh. See Appendix II.

the horrifying suggestion of chloroform for women in labour. He recommended 'the soothing comforts of religion' instead. He intensely disliked the presence of students on his rounds, so Elizabeth found herself, fortunately for her, handed over to the Resident Accoucheur for instruction. Nathaniel Heckford was five years younger than herself and already a gold medallist both in medicine and surgery, yet he did not conceal his boredom at the idea of fashionable patients or practising for money. He had a dark, clever face, untidy clothes and a passion for children and animals.[1] As a teacher he was immensely kind, took Elizabeth's part among the staff and students, and thought well enough of her ability to offer her an appointment at his own hospital in later years. His method of teaching suited her temperament. He put her in charge of a case, left her to form her own diagnosis, and was at hand to help only if she asked for him. Elizabeth Garrett's spirits rose to meet the challenge of responsibility, even when it meant staying up all night on

> my first case of operative midwifery. When I found the diffi-
> culty I made up my mind what I should like to do but thought
> it wiser to call in Mr Heckford. When he came he agreed to my
> plan of treatment and kindly left me everything to do except
> giving the chloroform. It was not a minor operation and I
> enjoyed it immensely.[2]

Elizabeth herself felt she had taken a great step forward in completing her anatomy and midwifery courses and was emboldened to write on 5 April to the President of the Royal College of Physicians for permission to sit for the L.R.C.P. Her letter, drafted and re-drafted with great pains, was, she told Emily Davies, a model of craft. She stressed that she 'wished above all things *not* to assist in lowering the standard of preliminary or professional education'.[3]

[1] *London Hospital Gazette*, Vol., LX, no. 3, pp. 82–4.
[2] Elizabeth Garrett to Emily Davies, 3 Feb. 1864. Fawcett Library.
[3] See Appendix III.

The letter was acknowledged by the Registrar with the note that 'your approach being of so singular and exceptional a nature', it would be laid before a meeting of the college. Elizabeth had to wait five weeks for a decisive reply. This communicated to her in the most formal terms that the college had consulted its legal advisers who were of opinion 'that by the terms of the Charter the College is precluded from admitting females and examination for a License to practise Physic'.[1] This opinion was sound, since one of the avowed aims of the Tudor founders of the college had been to exclude women from their profession. It made discouraging reading in Philpot Street. The L.R.C.P. had to follow the M.D. into the category of qualifications Elizabeth Garrett could not hope to possess.

Nor was her clinical practice at the hospital an unmixed happiness. The work was as satisfying as ever, and the thrill of standing on her own feet in the professional world buoyed her up, but once again her presence in hospital threatened to raise a storm. As at the Middlesex, many of the elder, more serious students were friendly and offered a helpful word as they met in the wards. Others, taking their lead from certain members of the staff, complained of the 'shabbiness' of a rival student pretending to be a nurse. 'I never saw the school in such an uproar about anything before,' Heckford warned her. 'It is not my fault,' said Elizabeth Garrett, smarting under the accusation of dishonesty. 'I gave them two chances of having me as a regular student!' Worse was to follow. Every day Elizabeth joined the morning round of beds with Dr Powell, the Resident Medical Officer, who described and discussed individual cases with her. One morning he took her into the privacy of the nurses' duty room instead. 'I have been officially ordered not to allow you to go round the wards with me,' he said apologetically. 'As I am only a subaltern here I am reluctantly obliged to obey.' 'Then I must peg away alone and do as well as I can,' replied Elizabeth, who had now learnt never to reveal

---

[1] The Secretary, The Royal College of Physicians, to Elizabeth Garrett, 13 May 1864. The Library of the Royal College of Physicians.

annoyance. She told herself that self-reliance was good, that it forced her to observe closely and develop her own judgment, even though the work was harder and duller alone.[1] In this spirit she worked through the long gas-lit evenings in her room at Philpot Street. She suffered nevertheless; though brave, she was not insensitive, and the feeling of continual hostility made her nervous whenever an enemy came into the ward. Any evidence of serious ability on her part only increased the 'obstructive interest' against her. It did not take Elizabeth long to find out that the leader of opposition to her presence at the London was Dr Parker, a Lecturer in Medicine to the School. They had never spoken, since he refused to allow her to follow his ward rounds, but it was he who had forbidden Powell to teach her, and his hostile remarks were repeated round the hospital. Three years ago, at the Middlesex Elizabeth had hoped that such prejudices would melt away of their own accord. Hard experience had taught her otherwise; now she nerved herself for 'a skirmish with the arch-enemy'.

Dr Parker lived, like many of the London's senior staff, in Finsbury Square at number 22. Here on the morning of 16 April 1864 Elizabeth Garrett presented herself by appointment. As she stood outside the door she was horrified by her errand, but once in the presence of the enemy she felt the familiar surge of courage, and heard her own voice speaking calmly as well as strongly.

She said she had heard of his remarks and was determined to stop them if possible. She would yield the point about going round the wards with him, if he would not order the resident medical officer to cut her. Dr Parker was taken aback, as well he might be, at the coolness of his small feminine opponent. 'I told him my mind,' reported Elizabeth with satisfaction, 'and I think he was ashamed.' Having trounced him, she set out to charm; their talk lasted more than half an hour and Dr Parker became wonderfully civil and pleasant before they finished.[2] She had

[1] Elizabeth Garrett to Emily Davies, 18 Feb. 1864. Fawcett Library.
[2] Elizabeth Garrett to Emily Davies, 16 April 1864. Fawcett Library.

chosen her tactics well. Dr Parker gave her no more trouble, and she remained at the hospital another three months, leaving at the end of July 1864 with a certificate that she had attended, on her own responsibility, fifty-five cases of labour.[1]

Outwardly, Elizabeth Garrett seemed quite unaffected by her solitary battle against circumstance. She still looked demure and young for her years. Less than three weeks after the battle with Dr Parker, Emily Davies was employing her as a stage property at a meeting of the Social Science Association to discuss the admission of girls to Oxford and Cambridge Local Examinations. Having banished the unattractive blue-stockings to the back row, she arranged in the front 'three lovely girls and Miss Garrett looking exactly like one of those girls whose instinct is to do what you tell them'.[2] This appearance was more than ever deceptive. Elizabeth Garrett's instinct was to do what she, and she alone, thought right. For years she had forced herself to ignore the sting of ridicule. She knew what it was 'to be sneered at as a woman by a stupid fool of a man', and to endure the insult behind the mask of a calm face. Such self-command is purchased at a high price and the discipline she imposed upon herself was dangerously rigid. There was little room in her life for friendship. She must have been lonely in the dingy surroundings of Philpot Street, yet when, in June 1864, a young woman turned up, eager to become a fellow-student, Elizabeth surveyed her critically. She was entertained to tea, summed up as 'crude and dogmatic' and politely dismissed.[3]

Elizabeth Garrett insisted on ordering her social life, like her working life, upon her own terms. She would go to parties, but leave early because the evening time was valuable for work. She loved to go for long fireside conversations with Mrs Gurney, but would leave when other guests broke in upon their intimacy.

---

[1] The next woman student, Miss G. M. Wauchope, was admitted as a wartime concession in 1918.
[2] Stephen, B., *Emily Davies and Girton College*, p. 90.
[3] Elizabeth Garrett to Emily Davies, 27 June 1864. Fawcett Library.

In these student years she formed only one relationship which went deeper than she had intended, with the most outstanding character in their circle. Henry Fawcett was three years older than Elizabeth, an immensely tall man, with massive head and ugly features. He had been blinded in a shooting accident, but within ten minutes of the disaster he had made up his mind to live life to the full. He was already Professor of Political Economy at Cambridge, and a brilliant Liberal speaker. Next he was determined to force his way into the House of Commons. Elizabeth respected his keen mind and honoured his courage. If one admired Henry Fawcett it was impossible not to enjoy him too. His zest for living, his gift for good talk, his incapacity for being awed by differences in status, made him a wonderful companion. He told of rowing with a crew of dons known as the Ancient Mariners, of walking on the Gogs at Cambridge, of skating out to Ely at fifteen miles an hour, when he felt but could not see, the Fenland sunset crimsoning the banks of snow.[1] They became close friends, and met whenever Henry Fawcett came to London from Cambridge, but they kept their meetings private, and because of his blindness no letters passed between them. There is therefore no record of the exact day, momentous for them both, when Harry asked Elizabeth to marry him.[2] Both were passionate reformers, both committed to public life, both incapable of conventional domesticity. Henry's blindness, which might have repelled some women, had for Elizabeth the attraction of a challenge. Marriage had no place in her rigorously planned life, but this was no ordinary suitor and for once she could not make up her mind. She said

[1] Stephen, L., *Henry Fawcett*, p. 51.

[2] MS. notes of Sir Alan Garrett Anderson. 'Among others Harry Fawcett asked Elizabeth to marry him, and when he afterwards proposed to Millie, Elizabeth voted con. whereas Louie, who had not wanted Elizabeth to marry him, encouraged Millie to accept. . . . Incidentally I never knew about this till I saw it in the letters.' He adds, 'As they are all dead I don't think there is any harm in knowing about it now!' The letters in question were those written to Mrs Garrett by her children and hoarded by her at Alde House over a period of fifty years. Nearly all of them were destroyed after her death, during a vigorous spring-cleaning.

nothing to the rest of her family, but turned for help to Louie, whom she loved and trusted. Louie, perhaps thinking their temperaments too nearly alike, advised Elizabeth not to marry Henry Fawcett. She was wise, as their lives were to show, but the decision to part from this exceptional man cost Elizabeth real pain.

This rejection was decisive. All Elizabeth's efforts, all her energies, were now concentrated upon success in her chosen career. She refused a further three or four proposals of marriage, apparently without regret.[1] Emily Davies noted with some disquiet the increasing self-sufficiency of her friend. Elizabeth could still charm when she pleased, but she made it clear that she did not need or welcome advice. 'My complaint', wrote Emily Davies forthrightly after some disagreement,[2] 'is that you *knew*, and did not want advice or help from anybody.' Apparently Elizabeth, in this as in other ways her father's daughter, had the habit of 'receiving a suggestion (advice is too large and strong a word) by contradiction'. This, as Emily Davies pointed out, might lead her into decisions she would afterwards regret. Elizabeth seems to have replied that she did not despise counsel 'when I acknowledge the fitness of the giver and feel in need of advice'. 'My regret', replied Emily Davies, 'is that you so seldom do either and especially the last . . . As far as I can see there is no one except Louie, and myself, with whom you are in the habit of discussing plans on quite free and equal terms (if you are with us?).' She ended with a sharp warning against the atmosphere of 'mutual admiration rather conspicuously manifested' in the Garrett family circle and the dangerous over-confidence it bred.

It says much for these remarkable women that their friendship continued after this exchange of letters. Nevertheless Emily Davies' insight had revealed an underlying danger. Intellectually Elizabeth Garrett's life was filled with interesting work and the exhilaration of knowing herself a pioneer. Emotionally she was

[1] Anderson, Sir A. G., MS.
[2] Anderson, L. G., op. cit. pp. 114–17.

too much alone. She had subdued a powerful temperament by deliberate self-control She had rejected light-hearted friendship or romantic love; now she could turn only to Louie for understanding.

In October 1864 Elizabeth Garrett entered upon her last year as a medical student. For her course in morbid anatomy she continued the private tuition with L. S. Little which had worked so well for dissection. For principles and practice of medicine she was able to renew her connection with the Middlesex Hospital. Dr Stewart, the learned but 'horribly unpunctual' physician who had offered to take her on his teaching rounds, had as joint-lecturer in medicine at the hospital S. J. Goodfellow, F.R.C.P. Dr Goodfellow knew of Elizabeth already, and consented to take her as private pupil in his house at Savile Row for the entire course. In this he may well have been encouraged by his own wife, a highly intelligent woman who helped him by translating foreign scientific journals and drawing exquisite diagrams to illustrate his lectures. Goodfellow delivered to Elizabeth privately the systematic course which he normally gave at the hospital and she found his teaching clear and interesting. Unusually for a physician of his times, he taught that one should explain the reason for his treatment to the patient, and his quiet manner won the confidence of the most nervous.[1]

While Adams's pupil, Elizabeth had secured entry to the London Hospital wards, and in the same way she used her connection with Goodfellow to re-enter the Middlesex. There was no question, of course, of her being accepted officially as a student, but in October 1864 she asked permission to enter the wards as a visitor. The committee gave no general authority but allowed her to attend certain wards by permission of the individual physicians and surgeons in charge. Elizabeth had been wise in restraining her father and refusing to quarrel with the senior staff at the time of her dismissal three years before. Personal goodwill now won her the entry to most departments of the hospital. She was, as always,

[1] *The Lancet*, 17 Aug. 1895.

the subject of masculine speculation and gossip, but this she had learnt to ignore.

There is a vivid picture of Elizabeth Garrett at twenty-eight, seen through the eyes of a young Scots doctor on the Middlesex staff. John Ford Anderson was twenty-four years old, a son of the manse, who had recently come, after his training at Aberdeen, to serve as Resident Medical Officer under Dr Stewart at the Middlesex. One day, in the course of his work, he went down to the pathological laboratory where he was discussing some tests with the pathologist when, to his great surprise, a cultivated woman's voice cut into the conversation. He turned round and saw a lady, elegantly dressed in the fashion of the day. He was still more surprised to learn that she knew all about the work of the laboratory, and as they left the room together, still talking, he was cudgelling his brains to think who she might be. Suddenly it dawned on him. 'This must be Miss Garrett!' The lady, when questioned, confirmed his suspicions, quite without embarrassment, and continued to talk to him in a natural, easy way until the rather cautious young Scotsman was won over. They became friends, and this chance meeting, as it proved, was fateful in Elizabeth Garrett's career.[1]

She visited for six months at the Middlesex and completed her last statutory period of clinical practice by the end of March 1865, when the medical committee ruled that her visits must cease. Probably they feared that if allowed to continue she would somehow dig herself into their hospital for good. Individual doctors wrote kindly in withdrawing their permission and several continued to follow her career with interest.

There was time in April for a spring holiday, staying at Grasmere and tramping over the fells, before Elizabeth returned to Manchester Square and her last course of lectures for the L.S.A. For these, in toxicology and forensic medicine, she obtained an introduction to George Harley, Professor of Medical Jurisprudence

[1] Anderson, Dr J. F., *A Pioneer*. Manuscript reminiscences. Anderson family papers.

at University College. Harley was a man of strength of character. A sudden severe attack of retinitis had threatened him with blindness. He decided to experiment by treating it with 'complete physiological rest' and remained for nine months in a darkened room without seeing even his own hands. He emerged, unable to distinguish colours, but cured, to publish an account of his own case in *The Lancet*. Harley had the freshness of true scientific curiosity and he was a stimulating companion and teacher.[1] With only one course of lectures to follow, and her clinical work completed, Elizabeth Garrett had time to spare in the summer of 1865. She used it to go with Louie to the first meetings of the Kensington Society, a group of about fifty ladies who met to discuss questions concerning women. There was no doubt who should lead the first discussion on 23 May; among the members no one had advanced so far towards full professional independence as Elizabeth Garrett. Elizabeth read a paper, choosing as her subject 'What is the Basis and what are the Limits of Parental Authority?' This subject aroused intense interest. Among the hearers were Miss Helen Taylor, Miss Sophia Jex-Blake, Miss Beale, Miss Buss, Miss Wolstenholme and Madame Bodichon. Elizabeth's views were of more than academic interest to these ladies since she had already bent parental authority to her own ends with notable success. In the same month Sophia Jex-Blake, after many parental protests, sailed for a long visit to America, where a friendship with Dr Lucy Sewell of the New England Hospital for Women and Children was to draw her in turn to a career in medicine.

By 4 August, Elizabeth's final course of lectures was finished and she had nothing more to do but go home to Suffolk and revise for her finals in eight weeks' time. It would have been out of character for the long struggle to end so quietly. Suddenly, with victory almost in sight, disaster threatened the work of five years. Too late the Society of Apothecaries realized that this determined young female actually intended to qualify, and that they would

[1] *Lives of the Fellows of the Royal College of Physicians*, Vol. IV, p. 141.

bear the blame for it throughout the medical profession. As a last resort the Court of Examiners wrote to Elizabeth ignoring their undertaking of 1862 and regretting that they could not examine her. Newson Garrett was incensed, and this time his daughter did not attempt to restrain him. He issued an ultimatum, threatening a lawsuit if they did not admit Elizabeth to the L.S.A. finals. Mr Garrett's reputation for truculence had reached London, and the Society hastily took Counsel's opinion. They too retained Mr Hannen, Q.C., whom the Garretts had already consulted about university charters. They were informed once more, as they had been in 1861, that the terms of their charter did not exclude women. Possibly Hannen also warned them against litigation with Newson Garrett.[1] The Society retired crestfallen and in danger of being boycotted by the medical profession for what it had done, to consider ways of altering its regulations as quickly as possible before any other woman could qualify.

Elizabeth Garrett, in Suffolk, calmly took a holiday before tackling her revision. She went to stay with some cousins at Wickham Market where the peal of bells cast by her ancestor, the Puritan pioneer Harmon Garrett, still rang over the town. Glemham Hall was a Tudor house, said to date from Henry VIII's reign. Elizabeth enjoyed roaming the overgrown garden and the big half-furnished rooms. 'I am still completely idle,' she wrote, 'except for working in the garden half the day and mending my clothes occasionally. I mean to shut myself up next week with my books.'[2] On her return, Alde House was noisy with the voices and boots of visiting grandchildren, so Elizabeth borrowed a room in an empty house facing the sea, and withdrew there every morning for the next week. 'Studys out of the house are such bless-

---

[1] Newson Garrett was at the peak of his career as litigant. Clodd, H. P., op. cit. pp. 133–5, relates the case in which he sued a summer visitor for leading a donkey on the Crag Path at Aldeburgh. The defendant remarked 'I was told I should be interfered with by Mr Garrett. I enquired who he was and was informed that Mr G. was the Corporation and the Magistrates and everything else.'

[2] Elizabeth Garrett to Emily Davies, 12 Sept. 1865. Fawcett Library.

ings when one wants to get through work quickly,' she wrote to Emily Davies. 'I am very placid about the exam. though I try to avoid unbecoming confidence.'[1] She had nothing to worry about, and she was too honest to pretend otherwise. The quality of her teachers, and the effort she had put into her work, lifted her out of the class of the routine L.S.A. candidate. Dr Louisa Garrett Anderson described her mother's training as 'desultory' and considered the best part of it over when she left the Middlesex in 1861,[2] having completed only four out of the eighteen prescribed courses. The Apothecaries' Hall registers do not support this view, for Elizabeth Garrett over-fulfilled their admittedly modest requirements. Among the lecturers who gave her individual coaching were an F.R.S. and Regius Professor, an F.R.C.S. and three F.R.C.P.s, and she spent five periods of statutory clinical practice at hospitals of high standing.

On 22 September Elizabeth came to London and stayed with her Dunnell grandparents in St John's Wood, making her way to Blackfriars at five o-clock on 28 September with seven other candidates for the examination. Apothecaries' Hall held no terrors for her. She already knew the courtyard with the black-and-gold-faced clock and the oaken staircase ascending to the hall with its long, shining table and portraits of bygone masters of the company upon the panelled walls. Elizabeth Garrett presented her schedule of lectures and practice, signed up with such stubborn persistence over the years which had changed her from a daughter at home to a woman of the world. She was directed to her examiner, Mr Wheeler. The examination was straightforward with no written papers and no clinical trials; Mr Wheeler's questions covered medicine, midwifery and medical pathology. She sailed through it telling herself that it was too easy to feel elated about. By half-past seven it was all over; Elizabeth was one of three who received a final certificate. Two of the examiners, con-

[1] Elizabeth Garrett to Emily Davies, 22 Sept. 1865. Fawcett Library.
[2] 'Thus ended the best and most consecutive part of Elizabeth's training.' Anderson, L. G., op. cit. p. 86.

ferring afterwards, agreed that it was a mercy they did not put the names in order of merit as in this case they must have put her first.

The Lancet, which had cheered Elizabeth's expulsion from the Middlesex four years before, hastened to congratulate her, although still in facetious terms, under the heading 'Frocks and Gowns'. It was impossible to deny her ability, her hard work and determination, the time, labour and money she had spent in the cause. 'No doubt', observed the writer, 'the examiners had due regard for her sex and omitted all those subjects of examination which would be shocking to the female mind.'[1] Such a patronizing tone had long lost its power to infuriate Elizabeth Garrett. For the first time in British history a woman had passed through a recognized course of medical training and secured a modern legal qualification in her own country. It was a unique achievement and she knew it. '*I was in the fortress* as it were, but alone and likely to be for a good long time.'[2]

[1] *The Lancet*, 7 Oct. 1865.
[2] Elizabeth Garrett Anderson, MS. draft for a speech, Royal Free Hospital School of Medicine.

PART TWO

The Physician

CHAPTER ELEVEN

Licentiate of the Society of Apothecaries
1866–1869

Life as a doctor was not going to be easy. Elizabeth Garrett was barred from any hospital appointment, from any army, navy or even poor-law post. She could hardly hope to be accepted as an assistant in general practice, or as the sole doctor in a country community. She was qualified and willing to attend male patients but decided not to do so for fear of scandal. Her best hope was to settle in London as consultant physician for women and children only, and hope that with time and patience her practice would pay its way. Many eminent men had done the same; Broadbent had lodged in a humble street and Paget had supplemented his earnings by writing for a Penny Encyclopaedia. Newson Garrett, who had already spent a great deal on this exceptional daughter, was willing to rent a house in London for her and to subsidize her over the early, inevitably difficult years.[1] After some searching Elizabeth had found a house discreetly on the fringe of fashionable medical London.

Upper Berkeley Street lay between the plane trees of Portman Square and the hansom cabs of the Edgware Road. Its quiet terraces, laid out about 1800, had faded to an even brown, a perspective of slender windows, wrought-iron balconies and delicate fanlights. Even now, on winter evenings, it keeps its lamplit

[1] Anderson, L. G., op. cit., p. 120, says 'she made a success of general practice', but it is plain that so far as private patients were concerned this success was only gradually built up. In Jan. 1867 Elizabeth told Emily Davies that she was still dependent on an allowance from home.

intimacy. In the 1860s it had its own church, the Brunswick
Episcopal Chapel, its own inn, the Portman Arms, its own dairy,
baker, cabinet maker and milliner, as well as a handful of physicians
and surgeons. In autumn 1865 these residents saw an addition to
their street, a night bell outside number 20 and a new brass plate
bearing the words 'Elizabeth Garrett, L.S.A.'[1]

They could not know how anxiously the wording of that plate
had been discussed, nor what pains the new tenant took to present
herself tactfully to her neighbours. To describe herself as 'Dr'
might seem pushing, and Emily Davies advised against it. 'I
should not consider it an act of friendship', she said, 'to present
anyone to strangers under a title which excites repugnance.'[2] On
the other hand, Elizabeth herself could not stomach 'Miss Garrett'
on the door. 'It is like a dressmaker,' she objected. In the end it
was Louie who found the tactful form of full name and qualification, with a night bell to attract custom.

Patients arriving at 20 Upper Berkeley Street were admitted by
a trim parlourmaid and passed upstairs to wait in the front
drawing room. A communicating door led to the back drawing
room where Elizabeth, elegant in brown velvet and Irish lace,
received them. The consultation over, another door of heavy
carved mahogany, excluding every sound, led them directly to
the landing. Elizabeth was determined that her practice should
conform to the most rigorous standards of dignity and professional etiquette. She avoided personal publicity although, as the
only woman doctor the British public could see at work, she was
an object of intense curiosity. She refused to have her photograph
taken for postcards though she allowed a woman artist, Laura
Herford, to paint her portrait, looking from the canvas with an air
of alert, composed interest. Nor did Elizabeth Garrett forget
that an L.S.A. was very far from the M.D. on which she had set
her heart. She refused to be addressed as 'Dr', and in replying to
an invitation wrote 'I am sorry I have no claim to the title of *Dr*

[1] *Post Office Directory for 1866*, p. 748.
[2] Stephen, B., *Emily Davies and Girton College*, p. 80.

Elizabeth, and I do not like to have that which does not of right belong to me.'[1] In September 1866 she entered herself as an L.S.A. in the Medical Register.

Her family reacted predictably to Elizabeth's success. Mrs Garrett accepted it, but did not pretend to like it; a career had no place in her scheme of things for her daughters. She sent hampers of garden produce, home baking and poultry to supplement the diet of Upper Berkeley Street, and Elizabeth in reply never failed to send a weekly account of her doings. The younger brothers and sisters were delighted, and Newson Garrett exultant. *The Victoria Magazine* published an article on Lady Doctors which applauded Elizabeth's L.S.A. Instantly Mr Garrett approached Mr W. H. Smith, the newsagent, and asked him to give a general order to '*push* it at the railway bookstalls'.[2]

At first patients were few and Elizabeth could enjoy some leisure. She went to concerts and picture galleries and found herself, as something of a celebrity, much in demand at dinner parties. Emily Davies had doubts about the wisdom of such junketings for herself, though approving of them for her friend.

> I felt directly that if I went to Lady Stanley's again, I must get a new bonnet [she wrote to a mutual friend]. And is it well to spend one's money in bonnets and flys instead of on instructive books? But on the whole I think the advantages preponderate.... Miss Garrett's case is different, because successful physicians always consort with the aristocracy, and she of course wants to make her way in the world.[3]

Elizabeth felt free to accept the invitations of those she disrespectfully called 'swells' as well as those of her own intimates. She dined at Blackheath with John Stuart Mill and returned in the carriage with Lady Amberley, daughter of the formidable Lady Stanley of Alderley. On a rainy day in March 1866 a group of

[1] Elizabeth Garrett to Mrs Lankester, June 1866. Wellcome Historical Medical Library.
[2] Stephen, B., op. cit. p. 77.
[3] ibid. pp. 110–11.

advanced ladies, including Mill's step-daughter, Harriet Taylor, Lady Amberley and fat, jovial Frances Power Cobbe the philanthropist, met at Elizabeth's house to hear her give a lecture on physiology. 'Everyone cared more for it than I did,' wrote Kate Amberley in her diary that evening, but she liked Elizabeth personally.[1]

For Elizabeth to live alone, unchaperoned, would have caused damaging scandal, so she invited her school friend, Jane Crow, to share her home. Jane Crow now worked as secretary at the Society for Promoting the Employment of Women, and the two young women, both busy, both independent, lived agreeably together. Their house formed the centre for a group of friends all living within walking distance, Louisa and James Smith, Llewelyn Davies and his wife, Emily Davies and Barbara Bodichon, who each summer deserted her Moorish villa for a long visit to London.

Barbara Bodichon's arrival in March 1866 coincided with the introduction of Gladstone's Reform Bill in the House of Commons. Barbara, quick to see an opportunity, went to John Stuart Mill and asked if he would submit a petition for extending the vote to certain women, as had been unofficially proposed by the Kensington Society. The Society did not suggest votes for all women, merely for women property owners.[2] Mill agreed to submit a petition on condition that the Kensington Society could find a hundred signatures. Barbara returned with the news, and a small working committee consisting of herself, Emily Davies, Rosamund Hill, Jessie Boucherett and Elizabeth Garrett was formed to collect signatures – the first Women's Suffrage Committee.[3]

Elizabeth Garrett as an independent woman householder offered accommodation in her dining room for the office work, and it was in her home that the first British suffrage society was born. For a fortnight the little committee worked with intense pleasure.

[1] Russell, B. and P., *The Amberley Papers*, Vol. I, p. 479.
[2] These were necessarily widows or spinsters, since a married woman's property passed to her husband; Mrs Gaskell recounts how she used to watch the Rev. William Gaskell pocketing her royalty cheques.
[3] Strachey, R., *The Cause*, p. 104.

Emily Davies was reluctant at first to be associated with too many radicals, but was reassured to find the signature of Mrs Alford, from an address The Deanery, Canterbury, then considered the height of respectability. Harriet Martineau, Mary Somerville and Josephine Butler signed and so, to the immense encouragement of the organizers, did 1,498 other women.

On 7 June 1866 Barbara Bodichon handed the document to Emily Davies to present to J. S. Mill. Emily Davies called on Elizabeth Garrett, and the two set out for Westminster Hall in a hansom-cab with the paper scroll. When they arrived, the first person they met was Henry Fawcett, who at once sent his secretary to find Mill. In the meantime the two women walked up and down the Hall, Elizabeth dandling the long scroll in her arms like a baby. An inquisitive crowd gathered around. The petition was too big to hide, and they turned for help to the only other female present, an old woman selling apples from a stall. She put it under her stall for them just as J. S. Mill appeared to find his petitioners empty-handed. He looked taken aback, but Elizabeth, choking with suppressed laughter, said 'We've put it down.' The roll was brought out from its hiding-place and Mill, waving its impressive bulk in the air, said, 'I can brandish this with effect.'[1] He was heard by the House with attention and respect, and seconded in a short speech by Henry Fawcett. The voting, 73 for changing the word in clause 4 from 'man' to 'person', and 196 against, pleased the women, who had expected overwhelming defeat.

The Suffrage Committee continued as a permanent organization with Louie Smith as secretary. Elizabeth Garrett supported its work, but felt it would prejudice the cause of women in medicine to be too openly associated with politics. Sending a subscription, she wrote:

I would rather not have my name advertised on the general committee. I think it is wiser as a medical woman to keep somewhat in the background as regards other movements. I do not

[1] Stephen, B., op. cit. pp. 111–12.

mind my name appearing in any list for private circulation, but I particularly wish it not to appear in public advertisements.[1]

Elizabeth's practice was slowly growing and by April 1868 she felt able to promise a hundred pounds to Emily Davies's proposed College for Women although she could only afford to pay by instalments. She was always afraid, she said, 'that patients will suddenly come to an end – all get well at once – or something as calamitous'. Nevertheless as a token of faith she undertook to pay twenty pounds a year.[2] The patients did not all recover as irrevocably as their physician feared, and slowly their numbers grew. Josephine Butler, whose life was a continuous struggle against ill health, and who distrusted most doctors, travelled from Liverpool in 1868 to consult her.

> But for Miss Garrett [she wrote to a friend], I must say of her that I gained more from her than from any other doctor, for she not only repeated what all the others had said, but entered much more into my mental state and way of life than they could do, because I was able to *tell* her so much more than I ever could or would tell to any *man*.[3]

Elizabeth could not promise Mrs Butler health, and she never offered patients unfounded hopes, but at least she had real insight into women's problems.

After six months in practice, seeking more clinical experience, she determined to found her own out-patients dispensary. She was strengthened by the approval of Llewelyn Davies, whose parish contained some thirty thousand souls in the horrifying slums round Lisson Grove. Davies worked himself to the bone for his poor, with pastoral visiting, schools, Sunday schools, a sewing club for women, a blanket club and a provident fund to save them from the extortions of moneylenders. All this effort was not enough to prevent the death of an old woman from

[1] Elizabeth Garrett to Millicent Fawcett, June 1867. Fawcett Library.
[2] Stephen, B., op. cit. p. 173.
[3] Bell, E. M., *Josephine Butler*, p. 47.

starvation on the steps of the Marylebone Workhouse on Christmas Day. To a sympathetic reporter the rector confessed that he was sometimes weighed down by the burden of so much human misery,[1] and the undeserved suffering of women and children particularly distressed him. When Elizabeth Garrett proposed a dispensary where poor women might receive medical advice free, or almost free, from a qualified woman, he promised his personal support. She could count on help from liberal friends like Mme Bodichon, the Russell Gurneys and Mill. General support for an all-woman venture was more doubtful and might not have been won without the accident of a cholera outbreak.

In 1865 there was an epidemic of Asiatic cholera in Egypt and by the early summer of 1866 individual cases arriving from the Continent caused a number of outbreaks in Britain, especially severe in Swansea and the East End of London.[2] Cholera spreading from poor to rich, hideous in its symptoms and lethal in its outcome, was the most dreaded disease of the century. Many Londoners still remembered with horror the outbreaks of 1831, 1847 and 1853. In this atmosphere of panic, hostility to women doctors was forgotten, and Elizabeth Garrett's proposal to open a dispensary in a poor and densely crowded part of Marylebone met with general goodwill. Nearly a hundred and fifty pounds was collected in subscriptions and donations, and she received letters of encouragement from Sir Harry Verney (Florence Nightingale's brother-in-law) and Lord Shaftesbury.[3] Elizabeth was quick to exploit a tactical advantage. The first London death from cholera took place at Poplar on 18 July 1866; but the St Mary's Dispensary for Women and Children had already opened its doors sixteen days earlier at 69 Seymour Place,[4] 'twice daily for the relief of persons suffering from premonitory symptoms'. The building,

[1] *Macmillan's Magazine*, Feb. 1861.
[2] Frazer, W., *A History of English Public Health*, p. 97.
[3] *British Medical Journal*, 14 July 1866.
[4] *Annual Report* of the St Mary's Dispensary, 1867. The house was later re-numbered 72.

a dingy shop on a street corner a few minutes' walk from Elizabeth's home, was scrubbed and the windows whitewashed for privacy, but remained otherwise unaltered.

The dispensary opened with the goodwill of the medical profession. Dr Billings, F.R.S., former Professor of Medicine at the London Hospital, agreed to act as one of the consultant physicians and spoke at the modest opening ceremony.

> Not only is the management mainly in the hands of ladies, but in Miss Garrett we have the first legally qualified female practitioner which England can boast. . . . I consider it very important that women who enter the profession should not profess to take medical supervision unless they have had a complete medical examination and training. This is what Miss Garrett has had . . . and what is of more consequence she has the knowledge which will qualify her to practise with skill and success.[1]

The future Sir William Broadbent, then living in Seymour Street, called on the young founder to wish her well. The honorary consulting staff of men included one physician of undoubted genius, the shy, eccentric Hughlings Jackson, three surgeons and three obstetricians. Elizabeth's former teachers, Little and Adams, sent subscriptions, while Nathaniel Heckford, who had recently married and was far from rich, sent sixteen guineas.

By the autumn of 1866, when the cholera epidemic and its attendant panic were dying away, the principle of a dispensary for women staffed by women had been established. Elizabeth attended three times a week, and found seventy or eighty women a day willing to pay a penny for her advice.[2] Pinched by respectable poverty, or battered and bedraggled, worn out by childbearing and the struggle against filth, they poured out their troubles to her as they never could to a man. Prostitutes, forced to follow their trade until they were too ill to walk the beat,

[1] *British Medical Journal*, 14 July 1866.
[2] *Annual Report* of the St Mary's Dispensary, 1867.

revealed their sufferings, because they found in 'the young lady doctor' a friend they could trust.

The conditions of practice a hundred years ago made heavy demands on her character and courage. There was no team of experts with the resources of bacteriology, X-rays and hospital laboratories behind her. She was forced to rely almost entirely on personal observation and experience and have the courage of her own opinions. Disease itself was dramatic in character and the crisis of an illness was often at hand with small warning. Deaths from appendicitis or pneumonia were a commonplace, and every doctor knew the anxiety of the week following a confinement, when he lay awake at night listening for the quick step of his patient's husband in the silent street, bringing the news of puerperal fever.[1] Elizabeth Garrett found this single-handed struggle exciting and satisfying. Moreover, it taught her medicine. In the first year she admitted 3,000 new cases, who made between them 9,300 visits to the dispensary. She visited those too ill to attend without extra charge. Her nights were often broken by maternity calls and she came to know the empty London streets under summer stars, or in winter when fog haloed the long rows of gas lamps, until sheer demand on her time forced her to limit the dispensary's midwifery cases. She learnt to recognize 'the immediate illness superadded to the depressed physical condition which poverty and ignorance tend to induce'. Before such social ills the doctor was helpless, apart from 'a liberal use of cod-liver oil, quinine and other expensive remedies'.[2] Already she needed beds, for 'the difference between the good nursing, the quiet and comfort of a well-ordered hospital and the opposite conditions too often inevitable in their own homes, involves to many the difference between recovery and death'.[3]

Medicines were made up by a salaried male dispenser; Elizabeth persuaded him to take two girls as paying pupils. She looked to

[1] Anderson, Dr J. F., 'Memories of a Medical Life'.
[2] *Annual Report* of the St Mary's Dispensary, 1867.
[3] ibid.

the future and intended that a trained woman should succeed him. There were also three young women studying for the Society of Apothecaries' qualification, whom Elizabeth had invited to attend for clinical training. The three, Frances Morgan, Louisa Atkins and Eliza Walker Dunbar, were making good progress when in May 1868 the Society of Apothecaries revised its constitution specifically to exclude them from examinations. Refusing to give up, they went to Zürich University, which had been open to women since 1865.

At the end of two years Elizabeth could judge that the dispensary had served both the women who worked there and those who came for help. To her it had brought professional experience and recognition. Her reputation was growing. In the last year she had been invited to read a paper to the Social Science Association on the administration of medical charities, and another, which was published in *Macmillan's Magazine* in 1867, on volunteer nursing.[1] This latter contrasted the often rough and ready hospital nursing she had seen in her student days with the work of the educated women who had nursed as volunteers during the cholera epidemic. She suggested that gentlewomen should be trained to supervise hospital nursing both day and night, and made the revolutionary suggestion that a qualified lady superintendent should be properly paid, not less than £150 with board and rooms.

It is not fair [she maintained] to the women for whom work is bread, for those to whom it is a luxury to come into the market and cheapen its price by giving what others have to sell. It should be a point of honour among women, as among professional men, to take the proper fee which belongs to any post.

This was a principle from which, in teaching and practice, she never departed, and it won her the respect of her colleagues. 'The doctors were delighted with E.G.,' reported Emily Davies from the meeting to Barbara Bodichon.[2]

[1] *Macmillan's Magazine*, April 1867.
[2] Stephen, B., op. cit. p. 178.

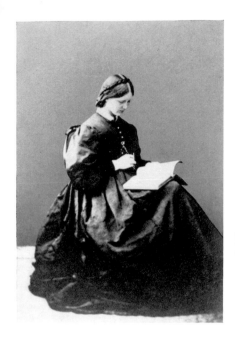

a. Louisa Smith
her elder sister

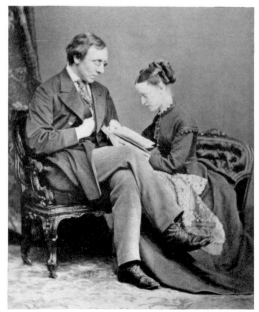

b. Millicent acting as
reader to her husband
Henry Fawcett, the
blind M.P.

5. Two sisters of Elizabeth Garrett

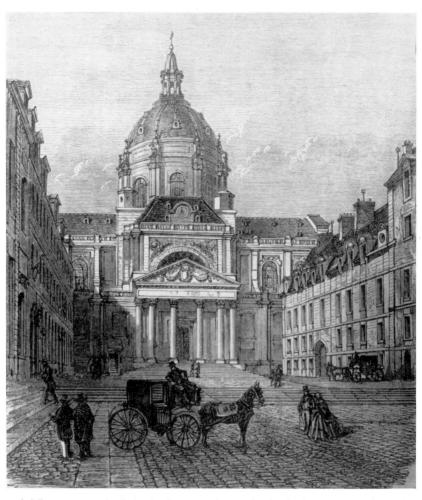

6. The courtyard of the Sorbonne where Elizabeth Garrett was cheered
by students as the first woman M.D. Paris

This growing professional reputation began to be reflected in Elizabeth's private practice. In the summer of 1867 she had acquired a new and aristocratic patient in Lady Amberley. Kate Amberley, daughter-in-law of Lord John Russell and mother of Bertrand Russell, was bravely progressive. She read a paper on women's suffrage to the Mechanics Institute in Stroud, causing the outraged Queen Victoria to write, 'Lady Amberley ought to get a *good whipping*,' a royal pronouncement successfully concealed for forty years. Kate Amberley was in fact a gentle creature devoted to her husband and children, who first consulted Elizabeth to know if she could safely travel to America with Amberley during a pregnancy. On 2 March 1868 she went suddenly into premature labour. Elizabeth was sent for, and found twins presenting by the foot, with contractions too strong and rapid to move the patient. Nothing was ready, there was no nurse, and when she sent in haste for Dr Priestley he was out and did not come. There was nothing to do but to deliver the babies herself. The first lived, but the second did not breathe although its heart beat for some time, and she did all in her power to revive it. Lord Stanley was openly angry that a woman was attending his daughter. The intimidating presence of Lady Stanley, who was sometimes heard to remark after a departing guest, 'Fools are so fatiguin' ', did not make the young doctor's position any easier. Anxiety and embarrassment increased Elizabeth's native brusqueness. She shocked the Stanleys by not appearing suitably distressed at the loss of one twin, and by remarking that 'she supposed Amberley did not mind as he was so Malthusian'. 'He did mind he told me,' wrote Kate Amberley in her journal.[1] After three weeks Elizabeth was still anxious about her patient and decided to call in James Paget. Paget, then Professor of Surgery at St Bartholomew's, had befriended Elizabeth Blackwell on her first visit

[1] Russell, B. and P., *The Amberley Papers*, Vol. II, pp. 84–6. Lord Amberley having said at a private gathering that birth control was a matter deserving the consideration of the medical profession, became the victim of a scurrilous election campaign, in which he was described as advocating infanticide. Elizabeth could hardly have made a more tactless remark.

to London in 1859. He was also a friend and medical adviser to George Eliot. The case ended happily; Lady Amberley recovered enough to go for a convalescent holiday to Worthing in June and to have 'a row with Mama', while Paget became one of Elizabeth's most valued medical friends. Lady Amberley remained her patient as long as she lived in London, and in August 1869 contributed £50 for three years to a medical scholarship for women.

The Langham Place circle was now entering its second decade. Emily Davies was at work for the proposed Women's College, managing with skilful generalship a committee which included two deans and three bishops. Sophia Jex-Blake returned to England after a year with Dr Lucy Sewell of the Women's and Children's Dispensary in Boston, afire with a new enthusiasm; she too would read medicine. Most of her friends encouraged her, but not Elizabeth. She had learnt by hard experience how much self-control a doctor needs; she knew Sophia's passionate nature, her ungovernable loves and hates, and her intolerance of any criticism. 'Frankly,' she said when asked for advice, 'I think you not specially suited.'[1] Accustomed to give and to get the truth herself, it did not occur to her that these words might wound. In the upshot, Sophia Jex-Blake, after an abortive start in New York, set out for Edinburgh University in March 1869, to begin the stormiest part of the medical women's struggle, with a resentful feeling that Elizabeth Garrett undervalued her.

The same outspokenness offended Elizabeth's friends in the women's movement on a subject which became the subject of bitter controversy during the years 1866–70. A series of Acts, under the title Contagious Diseases (Women) Acts,[2] applied the Continental system of regulated prostitution to British garrison towns, in order to control the sexual immorality which was considered essential for soldiers and sailors. Any woman living in certain garrison areas might be declared, on police accusation

---

[1] Todd, M., *The Life of Sophia Jex-Blake*, p. 186.
[2] The first was passed in 1864, and its provisions extended by amendments dated 1866, 1868, 1869.

alone, a common prostitute and as such forced on pain of imprisonment to undergo medical examination. With almost one voice the women's movement attacked the injustice of the new laws. 'By this law', wrote Josephine Butler, 'a crime has been *created* in order that it may be severely punished, but observe, that has been ruled to be a crime in women, which is not to be a crime in men.'[1]

In print and in public, those who demanded the repeal of the Contagious Diseases Acts did battle with those who believed they should be extended to cover the whole country. The British Medical Association praised the Acts; the women's crusade looked to Elizabeth Garrett, the one practising woman doctor, to attack them. They were disappointed; after three years' dispensary experience she did not believe that voluntary treatment or individual attempts at reform could defeat the dangers of venereal disease, and she was prepared to stand by this opinion in print. It has been suggested that she was rashly persuaded into writing on a subject about which she knew very little, or, by her detractors, that she was currying favour with the medical profession. A letter to the press, reprinted by the Society for the Extension of the Contagious Diseases Acts, makes it plain that she wrote from honest conviction.[2]

She regarded the Acts as an attempt to diminish an injury to public health and their aim, the relief of physical suffering, as one which should commend itself to a doctor. The evidence, she wrote, 'can only be fully appreciated by those who have had medical experience'. She believed compulsory treatment necessary because women refused to enter hospital early enough or to stay long enough. She thought powers of arrest a useful check on the ignorant girl of sixteen or seventeen who failed to see the danger of disease, and ridiculed the idea of police persecution: 'it is difficult to believe anyone can seriously credit women with such

[1] Butler, A. S. G., *Portrait of Josephine Butler*, p. 82.
[2] Garrett, E., 'An Enquiry into the nature of the Contagious Diseases Acts', *Pall Mall Gazette*, 25 Jan. 1870.

a degree of helplessness'. Elizabeth Garrett found it hard to put herself in the place of women without her own force of character.

She wrote with compassion of her prostitute patients. 'Hospitals do not as a rule admit them, dispensaries cannot cure them; missions and refuges reach but few of them; they are without their health, without character, without friends, without money. Could their position be more forlorn?' Compulsory hospital care, she felt, was their only hope.

Her main point, however, was the injustice of leaving innocent women and children to suffer from venereal disease. She quoted from her eminent friend James Paget on 'the number of children born subject to diseases which render them quite unfit for the work of life', and added, 'I have found that two thirds of the whole number of patients treated for this class of disease are suffering through no fault of their own. I believe that among the poor, the number of innocent people who suffer from the worst and most lasting forms is greater than the guilty.' Finally she had this to say, from her experience as a medical woman in the slums of Marylebone: 'Degradation cannot be taken by storm and the animal side of nature will outlive crusades.' Elizabeth Garrett's arguments were bandied to and fro in the twenty years' struggle which led finally to the repeal of the Acts in 1886, and some members of the women's movement never forgave her the part she had played in it.

At the same time, Elizabeth was also involved in a family quarrel. Her sister Millicent, a girl of seventeen whose fragile prettiness concealed a first-class brain, was taken by Louie to an evening party on 18 April 1865. There the stunned guests heard the news of Lincoln's assassination. 'It is the greatest misfortune that could have befallen the world,' exclaimed the young girl; 'greater than the loss of any of the crowned heads of Europe.' The blind Henry Fawcett, a fellow guest, instantly asked their hostess to introduce him to 'the owner of that voice'. For the next year he cultivated the society of the Garrett family. 'If you ask him to Alde House,' warned an acquaintance, 'he will want to marry Milly.' 'Stuff and nonsense!' replied Newson Garrett, and promptly invited him. The invitation settled his daughter's life, for in October 1866 Millicent and Henry Fawcett became engaged.[1]

At first Elizabeth did not believe it. When she realized the situation this put her in, she was appalled. Pride and reticence would not allow her to speak of the offer of marriage she had received from the same man, nor what she had suffered in refusing it. Moreover Elizabeth still thought of her sister as a child. She wrote sharply to Millicent about Harry's poverty, his blindness and the impossibility of his ever supporting a family. Desperately trying to add weight to her arguments, she offered to get the opinion of Jane Crow or Barbara Bodichon. Millicent, a true Garrett, refused since 'judging from Dr Bodichon's appearance, I should say that it was improbable that we should agree in the choice of husbands'. As a last resort Elizabeth threatened to come down to Alde House and speak her mind in family council. To this Millicent reacted promptly and with spirit, enlisting the help of the one person in the world who could manage Elizabeth.

I have been rather heavily jumped on by dear old Lizzie and the parents during the last few days [she wrote to Louie]. I had a most awful letter from Liz on Sunday morning . . . I have not written for fear of vexing her which I should be dreadfully sorry to do, for I know that it is out of pure love for me and anxiety for my future that she wrote as she did . . . I believe she would think we were throwing ourselves away if we married the Archangel Michael with twenty thousand a year . . . If you see her before Saturday, give her my love and try to talk her over, at least so far as to refrain from further jumping when she comes down here.

Louie Smith, whose judgment they all trusted, decided that just as Henry Fawcett had been the wrong husband for the determined elder sister, he was right for the younger. She wrote quickly to

---

[1] Strachey, R., *Millicent Garrett Fawcett*, p. 26.

calm Millicent's fears and to reassure her about Elizabeth's motives. 'I believe that dear old Lizzie is as wrong as ever she was right in being afraid, and I am quite sure that no one will be more glad than she will to have it proved so.'[1] Louie saw Elizabeth, reasoned with her about the engagement and persuaded her to accept Harry as a brother. By mutual consent they did not speak of the earlier proposal; it even seems possible that Millicent never knew of it.

Millicent and Henry Fawcett were married on 23 April 1867, but Louie was not there to see their wedding. In smoothing the way to Millicent's marriage she had used her magical touch for the last time. During the first days of February 1867 Elizabeth was suddenly called to Manchester Square, where Louie had been taken ill with pain and nausea. Elizabeth left home, patients and dispensary to nurse her sister, only to see the pain and fever increase. Night and day she applied hot fomentations, and measured out drops of opium, without result. It was appendicitis, for which there was then no surgical treatment and small hope of recovery. By 5 February Louisa was sinking.

She suffered bitterly at the thought of leaving her four young children. 'It *does* make one dread death', she had once written to her mother, 'to contemplate the possibility of it bringing such a loss to one's children . . . how much better to have a dear child taken into God's good keeping than to be taken from them thus.'[2] Elizabeth, practical even in her grief, felt that to care for the children was the only way she could help her sister. 'Don't be unhappy about the children', she urged the dying Louie. 'Your children shall be mine, even if I have my own.' Next day, 6 February 1867, Louisa died.

For her sisters it was if a light had gone out. 'Whenever I try to describe Louie to myself,' wrote Alice years later, 'I think of *flame*: hers was such a bright splendid fiery spirit . . . Louie was a bright, shining star – a more wonderful woman, in a wholly

[1] Strachey, R., *Millicent Garrett Fawcett*, pp. 28–9.
[2] Louisa Smith to Mrs Garrett, 29 April 1862. Anderson family papers.

different way, even than Elizabeth.'[1] Elizabeth was heartbroken. 'Our darling is gone', she cried, 'and we can never get a word or a look from her again!' With Louie's death went the affection, companionship, tenderness and good counsel of years; her favourite sister was left in spiritual desolation. Everything conspired to remind her of the qualities Louie possessed, and which she herself lacked. 'I think you know how much I cared for your sister and how highly I prized her friendship', wrote Sophia Jex-Blake. 'Perhaps you and I have not always understood each other so well as she and I did, but I want you to know how heartily and painfully I sympathize with you.'[2]

Now Elizabeth Garrett was forced to see how the years which had enriched her career had robbed her affections. Her friendships, largely impersonal, had been based on shared work for the women's movement, and her attitude over the Contagious Diseases Acts had alienated the Langham Place circle. On this even Millicent and their favourite cousin Rhoda Garrett disagreed with her to the distress of all three. Her mother was out of sympathy with the whole tenor of her life. She had achieved her career, but at a very high price. She was warm, affectionate, even passionate, yet she was forced to live alone. She was gay, spontaneous, unselfconscious, yet for years she had forced herself to the 'distressingly nervous work' of behaving discreetly under hostile eyes. She was self-willed with plenty of her father's impatience, yet she had learnt to repress her natural fire. Someone who knew her very well saw that 'with her the effort was constant to keep reason in command as the controlling power'.[3] However much one admires such self-discipline, it imposes great strain on the personality. In the years after Louisa's death this strain began to show itself in Elizabeth. She sometimes spoke or wrote sharply; she could not endure the stupidity of those who disagreed with her. She was

---

[1] Alice Cowell to Alan Garrett Anderson, 26 Dec. 1917. Anderson family papers.
[2] Sophia Jex-Blake to Elizabeth Garrett, 10 April 1867.
[3] Anderson, J. F., *A Pioneer*. MS.

kind to her patients, but curt with their relatives. To Louie's children, the girls especially, she was devoted, but dangerously possessive, calling them '*my* children' though their father was still living. She claimed jurisdiction over their outings, treats and discipline, although they lived with the Smith family at Suffolk Lodge, Acton. For herself she had only one remedy, work and more work.

In June 1868 M. Wurtz, Dean of the Faculty of Medicine at Paris, having heard of the women medical students at Zürich, requested a report on the admission of women to European medical schools. Dr Dureau investigated the question both at home and abroad, and gave his informed opinion, 'En France, aucun texte de loi ne pouvait s'opposer a cette admission . . . mais la grande difficulté était d'exiger des étudiantes les formalités préalables, diplômes, certificates etc., enfin toutes les études de scolarité qu'on exigeait des étudiants.'[1] The challenge to be once again first in the field was irresistible; Elizabeth determined to take a Paris M.D., if she could do so without keeping residence. As a preliminary, she withdrew from the women's suffrage committee and from all social engagements to devote herself to medical revision. 'It is not easy to work up for examinations amid the distractions of practical work,' she wrote to Helen Taylor. 'I am giving up all society in order to keep the evenings free for work, as this saves both time and energy.'[2] Every evening she sat alone with her books, and got up early in the morning to study before breakfast. During the day she studied in a cab as she drove on her rounds. She was, at thirty-two, assured, successful, respected though not always liked, but above all alone.

[1] Lipinska, M., *Histoire des Femmes Médecins*, p. 412.
[2] Strachey, R., *The Cause*, p. 172.

CHAPTER TWELVE

M.D. Paris
January 1869 – September 1870

News that Elizabeth Garrett was now working for the Paris M.D. spread through the women's movement. It reached the ears of the Hon. Amelia Murray, a royal lady-in-waiting who had founded the Governesses Benevolent Association and now summoned Elizabeth to the Palace to give an account of her work.

'My dear,' said Miss Murray at the end of it, 'I think what you are doing quite right, and I really believe that if I were a woman myself I would do the same.'

'If you were a woman yourself?' said Elizabeth, surprised.

'I mean, of course,' said Miss Murray, as though the distinction were self-evident, 'if I were in that station of life.'[1]

The lady-in-waiting apparently mentioned women doctors at the Palace, for one afternoon, when Elizabeth Garrett was on a step-ladder in the consulting room, economizing by hanging her own wall-paper, the door was thrown open and a flustered parlourmaid announced, 'Her Royal Highness, the Princess Louise.' There was no need to apologize for old clothes, piles of books or the articulated skeleton lying on the desk for Elizabeth's anatomy revision. The twenty-one-year-old princess, the most intelligent and least conventional of Queen Victoria's daughters, talked eagerly and without restraint. Only in parting did she ask Elizabeth '*please* not to tell her mother she had called, as she would not

---

[1] Strachey, R., *The Cause*, pp. 60–1.

approve'.[1] Queen Victoria learnt of the visit and was reported to be extremely annoyed. Meanwhile, regardless of royal approval or disapproval, Elizabeth Garrett worked at the Paris syllabus in hopes of an M.D. at last. She had never changed the judgment of six years before. 'My own feeling is in favour of having the M.D.; though it should be a foreign one I believe it would command more respect than the license from the Hall alone.'[2]

Since 1866 a young American, Mary Putnam, daughter of the New York publisher, and a graduate of the Women's Medical College of Philadelphia, had been working in the Paris hospitals, though for eighteen months she was refused admission to the medical faculty from lack of precedent.[3] In 1868, as a result of her persistence, she was at last admitted, and Elizabeth Garrett always insisted that the opening of the Sorbonne to women was due to Mary Putnam. Elizabeth herself had no desire for further lectures; what she wanted was permission to sit the six examinations of the Paris M.D. without keeping residence or presenting French certificates of study.

She approached Lord Lyons, the British Ambassador in Paris, who submitted her request through the Minister of Public Instruction to the Faculty of Medicine. The Ambassador's task was not easy, for the University, jealous of its traditions, was not disposed to lower its admission requirements.[4] Lord Lyons could only advance Elizabeth Garrett's claims as a practising physician of three years' standing. She was well known in liberal French circles because of the interest aroused by the St Andrews case, and the Dean of the Faculty of Medicine was her enthusiastic supporter. Unfortunately two other foreign women applied for admission at the same time, and the faculty council, fearing an influx of women

[1] Anderson, J. F., *A Pioneer*. MS. Anderson family papers.
[2] Elizabeth Garrett to Elizabeth Blackwell, 8 May 1862, quoted Blackwell, E., op. cit. p. 185.
[3] One professor suggested she should attend lectures disguised as a man.
[4] 'La Faculté avec raison', noted a professor, 'ne voulait plus d'équivalentes.'

not only in medicine but in law, arts and science, voted against accepting Elizabeth Garrett.[1]

In Britain a hostile vote by a university had always meant the end of Elizabeth's hopes, but in centralized France the case was different. The Dean of Medicine reported his difficulty to the Minister of Public Instruction, Victor Duruy, who in turn referred it to the Council of Ministers. The position was delicate. Lord Lyons was a diplomat of repute, enjoying the personal confidence of Napoleon III, and a much-needed friend of France in international negotiations. The Council of Ministers prepared to debate the case, when it was abruptly taken out of their hands. The Empress Eugénie, presiding over them during the illness of the Emperor, approved the inscription of the candidates on her own authority, adding, 'I hope these young women will find imitators, now that the way is open.' She even hoped to open a medical college for women herself in the autumn of 1870, 'but alas by then,' as Duruy wrote, 'the invalid was France'.[2]

The Empress Eugénie's intervention won the battle for Elizabeth Garrett. On 18 February 1869 Lord Lyons received a personal letter from Duruy reporting that by a special ministerial edict Miss Garrett could inscribe herself for the Paris M.D. without producing certificates of preliminary studies at the Sorbonne.[3] The M.D. which had been the goal of Elizabeth's ambition for ten years was at last within her grasp. She prepared to go to Paris for the first examination next month.

For anyone with a dislike of personal publicity the Paris viva voce was an ordeal, and Elizabeth entered the examination theatre on 15 March 1869 with some dread. Before her at a long table sat three examiners, stately in black robes lined with crimson.

[1] Anderson, Elizabeth Garrett, *Fortnightly Review*, March 1895.

[2] Duruy, V., *Notes et Souvenirs*, pp. 197–216. The Empress Eugénie was much more liberal in her views on education than has been commonly supposed. She was already supporting Duruy, in the face of sharp clerical opposition, in his plan to open lycées for the secondary education of French girls. Cf. Harold Kurtz, *The Empress Eugénie* pp. 196–7.

[3] Lipinska, M., *Histoire des Femmes Médecins*, p. 450.

Behind her, separated only by a wooden balustrade, male students and lecturers filled the tiers of benches almost to the roof.[1] The novelty of seeing this adventurous young Englishwoman in person had packed the room. Nothing was so hard for Elizabeth Garrett as waiting in apprehension, and nothing more challenging than the moment of action when it came. Nervousness quickened the tempo of her thoughts and faculties; afterwards she might be spent with exhaustion, but in a crisis she had courage. She answered the examiners in turn so promptly and clearly that the spectators broke into clapping at each reply. The hours spent parsing medical Greek and Latin with Joshua Plaskitt, the ludicrous French conversations at Miss Browning's Boarding School for Ladies, the hundreds of dispensary patients she had examined, all stood her in good stead now. Elizabeth Garrett passed the first examination with triumph, and the words of compliment addressed her by M. Broca, President of the Examiners, were cheered by the students and onlookers.[2] It was encouraging to Elizabeth after her English experiences to find this room full of young Frenchmen wholeheartedly on her side, still better after the anger of Queen Victoria to receive the personal good wishes of the Emperor and Empress. Elizabeth boarded with the family of a professor at the Sorbonne, and found that Paris welcomed a woman doctor if she was well dressed, well read, well mannered and witty. She enjoyed Paris but had to hurry back to London where there was still no qualified woman to act as her locum.

In June 1869 she returned to Paris for the second part of the M.D. in surgery and pathology.

Each candidate had to perform two operations before the judges and a crowd of spectators and then go through a long viva voce examination [she wrote to Helen Taylor]. Two men were examined with me. One of them passed in the *bien satisfait* class, as I did, the other was three degrees lower in the *passable*.

[1] Fontanges, H., *Les Femmes Docteurs*, pp. 69–72.
[2] *British Medical Journal*, 20 March 1869.

I can do no more till November as there is a long vacation, but I shall be ready then for the third and fourth and I hope also with the thesis in the interval. I have chosen Headache as its subject. I had to find a subject which could be well studied without post-mortem observations, of which I can have but very few in either private or dispensary practice; and I wished also to take a large subject, one that demanded some insight into the harmony which exists between the main physiological functions.[1]

While collecting and translating material for her thesis, Elizabeth Garrett was encouraged by the support of Elizabeth Blackwell, who had returned to settle and practise in London. Emily Davies also brought a new interest into Elizabeth's life, and the opportunity to repay in part a ten years' debt of gratitude, when she asked her friend to serve on the House Committee of the Cambridge College for Women, which opened in October 1869 at the reassuring distance of Hitchin. Remembering her own solitary student days in the little pantry-like room at the Middlesex Hospital, Elizabeth took a warm-hearted interest in the six 'real girls' who were finally installed for the Michaelmas term. 'If not numerous', noted Emily Davies with satisfaction, 'they are certainly select.'

A month after the new college opened, Elizabeth Garrett returned to Paris. On 4 December she took the third M.D. examination in chemistry, zoology, natural philosophy – the usual term for physics – and botany. The three examiners, one of whom was her supporter Wurtz, Dean of the Faculty, declared themselves 'bien satisfait', the highest class gained in these subjects since the beginning of the session.[2] On Christmas Eve Elizabeth faced three fresh examiners, this time in medical jurisprudence, materia medica and hygiene, and once again they were 'bien satisfait'.[3] Her Christmas holiday was brief, for on 4 January 1870

[1] Quoted, Strachey, R., op. cit. p. 172.
[2] *The Pall Mall Gazette*, 20 Dec. 1869.
[3] *British Medical Journal*, 1 Jan. 1870.

she sat the fifth examination, the last before the thesis, in clinical medicine, midwifery and surgery.[1] She had gained confidence now, and felt at home in the crowded examination theatre. On her return to London she told her Middlesex Hospital friend Ford Anderson of a successful riposte during the viva. She had been unable fully to answer a question on the great Dr Graves of Dublin.

'Mademoiselle,' expostulated the examiner, 'vous ne connaissez pas donc vos grands hommes?'

'Mais, Monsieur,' she replied undismayed, 'nous en avons tant!'

There was a burst of laughter in which the examiners joined, and once again they passed her.[2]

On 15 January 1870 Elizabeth submitted her thesis to the medical jury, Axenfeld, medical pathologist, Broca, surgeon, Cornil and Duplay, agrégés en exercise. Only their verdict and the final public disputation separated her from her M.D. diploma. In six weeks she had passed with credit three major professional examinations in a foreign language, a considerable feat of stamina and concentration.

'Sur la Migraine', Elizabeth Garrett's M.D. thesis, runs to thirty pages in print.[3] It is plain that her clinical observations were not devoted to mere headache, but to the severe disability of migraine proper; 'une vive douleur à la tête qui se fait sentir de temps en temps . . . presque toujours accompagné de vertiges, de nausées et de vomissements'. She describes the symptoms clearly and at length, showing the interdependent relationship between the pains in the head and the gastric disturbances, and attempting to distinguish between the immediate and underlying causes of the attacks. 'La migraine', she observes, 'est une nevrose réelle et non pas un embarras digestif,' and remarks that among her

[1] *The Lancet*, 8 Jan. 1870.
[2] Anderson, J. F., *A Pioneer*, MS. Anderson family papers.
[3] Faculté de Médecine de Paris: *Collection de Thèses pour le Doctorat en Médecine*, an 1870, tome 5. 'Sur la Migraine'. See also Appendix IV.

patients it was often the most gifted and intelligent who were sufferers.

In considering the pathology of migraine she concludes that 'la lésion centrale consiste dans la nutrition imparfaite des tissus nerveux. Le resultat immédiat est une trop rapide décharge de l'électricité inherente aux molecules nerveux.' To reduce the frequence and severity of attacks she recommends simple food and the avoidance of alcohol, plenty of exercise, good ventilation in bedrooms and as many hours as possible in the fresh air, rather than 'tonics' of dubious usefulness. The only experimental treatment she can suggest to avert repeated attacks is a course of faradization, which she had successfully administered to her own patients by means of portable electric apparatus. Her advice on the treatment of a migraine attack once it has started is cautious; it also reveals a sympathetic understanding of the patient's needs.

On ne doit presque jamais recourir à un traitement quelconque pendant la durée de l'accès. L'empressement des amis à faire prendre de la nourriture, des stimulants ou des remèdes ne fait qu'augmenter les souffrances. Généralement, il ne faut au malade que de l'air, de la tranquillité, la solitude et de l'obscurité. Tout mouvement le torture, ne fût-ce que le bruit des pas ou le tic-tac d'une montre . . . Le thé en grande quantité et très chaude est recommandé, soit qu'il agisse comme émétique ou purgatif, ou par l'action sédative de la chaleur sur les nerfs gastriques et duodénaux.

The Paris faculty apparently found no fault in this apotheosis of the British cup of tea and in June 1870 Elizabeth Garrett was summoned to Paris to hear their verdict. The likelihood of her success, and the approach of the mortifying moment when the diploma of M.D. would be placed for the first time in the hands of a woman, roused the hostile party in the Sorbonne to a final protest. Once again they were overruled by the Minister of Public Instruction. On 15 June 1870 Elizabeth Garrett presented herself at the Faculty, dressed, as custom demanded, in a long gown of black wool with starched bands, bare head and rolled thesis in hand.[1] She read the thesis aloud and answered a final viva covering the whole M.D. course. This was a test of mental agility. The questions ranged from the classification of species of fish through the preparation of arsenical compounds, the treatment of pneumonia and the taking of footprints in police cases, to the management of extra-uterine pregnancy.[2] The candidate and the spectators were then ordered to withdraw, while double doors closed on the final deliberations of the judges. When they reopened, a chamberlain announced in a loud voice that the thesis had been 'lue et soutenue', and Elizabeth Garrett, the first woman M.D. of the Sorbonne, was invited to receive the congratulations of her examiners.

The excitement that followed was described by the Paris correspondent of *The Lancet*.

In great haste I write you a few lines touching the medical event of the day – to wit the reception of Miss Garrett as an M.D. of the Paris Faculty, which has just this instant taken place and in which I had the pleasure of assisting. . . . The hall was literally crowded with students, and, on Miss Garrett's crossing the courtyard to leave the school, I observed with pleasure that almost all the students gallantly bowed to their lady confrère. All the judges, on complimenting Miss Garrett, more or less expressed liberal opinions on the subject of lady doctors, and one Professor M. Broca was especially energetic and enthusiastic. Altogether there was really an air of fête about the Faculty.[3]

The whole tone of the press towards Elizabeth had changed during her years in practice. Even the *British Medical Journal*, which abated none of its hostility to the whole idea of women in medicine, admitted that 'everyone must admire the indomitable perseverance and pluck which Miss Garrett has shown'.[4] Congratulations poured in, from family, from friends, from the medical

[1] Fontanges, H., op. cit. pp. 69–72.
[2] See Appendix IV.
[3] *The Lancet*, 18 June 1870.
[4] *British Medical Journal*, 18 June 1870.

profession. Sophia Jex-Blake wrote stiffly but sincerely on 'the brilliant success at Paris which has at length crowned your many years of arduous work'. Mrs Gurney wrote in affectionate reminiscence. 'How you have prospered and how you have worked and willed since I saw you as a bud ten years ago—was it? Now the fowls of the air may lodge in your branches.' Elizabeth Garrett was delighted and touched, but soon grew bored with the flood of compliments. When forced to draft an account of her success for a newspaper article she added an emphatic private footnote for her own satisfaction: 'P.S. Spite of all this *absurd bunkum* E.G. does not when free to be candid think much of herself.'[1] She was emerging finally from her grief and loneliness after Louisa's death, and the Paris triumph marked the beginning of a new maturity.

During the past few months both her professional and private life had undergone a change. The first was recorded by a headline in *The Times:* 'Miss Garrett admitted on a Regular Medical Staff'.[2] Nathaniel Heckford of the London Hospital had never forgotten his friendship for Elizabeth. During the cholera epidemic of 1866, when she was opening the St Mary's Dispensary, he had served at the Wapping District Cholera Hospital, where he met and married Sarah Goff, an Irish heiress and a volunteer 'lady nurse'. Everyone expected him to settle as a consultant surgeon in the West End, but he could not conceal his boredom at the prospect. 'I tell you what we *must* do,' he told his wife finally, 'we must start a children's hospital. It is the great need of the East End. We must do that and nothing else!'[3] They tramped the riverside parishes looking for a house and on the first anniversary of their wedding day moved into a sail-maker's warehouse, squeezed between a gin-shop and a coal yard on the bank of the river at Ratcliffe Cross, Shadwell. Mrs Heckford painted a board with the words 'East London Hospital for Children' which they fixed above the door.

[1] MS. draft for an article in *The Hampstead and Highgate Express.* Fawcett Library.
[2] *The Times,* 22 March 1870.
[3] Heckford, S., *Voluntaries for an East London Hospital.* Introduction.

Soon the ten little iron bedsteads in the loft were full of children and the ground floor crowded with out-patients. Heckford cheerfully gave up private practice and went alone through Butchers Row and Gin Alley, where the police feared to enter, visiting sick children. He converted two more wards, a babies' ward, the first of its kind in London, and a home for his wife to train girls as sick children's nurses. In December 1868 Charles Dickens visited the hospital to write an article for *All the Year Round* and saw in its chief 'in his pensive face, in the flow of his dark hair, in his eyelashes, in the very turn of his moustache' the ideal figure of the Children's Doctor.[1]

Subscriptions poured in from readers of *All the Year Round*, and the impromptu hospital acquired a Board of Management. To this body in February 1870 Heckford proposed Miss Garrett as visiting Medical Officer to the hospital. The members were doubtful; there was, recorded the Minutes, 'conversation as to whether or not advisable to make any innovation by introduction of female physicians, which would be a grave step for a Hospital in its infancy'. A month later Heckford returned to the subject of Miss Garrett again. He argued that her contact would be of great service to the hospital in strengthening its body of supporters, and urged that the committee should 'strike out a *new* path in expectation of gaining the suffrages of the public'. Dr Barnes said doubtfully that he 'would be glad to propose or second Miss Garrett on the grounds of her individual character'. He was not sure, though, that if the hospital were committed to the support of Miss Garrett's views the medical profession would not be alienated. Several other members, both doctors and laymen, were strongly in favour. Among those who hesitated was J. G. S. Anderson, the vice-chairman. He was financial adviser to the hospital and also represented his uncle's shipping firm, Anderson, Anderson & Co.,[2] important employers in this dockland district.

[1] Dickens, C., 'A small Star in the East', *All the Year Round*, 19 Dec. 1868.
[2] East London Children's Hospital, *Weekly Board Minutes*, 2 Feb. and 16 March 1870. Queen Elizabeth Hospital for Children, London.

He had not intended to support a woman's application for this very tough job. However, he was present at the meeting on 16 March when Elizabeth Garrett appeared before the Board. After watching her and hearing her replies to questions, he changed his mind. Not only did he help to vote Elizabeth Garrett in as the first woman honorary at any British hospital, but on an impulse he hurried after her and spoke to her on her way downstairs. Elizabeth saw a tall man of about her own age with the fair colouring of a Lowland Scot, strong, clear-cut features and steady eyes. He introduced himself as James Skelton Anderson, brother and housemate of her old acquaintance Ford Anderson of the Middlesex Hospital. Even more interesting to her, he had a sister who hoped to study medicine. Everyone who knew Skelton Anderson agreed on his good looks and charm of manner; Elizabeth Garrett went away across the city square feeling that she had found a friend.

On 23 March 1870 she took up her duties at the children's hospital. The repeated journeys were time-consuming but she refused to make them by cab, preferring the underground railway to Moorgate, a walk across the city in all weathers and a train from Fenchurch Street to Shadwell. Conditions there were a shock. To the people of Shadwell it was indeed 'an ark in the midst of a dreary sea of suffering, hunger and cold', but it was nothing like Elizabeth's idea of a hospital. Below the windows the river rose and fell with the tides; the wards had trap-doors in the flooring where goods had been hoisted, balks, beams and ladder-like staircases.[1] The staff were, as Dickens said, 'put to shifts for room like passengers in a ship'. The dispenser slept in the dining room and kept his spongebag in the sideboard cupboard. Trotting among the children's beds was a comical mongrel dog named Poodles, whom Heckford had found starving on the doorstep and taken in. The medical work was brilliant and children throve in this uninstitutional atmosphere, but a prospective matron, offered the then generous salary of £70 a year, said 'the inconvenience and bad

[1] *The Dickensian*, Autumn Issue, 1934, pp. 287–91.

arrangements were so overwhelming that she could not undertake the office'. The medical work was gruelling: many of the child patients were half starved and half clothed.[1] In nearly every family one or more children had died; it was heartbreaking to return a child saved by skill and devoted nursing to squalor and misery in which his chances of survival were small.[2]

Elizabeth willingly shouldered the burden of the work. She rebelled, however, against the hospital's haphazard administration. Both the Heckfords were incurably unbusinesslike. Nathaniel Heckford refused to kill even a black-beetle, on the grounds that 'death would probably be as disagreeable to the beetle as it would be to me', while Sarah felt 'the life of fun and frolic fading away like the dew of the morning' before the necessities of institutional management. They gloried in giving a Christmas party, with Punch and Judy show and hired barrel organ, for all the children of Ratcliffe Cross when there were only two or three pounds in the bank. To Elizabeth Garrett, who had accounted personally for every guinea subscribed to the St Mary's Dispensary, this attitude was incomprehensible and she turned for support in her criticism to the vice-chairman. James Skelton Anderson, who had anticipated a visionary pioneer, found himself supported on the committee by a woman as clear-headed and competent as he could wish. Elizabeth, as she met Mr Anderson more frequently, liked him increasingly. By June 1870 she was writing to him as an ally before she left for Paris, 'Drink to my becoming a great physician on the 15th, with 30 years of vigour before me.' When she returned in triumph, he was among the first to congratulate her. With the ordeal of examinations finally behind her, Elizabeth could afford to give more time to the children's hospital, and the friendship between them grew.

Soon after her return from Paris she proposed a practical reform

[1] Of 950 children admitted in one year 209 died, 144 of them being children under two years, of whom 56 died on the first day of admission.
[2] *British Medical Journal*, 1954, Vol. II, pp. 406–8. Back, E. H., and Levin, S., present a number of early case records.

to the Weekly Board: 'two members of the committee should be appointed visiting governors and they should make eight visits per month'.[1] The first pair chosen was herself and Mrs Heckford, and she reported to the Board on changes she considered essential. When her report was presented, Skelton Anderson moved that it should be accepted and put into action.

Nothing was too large for the new visiting officer to tackle, nor too small for her to notice. In spite of opposition from the committee, she insisted on forming a sub-committee to bring order into the noisy, jostling crowd of out-patients. She scorned the idea that a man was necessary to control them. 'I think that the out-patients could easily be kept in order by a woman,' she said, 'especially as there will not be the same crowd under our new system.' She declared war on vermin brought into the hospital by patients. 'Dr Walker stood out a little against my proposal,' she reported after a stormy meeting, 'but as he gleefully owned that fleas were nothing to him, his less happy confrères were allowed to carry their point.'[2] She penetrated departments which were closed to lay members of the Board. 'I am very much dissatisfied with the way in which drugs are bought and kept,' she wrote to Skelton Anderson. 'I shall move to have this department set in order. The dispenser does not know his business and there is no supervision, no check either upon him or the wholesale druggist.'[3] The hospital committee made attempts to subdue Miss Garrett. In October 1870 they censured her for admitting an infectious case, a child with dropsy following scarlatina. She apologized politely, but maintained 'there was no risk in admitting the case under notice, some weeks having elapsed since the patient's recovery from scarlatina'. At the next meeting she was still demanding 'an enquiry by some competent person into the hospital's supply of drugs'.

Elizabeth Garrett believed that administrative muddles were

[1] *Weekly Board Minutes*, 21 June 1870.
[2] Elizabeth Garrett to Skelton Anderson, 5 Sept. 1870. Fawcett Library.
[3] Elizabeth Garrett to Skelton Anderson, 20 Aug. 1870. Fawcett Library.

harming the work of the children's hospital. She warned Skelton Anderson that if the reforms she demanded were not forthcoming she was prepared to resign rather than consume her energies in a futile struggle.

> For the moment I cannot afford to waste time and strength in merely being kind to the miserable people at the Hospital. . . . It almost breaks one's heart to realize what their lives are, what they must be whatever one gave up in order to help them, but this is no reason for allowing them to interfere with more important objects. Mr Heckford thinks this sort of thing is mere selfishness. He is wrong . . . but even if he were right, I almost think I would go on and sell my soul for the cause I care most to help. It is my business to become a great physician, nothing else I could do would help women so much as this, therefore if the hospital helps it is welcome, if it hinders, away with it![1]

In December 1870 a more serious committee battle began, in which Elizabeth and the vice-chairman found themselves firm allies. Heckford, the most friendly person imaginable, had met a German doctor, Dr Baron von Seidewitz, and invited him 'to see out-patients for the present'. Soon Elizabeth was writing to James Skelton Anderson with extreme bluntness.

> I ought to have spoken to you about the Baron. Dr Leonard the house surgeon has a very poor opinion of him . . . he is exceedingly slow and takes about six hours over the out-patients on Monday. Whatever may be thought of the Heckfords' right to put a private friend in as *consulting* physician . . . it seems to me quite clear that no one so appointed shd. have the actual charge of the patients.

Moreover Heckford, whose health was bad, intended to go on holiday leaving von Seidewitz in charge as consultant. 'This, if he is incompetent, will seriously injure the hospital,' Elizabeth warned. On 13 December she moved on behalf of J. G. S. Ander-

[1] ibid.

son that the Baron's appointment had been irregularly made and should lapse. This was not seconded but von Seidewitz was told it was 'absolutely necessary for him to be registered as a qualified medical practitioner in the United Kingdom'. Thereafter at every meeting either Elizabeth or Anderson inquired after the unfortunate Baron's registration. In April 1871 he was warned by the committee that he must obtain a British diploma or forfeit his appointment. Attempts to trace the Paris M.D., which he claimed, were unsuccessful. The Heckfords were hurt and embarrassed but helpless. A year after their original invitation the Baron von Seidewitz sent a letter of resignation through his solicitor.[1] The committee were relieved to be rid of him, and convinced that Elizabeth's judgment had been sound.

Skelton Anderson admired Elizabeth Garrett's gifts and ambition, but thought her self-willed, as indeed she was. He supported her on the committee but warned her in private about the harm flattery did to her judgment, 'too much butter' as he frankly called it. Elizabeth accepted this correction with surprising meekness. Her career had been conducted in such an atmosphere of struggle that her family and friends were wholly partisan. To be criticized by a man, with the applause of Paris still ringing in her ears, was a stimulating experience. Moreover she was honest enough to see the truth in his words.

> I *do* rejoice in every gift however trifling that makes me more fit for the special niche I am meant to fill! [she admitted], but I don't think this really hurts me. The corrective is found in life, in caring for great things and in an enthusiasm of admiration for those before whom one's self is pigmied. It is only in Lilliput land that I could be stuck up and thank heaven I am not living there yet.[2]

Plain speaking strengthened friendship. James Skelton Anderson was an officer in the London Scottish, and that summer of

[1] *Weekly Board Minutes*, 13 and 20 Dec. 1870; 19 April and 12 Dec. 1871.
[2] Elizabeth Garrett to Skelton Anderson, 20 Aug. 1870. Fawcett Library.

1870, when his regiment was under canvas on Wimbledon Common, he invited Elizabeth Garrett to visit him. She went, chaperoned by Emily Davies and carrying a volume of Wordsworth to read aloud; this was a significant choice, for these were poems she had formerly read with Louisa. Their host in kilt and bonnet looked both gallant and handsome and she accepted a photograph of him in uniform. Emily Davies, who could tell a hawk from a handsaw better than most people, observed them together on this outing and wrote with uncommon tact 'of all your friends I like Mr Anderson the best!' He was indeed a remarkable man. The Garrett character might be Suffolk crag, but the Anderson character was pure Aberdeen granite. Elizabeth realized this as gradually she learned from Skelton and Ford Anderson the story of their childhood.

Their father, the Rev. Alexander Anderson, had been a minister of the Presbyterian church of Scotland. Finding himself unable to accept its system of patronage or establishment, he was the first of all its servants to abandon home and income for conscience's sake. On a winter's day in 1842 he had left his manse and set out on foot through sleet and snow with seven young children, to shelter in a fisherman's cottage on the bleak Aberdeenshire coast. The children thought they saw 'Tibby Tap', the witch of the parish, beating the clouds with her broomstick, but were consoled by the kindly fisherwives and the fascination of watching haddock cured in the cottage chimneys. Next year the Great Disruption, when their father with many others left the Church of Scotland for the Free Kirk, made their exile final. 'Where and how are we to live?' asked their mother, to which their father replied sternly, 'The Lord will provide; butter we may not get, but God will make us sure of bread.'[1]

By 1848 Alexander Anderson had been expelled from the ministry and had started, at the age of forty, a second career as founder and headmaster of Chanonry House School, Old Aberdeen. His

[1] Anderson, J. F., 'A Scotsman's Memories of the Forties', broadcast on 21 May 1931.

family grew to twelve, and for many years money was exceedingly
short. The elder boys learnt to rely upon themselves. At the age
of sixteen James Skelton had been sent to London to enter his
uncle's shipping firm with a salary of £2 per week, from which
he sent a contribution home. He was an able boy, with a love
of ships and the sea in his blood; by 1869 he had been made
a junior partner. He was now responsible for supporting a
brother and his youngest sister Nellie, whom he fitted out for
boarding school, even struggling to choose her hats himself.[1]
He and his brother John Ford lived together in bachelor content-
ment at 28 Buckland Crescent, Belsize Park. Their standards of
conduct were high, their friendships selective, their loyalties
absolute.

Skelton Anderson, indifferent to conventional feminine charm,
was drawn to the gifted and strong-willed Elizabeth. He had met
his share of match-making mothers and dutiful daughters; it was
refreshing to meet a woman who had other things than marriage
in mind. The outbreak of the Franco-Prussian War in August 1870
roused in her a passionate sympathy for the French cause. She
found it hard to do anything but read the newspapers and look at
the map, and when she planned a much-needed holiday she chose
the most adventurous possible, a visit to the battle-front. Undismayed by the capture of 82,000 French troops at Sedan on 1
September, she set off on the 5th, taking her brother Sam, a Cambridge undergraduate of twenty, and her lively eighteen-year-old
sister Josephine. A ten-page letter, scribbled a week later 'on an
ambulance waggon from Bouillon to Sedan', told Skelton Anderson some of their adventures. He learnt that this surprising
woman was cheerfully prepared to travel twenty-four hours in the
straw of a baggage waggon on a diet of dry bread and raisins, and
take her chance of lodging in ransacked Bouillon for the chance
of seeing the field hospitals and helping to dress the wounded.
'The soldiers were beautifully patient while their wounds were

[1] Geddes, A. C., *The Forging of a Family*, pp. 86–7. The author was Nellie
Anderson's son.

dressed,' she wrote, and there was an unexpected strain of poetry in her description of an ambulance train at night.

> At a quiet country station in the bright moonlight, rows of stretchers on the ground were being carefully lifted one by one into carriages, with here and there a figure just able to walk being helped along by red-cross bearers. The moon was bright enough to make everything clear, and in addition there were torches increasing the contrast between the scene on the platform and the still beauty outside.[1]

Sedan was so crowded that they were almost reduced to sleeping in a church beside a dead man, until a kindly Prussian officer of the occupying forces gave up his own rooms to the two women. They made their way back through the battle zone, and reached London just as the siege of Paris began.

[1] Elizabeth Garrett to Skelton Anderson, 12 Sept 1870. Fawcett Library.

CHAPTER THIRTEEN

Miss Garrett and Mr Anderson
October 1870–February 1871

On 12 October 1870 Elizabeth Garrett found a deputation of men awaiting her at her house. They were husbands and fathers of her dispensary patients, and they had come from the Marylebone Working Men's Association to invite her to stand for election to the new London School Board. The Forster Education Act of 1870, which required public elementary schools with School Boards to administer them, admitted women for the first time both as electors and candidates. The choice of Marylebone families had fallen on a woman they knew and trusted, Elizabeth Garrett, and the men assured her she was certain to be elected.

Elizabeth was genuinely surprised. 'It's queer why they want me', she wrote to Emily Davies, who had also been invited to stand for Greenwich. Elizabeth was already working hard and dreaded public speaking, but decided she ought not to refuse:

> I dare say when it has to be done I can do it, and it is no use asking for women to be taken into public work and yet wish them to avoid publicity. . . . Still I am very sorry it is necessary, especially as I can't think of anything to say for four speeches: and after Huxley too, who speaks in epigrams![1]

By the end of the month she had agreed to stand on one condition.

> I have an idea [she wrote rather ingenuously to a committee member]. How would it be to depose Mr Christie from the

---

[1] Stephen, B., *Emily Davies and Girton College*, pp. 120-1.

executive, leaving him still chairman of the general committee, put *Mr Anderson* in his place and let him give all the orders. . . . Mr Anderson is quite to be trusted in all questions that require decision, energy and sound sense.[1]

The new chairman lived up to this recommendation. Since Elizabeth's days were filled by dispensary, consultations and rounds, he took upon himself the strategy of her election campaign. He wrote her leaflet, with the note 'cut and carve to your own liking', and arranged distribution in Marylebone, Hampstead and St Pancras, as well as briefing volunteers to canvass the ratepayers in these districts. He rallied supporters: Llewelyn Davies, Octavia Hill, Barbara Bodichon, Miss Buss, Henry Fawcett, Dr Andrew Clark, Elizabeth's own physician, and the Rev. Samuel Barnett, future founder of Toynbee Hall, at this time curate of St Mary, Bryanston Square. To these were added some influential names, Sir Frederick Pollock, Sir Henry Thompson, the Hon. Mr Justice Hannen[2] and Robert Browning, who was an enthusiastic supporter. Skelton Anderson persuaded Elizabeth, though she protested vigorously, to draw up notes on her career, from which he drafted an article for the *Hampstead and Highgate Express* concluding, 'It will be a matter of great regret if there is not one woman on a board which will have to deal so largely with questions relating to girls.'[3] On the same date *The Lancet*, converted by the Paris triumph to firm friendship, congratulated Elizabeth on her candidature and pronounced finally, 'Miss Garrett's abilities are so exceptionally great when tested by the standard of either sex that we will in her case at once put aside all controversy about women doctors and say that she is an ornament to the calling that she has embraced.'[4]

[1] Anderson, L. G., *Elizabeth Garrett Anderson*, p. 148.
[2] This was Sir James Hannen, who as a Q.C. had advised Elizabeth on the Apothecaries' charter. He was now a judge of Queen's Bench.
[3] *Hampstead and Highgate Express*, 29 Oct. 1870.
[4] *The Lancet*, 29 Oct. 1870.

November 1870 was a month of meetings and campaigning, also for Elizabeth Garrett a month of continual association with her chairman. Between 8 November and 8 December she wrote him at least fourteen 'headless and tailless notes', and they met to discuss election business over hasty early suppers at Upper Berkeley Street before meetings. 'Don't think of either answering or dressing!' she wrote in a note of invitation on 16 November. She handed over to him on 8 November a hundred pounds to meet campaign expenses, and he undertook to set her mind at rest, since she hated debt as much as she distrusted extravagance, by paying all bills as they arose.[1]

On 11 November Elizabeth held her first public meeting, at which she was formally proposed as candidate by the headmaster of the City of London School. She was no orator, confessing to 'an almost morbid love of brevity', and her low voice, pleasant in the sickroom, was unsuited to large halls. However, she answered questions straightforwardly and her honesty won support. At this first meeting she was asked if she considered physical training, for example swimming, really necessary for girls. She replied without hesitation 'she thought physical education *especially* necessary for girls and swimming so useful she had practised herself for many years to perfect the art'.[2] She often returned to the question of sports for girls in future years, always with the same forthrightness.

She held meetings almost every other evening, speaking at the Eyre Arms public house, where she was dissatisfied with her performance, and at the Grafton Hall ('costs £3' she noted) where the meeting was chaired by a St Pancras undertaker, an important vestry man whom, she reported with some satisfaction, she had 'knocked under completely'.[3] As Elizabeth Garrett gained confidence she began to speak in the open air, to workmen in their

[1] Elizabeth Garrett to Skelton Anderson, 8 Nov. 1870. Fawcett Library.
[2] *The Times*, 12 Nov. 1870.
[3] Elizabeth Garrett to Skelton Anderson, undated postcard. Fawcett Library.

dinner hour, and to three hundred employees of Collard's piano factory, who stood her on some steps leading from a balcony into the yard and were quite won over by the end of the meeting.[1] With practice she became a ready and reliable speaker; by 25 November she was able to address a crowd of a thousand people at Greenwich on Emily Davies's behalf and rouse them to enthusiasm. This was an achievement at a time when it was customary to ask a gentleman to read even a learned paper written by a woman. Elizabeth also learnt to deal with hecklers, particularly supporters of denominational control in religious education. Once she let herself be tempted to answer indiscreetly, and Skelton Anderson did not spare her feelings. 'You have lost yourself thousands of votes, you have taken the guidance of your affairs out of the hands of the committee, and you have shown as you say weakness and vacillation. It was most unfortunate,' he wrote sharply. Elizabeth Garrett seemed positively to enjoy such unaccustomed criticism. She knuckled under, apologized and merely begged him in his own speeches, not to call her energetic. 'I should dislike anyone extremely whose chief recommendation was energy', she said, 'and in a woman it is peculiarly unattractive. It suggests hurry and bustle.'[2]

Elizabeth Garrett's election campaign worked up to a climax in its last week, encouraged by a front-page article in *Punch*, recommending her as an invaluable acquisition to the Board. Cultivating social graces had not been a waste of time, for the article stressed particularly that 'Miss Garrett and the other ladies profess no "strong-minded women's" doctrines, but those which all rational men would teach.'[3] By polling day, 30 November, in spite of occasional attacks of election nerves, Elizabeth felt reasonably confident of success. Yet she and everyone else was unprepared for the result when the votes were finally counted. She slipped out at midnight on 30 November to send a card to Skelton

[1] Elizabeth Garrett to Skelton Anderson, 20 Nov. 1870. Fawcett Library.
[2] Anderson, L. G., op. cit. p. 153.
[3] *Punch*, 28 Nov. 1870.

Anderson consisting of names and figures which spoke for themselves:

12 p.m. Nov. 30th

Garrett	47,858
Huxley	13,494
Thorold	12,186
Angus	11,472
Hutchins	9,243
Dixon	9,031
Watson	8,355

Elizabeth Garrett was not merely top of the poll for Marylebone, but received more votes than any other candidate in London. Lord John Russell declared that she deserved a vote for Westminster.[1] *The Times* commented on her victory as a 'crowning reward. The interval which separated the six other runners in this remarkable electoral race was but trifling – a matter of only a poor thousand or two of votes – in comparison with the crushing way in which Miss Garrett beat every masculine rival.' *The Englishwoman's Review* had a simple explanation of her success. 'For several years Miss Garrett has attended a dispensary for women and children. Her kindness and attention to her poor patients has been great and her skill, we believe, not small.' Even *The Telegraph*, avowedly hostile, could only attempt a nervous jocularity.

Miss Garrett, if a motion of hers is rejected, may burst into tears, though those who know the lady deny the probability. But if such things do not occur – if the ladies[2] are calm, businesslike and useful and keep to the point in public debate – what is to become of us men! . . . If Miss Garrett once enters the House of Commons, taking the oath and her seat with a little rustle of her dress, then the supremacy of man is at an end.[3]

The words, written in jest, were prophetic in earnest. More

[1] Russell, B. and P., *The Amberley Papers*, Vol. II, p. 386.
[2] Emily Davies had also been elected.
[3] Quoted in *The Englishwoman's Review*, Jan. 1871.

decisively even than her L.S.A. or her Paris M.D., which remained individual achievements, Elizabeth Garrett's triumph in the London School Board elections marked a stage in the progress of feminism. It established for the first time a general principle of extreme importance. In future, where women were subject to administration as employees, pupils, prisoners, patients or paupers, women, and qualified women, must be represented among the administrators. From there the distance was merely a step, logical however long, to political enfranchisement.

Elizabeth Garrett was in no doubt that she owed much of her success to the skill with which her campaign had been managed. When all bills were settled, the deficit to be met out of her own pocket was 'not much over £100, a very moderate price to pay for such a pinnacle!' On 2 and 3 December she sat down to write 136 letters of thanks to volunteer workers in the Marylebone division. One of these has survived, a conventional but charming note in her own hand, showing not the slightest sign of haste or stress.[1] 'I am very glad and happy, both for the victory itself and also for its having been given to me to have a share in it. I am sure it will do the women's cause great good.' Elizabeth had already written to her chairman and helper-in-chief, James Skelton Anderson:

> I wish very much that I could find some adequate way of thanking you and all my other zealous friends. But I am quite beggared; I can find no words that do not seem either too small or too common or too formal. It is not however difficult to me to take help of any kind from friends, it does not burden me so long as I know I would do as much for them or more if I could.

Unforeseen problems arose when two women sat for the first time in the Guildhall as members of an elected body.[2] One was the suggestion that Miss Garrett, as the member with the largest

[1] Elizabeth Garrett to Mrs Boyce, 3 Dec. 1870. Wellcome Historical Medical Library.
[2] Emily Davies was elected for Greenwich.

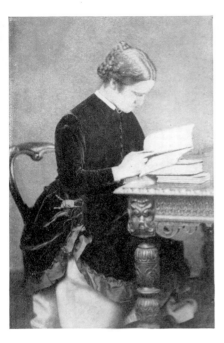

7a. Elizabeth Garrett M.D. in 1870: the photograph she wished to show to James Skelton Anderson

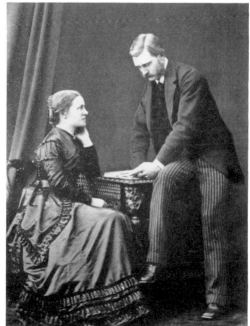

7b. Elizabeth Garrett and James Skelton Anderson: their engagement photograph

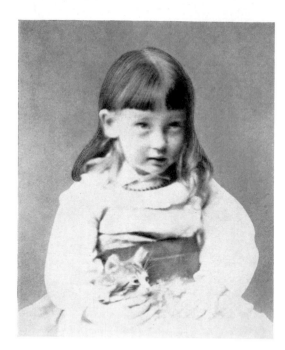

8a. Louisa Garrett Anderson with her pet kitten

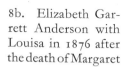

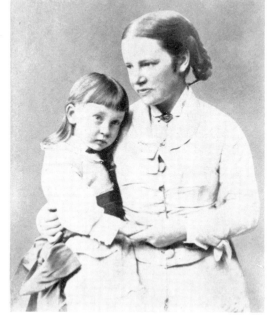

8b. Elizabeth Garrett Anderson with Louisa in 1876 after the death of Margaret

majority, should take the chair. Elizabeth, amused at the title of chairman, laughingly agreed, a piece of levity which caused Miss Davies to write severely:

> It is not being a woman (though that probably enhances it) but your youth and inexperience[1] that makes it strike me as almost indecorous to think of presiding over men like Lord Lawrence etc. . . . . I should be sorry for you to do anything which might give colour to the charge of being 'cheeky', which has been brought against you lately. It is true that your jokes are many and reckless. They do more harm than you know.[2]

Miss Davies in this vein had power to wither generations of female undergraduates, but Elizabeth in her growing happiness was quite unabashed; she sent the letter on to Skelton Anderson with a comment which shows new powers of self-criticism. 'I do not mind a little North East wind, and I know it is good to have it as a check on any tendency of uppishness which 47,000 might induce.'[3]

The chairman question was solved by the election of Lord Lawrence, but more serious was the suggestion that the two lady members should take seats apart. This they resisted and took their seats, with Russell Gurney's support, at the long council table facing the hall, although they felt the atmosphere decidedly hostile. Elizabeth for once was somewhat overawed 'by the whole thing being so extremely like Parliament and by having to spring up so quickly to get a hearing after someone else had finished. The whole difficulty of speaking is concentrated in that moment of swift self-assertion.' She managed to assert herself, however, to say a word or two in a good-humoured way at the first meeting, so honour was satisfied.[4]

As the triumphant candidate, she found herself everywhere in

---

[1] Elizabeth Garrett was thirty-four and had been a general practitioner for five years.

[2] Stephen, B., op. cit. p. 124.

[3] Elizabeth Garrett to Skelton Anderson, 8 Dec. 1870. Fawcett Library.

[4] Elizabeth Garrett to Skelton Anderson, 18 Dec. 1870. Fawcett Library.

demand. During December she visited her brothers, Sam at Cambridge and Edmund at Bow, thereby missing Skelton Anderson who called at Upper Berkeley Street in full glory of tartan and cairngorms on his way to a Scottish dinner. She dined with Browning, Jenny Lind, Dean Stanley and Lady Augusta, Professor Mohl, the artist Armitage and 'plenty of French dons'. There was barely time to scramble into evening dress to eat the unwholesome number of good dinners, and Elizabeth felt she needed a cloak of darkness to slip out and catch the midnight post with her last letters before going to bed. She found herself envying the wearers of dress coats, 'so changeless and easy to hide and walk out in!' She was perplexed by an invitation to stay in state with Lord Houghton at Fryston and confided in Skelton Anderson her reasons for refusing.

I shall decline tho' I dare say it would be more politic to go. I never enjoy being with swells, and in their houses, unless I sincerely like them personally; if I do the swelldom adds a little to the pleasure, but if I do not it crushes and depresses me and makes me feel like a snob. And till one knows how much would be possible in the way of real friendship, the difference of position is against one's liking them.[1]

After Christmas, she told him she would shut herself up in the evenings and live like a hermit with excursions only to the Guildhall Library until she had finished a medical textbook she had just contracted to write for Macmillan's.

This news acted as a spur to James Skelton Anderson, and on 23 December he wrote to ask if he might come to call after dinner. Elizabeth was a little uneasy at the thought of this, since Jane Crow would not be there. 'I shall be at home this evening', she wrote, 'but *perhaps* it would be better for you not to come. I should not like to confuse my maid's sense of decorum and I am afraid it might.' As she was writing, however, a messenger delivered some new photographs of herself from Caldesi, the Pall Mall

[1] Elizabeth Garrett to Skelton Anderson, 21 Dec. 1870. Fawcett Library.

photographers, on which she was anxious to have his opinion, and she added, 'Perhaps you might compromise with Mrs Grundy if you come tonight, by not staying so long.'[1] This was encouragement enough for the decisive Skelton Anderson. He came; how long he stayed and how far he compromised with Mrs Grundy is not revealed, but when he left they were engaged to be married.

Next day was Christmas Eve and Elizabeth was expected at Aldeburgh, where she must break the news of the engagement to her family and especially to her father. Deciding that bold tactics were best, she left on an early train, Skelton having promised to follow later in the day. At Alde House there was consternation at her news, and on Newson Garrett's part profound gloom. He was not favourable towards sons-in-law at any time, and felt convinced that marriage must ruin the career of his brilliant, favourite daughter. Luckily there was little time for family arguments since the visitor would soon be upon them, and Elizabeth must meet him at the station. The scene that followed passed into Garrett Anderson mythology. Parents and children waited in the hall where mistletoe and holly decorated the staircase, the grandfather clock and the ormolu cabinets. Newson was gloomy, the young sisters Agnes and Josephine critical and alert. The wheels of the brougham were heard muffled by the snow in the drive. They had arrived. A circle of light fell on the old mare and Lambert, the family coachman. Elizabeth, radiant and self-possessed, appeared first, followed by a tall man.[2]

Before James Skelton Anderson had been twenty-four hours in the house he had won over the entire family, with the exception of Newson. Mrs Garrett capitulated to the Biblical knowledge and doctrinal grasp of a son of the manse. Skelton charmed the girls by telling them amusing stories in his soft Scots accent, by dancing reels and acting charades, and by his unaccompanied singing of 'John Anderson My Jo' and the Skye Boat Song. Aldeburgh, having peered in vain for a sight of him in the depths

[1] Elizabeth Garrett to Skelton Anderson, 23 Dec. 1870. Fawcett Library.
[2] Anderson, L. G., op. cit. p. 166.

of the Corporation pew on Christmas morning, was able to watch him in the afternoon skating on the frozen marshes, where he cut figures on the ice to the admiration of all beholders.[1]

The engaged couple returned to London and a shower of congratulations. The Rev. Alexander Anderson, writing to Elizabeth for the first time, gave his son a testimonial of truly Aberdonian caution: 'James George possesses very superior abilities, an unfailing fund of wit and humour, an equal and most pleasant temper, and his life – as far as is known to me – has been pure and honourable.'[2] Emily Davies wrote with complete unselfishness: 'It is very sweet to me to be able to be so happy about it. It does not make me feel as if I should lose you. You must let me talk about it as soon as you can for I want to tell everybody how nice he is; they will know that I should not say so if it was not *very* true.' Old friends on the Dispensary committee, like Henry Mather Jackson, M.P., to whom Elizabeth broke the news by word of mouth, were surprised and delighted. 'You happy creature how pleased I am!' he shouted, beaming. 'Good Heavens! how cocky the fellar must be! Does the rascal know his luck?' Then he took her hands, and added, 'But my dear, he's a real fine fellow, you are quite right, as right as he is.' Finally he kissed her resoundingly. 'I never was so pleased,' wrote Elizabeth, relating the scene to Skelton.[3]

Even more precious were the congratulations of Sir James Paget, whom she happened to meet in consultation. 'Which do you like best, Miss Garrett – being the elect of fifty thousand or of one?' 'I rather despise the fifty thousand,' confessed Elizabeth. 'Then I think nothing could be happier in beginning public life than to have fifty thousand and despise them in comparison with one,' said the great surgeon.[4]

[1] Elizabeth Garrett to Millicent Fawcett, 25 Dec. 1870.
[2] Anderson, L. G., op. cit. p. 165.
[3] Elizabeth Garrett to Skelton Anderson, 28 Dec. 1870. Fawcett Library.
[4] Paget's own marriage was of legendary happiness. He described how his wife copied his manuscripts 'sitting with me till midnight or far into the morning, with the baby brought down in its cradle and watched and fed'.

Elizabeth Garrett was grateful for the understanding of these friends. She was, for the first time in her life, intensely in love, but she did not believe that marriage must mean the end of her vocation. Indeed two days after her engagement she had written to Millicent,

> I do hope my dear you will not think I have meanly deserted my post. I think it need not prove to be so and I believe that he would regret it as much as I or you would. I am sure that the woman question will never be solved in any complete way so long as marriage is thought to be incompatible with freedom and with an independent career, and I think there is a very good chance that we may be able to do something to discourage this notion.[1]

Very few other people had power to see so far into the future. Newson Garrett prophesied that her career was at an end. The Langham Place circle was thrown into confusion. Was the fortress of medicine, so long besieged and so hardly won, to be abandoned? An unnamed friend wrote: 'You will not expect me to deny that it is a blow to hear of such a defection.' Dr Murchison of the Middlesex was 'very gloomy'. A Dr Dudgeon publicly claimed that Skelton Anderson had told him he would not allow Elizabeth to go on with her practice. In her new mood of passionate responsiveness, doubt and criticism had power to wound Elizabeth deeply. 'You *must* not make me justify their want of trust,' says a note scribbled to Skelton at two in the morning[2] when she was attempting to deal with a pile of fifty letters.

Elizabeth hated to be an object of public curiosity and gossip. She heard two men discussing her engagement in the underground railway and wondering 'what the fellow was like'. She attempted to protect her feelings by never reading anything about herself in the newspapers, but it was impossible to shut out all comment. *The Times* queried whether Miss Garrett should not be deprived

[1] Elizabeth Garrett to Millicent Fawcett, 25 Dec. 1870.
[2] Elizabeth Garrett to Skelton Anderson, 5 Jan. 1871. Fawcett Library.

of her School Board seat on marriage 'since a conflict might arise between the right of the husband and the duties of the wife'.[1] The *British Medical Journal* commented on the engagement in dour but unanswerable terms: 'It is announced that Miss Elizabeth Garrett M.D. is about to marry. The problem of the compatibility of marriage with female medical practice, which has been much discussed, will thus be partly tested.'[2] This put Elizabeth's deepest fears into the black and white of newsprint. She had reconciled hostile institutions; would she be able to reconcile conflicts within herself? She was feminine; she wanted to love and be loved and bear children. Yet the habit of putting work and duty first was so deeply ingrained that she could hardly believe herself entitled, even at thirty-four after the struggles and labours of eleven years, to a measure of woman's ordinary happiness. She was haunted by George Eliot's *Spanish Gypsy*, who could not desert a cause even for her love:

> *if she gave herself*
> *'Twould be a self corrupt with stifled thoughts*
> *Of a forsaken better.*

Lying awake at night, she felt she would almost die of the sense of something akin to guilt if she found herself, after two or three years of marriage, out of the medical field.[3] The least failure in the gruelling schedule of her daily life, dispensary, hospital, consultations, accounts, visits in all parts of London, confinements, night calls, Louisa's children at Acton and School Board meetings, brought 'a rush of doubt as to the rightness of taking such absorbing happiness'. She confessed to 'a dread lest I may be choosing my own happiness at the price of the duty I owe to women who need something which I as one of their leaders can give them'.[4] She was passionately happy when she was with Skelton, but when she was alone doubt tormented her again and

[1] *The Times*, 7 Jan. 1871.
[2] *British Medical Journal*, 7 Jan. 1871.
[3] Elizabeth Garrett to Skelton Anderson, 31 Dec. 1870. Fawcett Library.
[4] Elizabeth Garrett to Skelton Anderson, 4 Jan. 1871. Fawcett Library.

again. She had to starve herself of his presence to get through the day's work, to be content with a brief wave up at his office window as she passed along Cornhill on her way to the children's hospital or a snatched meeting on Saturday afternoons 'at the Old Masters opposite the small Gainsborough blue boy'.[1] At the same time the revelation of love, coming in maturity after years of struggle, was overwhelming. Physically Elizabeth found this handsome, virile man intensely attractive. She refused to be chaperoned, gloried in the strong grasp of his arm round her waist as they drove home after evening parties, and found herself blushing like a young girl when she spoke his Christian name. 'I love you more than I thought I was made to love anyone,' she confessed. 'Life is *intolerable* apart!'[2]

James Skelton Anderson's reaction to this emotional conflict was swift and decisive. Once married, he was sure, Elizabeth would resolve her doubts. The wedding, which had been planned for Easter, was moved forward to the beginning of February, as soon as 'the Bishop', an impressive clerical cousin on the Anderson side, could come to London to marry them. Their plans were of a simplicity most unusual in their times. Their joint income was considerable and they would have a common purse, to which each contributed and from which each could draw for current expenses. Earlier in the year the first of the Married Women's Property Acts had at last been passed; by its terms a woman's earnings, though not her capital, could be legally secured to her, and Elizabeth insisted that this should be done in her case. Skelton, who approved of the Act in principle, was illogically hurt. Surely Elizabeth did not think he intended to rob her of her patients' fees? But she felt it was her duty to the women's movement and it was done. It helped to salve her conscience for falling in love and marrying at all. For the sake of the practice she pleaded to start married life at 20 Upper Berkeley Street, with the addition of a third maid, new red curtains in the dining room and an

[1] Elizabeth Garrett to Skelton Anderson, 19 Jan. 1871. Fawcett Library.
[2] Elizabeth Garrett to Skelton Anderson, 9 Jan. 1871. Fawcett Library.

essential smoking room for the master of the house on the top
storey.[1] Skelton, seeing Elizabeth trudge out through mud and
winter weather to calls by day and night, insisted on giving her
a carriage as a wedding present, to which he added a sealskin jacket
to keep out the cold. Elizabeth had a weakness for clothes. 'If it
would not be ruinous or greedy I *should* like a not very wide sable
border,' she confessed, and the fur jacket was made accordingly.

Both were united in horror of the conventional wedding, to
the distress of Mrs Garrett, who pleaded in vain for due form and
ceremony.

> It would be absurd as applied to me [wrote Elizabeth]. For
> instance fancy my being 'given away'. Monstrous and ludicrous
> notion! It's lucky no one has ever tried to do it. Might we not
> have the Bishop to marry us here with just our nearest friends
> present and plenty of wine and cold meat downstairs? On this
> plan of course the torture of speeches would be avoided.'[2]

Their honeymoon plans were also of refreshing simplicity, to stay
at the inn under Box Hill for a week-end, where no one would
suspect them of being a honeymoon couple 'however happy we
were, if we walk in without luggage. We should probably be
thought lunatics instead.'[3] They finally allowed themselves a
week in North Wales.

Skelton had acted wisely. To have the future firmly settled
calmed Elizabeth's doubts, and the last of her engagement letters
was hopeful and serene.

> If I thought you incapable of responding to the demands which
> the common weal makes on everyone, and perhaps in some
> special measure on me, incapable of preferring them, if need be
> to personal indulgence, you could not be to me what you
> are. . . . The only foregone conclusion is that we must not be
> made selfish by love.[4]

[1] Elizabeth Garrett to Skelton Anderson, 30 Dec. 1870. Fawcett Library.
[2] Elizabeth Garrett to Skelton Anderson, 13 Jan. 1871. Fawcett Library.
[3] Elizabeth Garrett to Skelton Anderson, 3 Jan. 1871. Fawcett Library.
[4] Elizabeth Garrett to Skelton Anderson, 22 Jan. 1871. Fawcett Library.

She continued to work steadily and on 8 February, the eve of her wedding day, attended, as well as her usual patients, a consultation at Wimbledon, and a meeting of the School Board at the Guildhall. That evening, Ford Anderson gave a dinner party with champagne at 27 Buckland Crescent for Elizabeth to meet the members of the Anderson family, including his father, who had made the journey from Aberdeen. At dinner Elizabeth sat next to 'the Bishop', the Rev. James Anderson, D.D., of Morpeth, an impressive cleric of seventy-eight, who was startled to find that the bride he was to marry next morning had already been wearing her wedding ring for two or three days. Perhaps she felt married already in intention, or perhaps she merely feared that Skelton would lose it. Elizabeth made herself very agreeable to the old clergyman, but declared she would not promise to obey in the marriage service. 'Now there must be nothing of that sort! If I thought you would insist, you should be packed right off to Morpeth again!' 'The Bishop', severe with other brides in the family, was delighted to be teased in this fashion. As the ladies withdrew from the dining room he was heard to pronounce, 'She's a nice creature, and a sensible. They're a clever pair. What *will* the bairns be!'[1]

Next morning on 9 February 1871, while the guests were complaining of the 'very objectionable hour' of 8.30 for a wedding, Elizabeth was up and writing her last letters of thanks at eight o'clock. She had chosen to be married early, 'without millinery and almost without cookery', to avoid a crowd. Of the thirty guests gathered at the Scottish Presbyterian Church, Upper George Street, Emily Davies was the only one who was not a relation of either family. It was a fine, bright day, the finest for weeks, and the sun streamed in upon the assembled Garretts and Andersons. The Bishop looked splendid in gown and bands, the Rev.

[1] Mrs Gavin Anderson of Hampstead to the Anderson family in Aberdeen, 9 Feb. 1871. This family letter of fourteen closely written pages describes the wedding festivities in detail, faithfully depicting the guests, their costumes, their comments and the unconscious prejudices of the writer. Anderson family papers.

Alexander Anderson pensive with an enormous black-and-white comforter, which he was too absent-minded to remove, wound innumerable times round his throat. Mr Garrett, torn between pride and resentment, sat in a front pew. The Andersons noted with interest that he wept profusely most of the time 'much more so than his wife'. Elizabeth appeared, a little tired but composed, in a wedding dress of stone-grey velvet, with a matching velvet bonnet and a pink rose under the brim. She walked quietly to her bridegroom, gave him the ring, which she had been so unorthodoxly keeping, and promised in a firm, distinct voice to be 'a faithful, loving and dutiful wife'. As 'the Bishop' pronounced his last Amen, she touched her husband's hand and lifted her face to be kissed, as though they were alone together.

At the breakfast, held downstairs in the panelled dining-room of her own house, she played her part as hostess calmly, forgetting nothing and nobody, and departing without fuss for their brief wedding journey. At the station they found they had missed their train, but filled the time until the next one quite cheerfully by driving to Marshall & Snelgrove to buy some stockings, which had somehow been forgotten during the wedding preparations. The simplicity of the whole occasion struck the guests almost with consternation. 'Are they not an *original* couple!' exclaimed an Anderson aunt as they finally departed.

To the bridal pair outward forms meant very little and their new relationship everything. 'The only possible basis for us', Skelton had written, 'is warm personal love and utter truth and outspokenness.' By this exacting ideal they were to live thirty-six years together. In its light Elizabeth Garrett Anderson saw the last of her fears vanish. A week after their wedding she wrote to her brother-in-law Ford, 'This week has made me know more than I did even on the 9th what a prize I have, so you will not wonder if I hold it with a somewhat nervous grasp. It is so much more than I deserve to have such a blessing for all the rest of our lives.'[1]

[1] Anderson, L. G., op. cit. p. 189.

CHAPTER FOURTEEN

Mr and Mrs Anderson
February 1871–August 1874

It was Elizabeth Garrett Anderson's special talent to combine the exceptional with the normal. From the day she returned from her brief honeymoon she was hard at work. She breakfasted punctually at eight o'clock with her walking boots on, and they were not unlaced until she dressed for dinner in the evening. Her public work, her private practice, her standing in the medical world grew until her days were filled with a round of meetings, visits and consultations. After dinner she answered letters by return of post and in her own hand, wrote up case notes or drafted lectures. In this exacting life she turned gratefully for advice and support to Skelton, her 'best counsellor'. To a strong-willed woman there is profound reassurance in the companionship of an even stronger-willed man. Skelton Anderson was master in his own house, and when his wife was over-serious he laughed at her, affectionately, without mockery. At the same time he delighted in her professional interests and was ready, when asked, with efficient help. Jealousy had no part in his nature; he had brains, character and determination, with charm and a sense of humour. Secure in his love, Elizabeth developed a breadth in her work which she might otherwise have missed.

At the same time she fulfilled, and enjoyed, the duties of an ordinary housewife.[1] The twentieth century, faced with the

[1] Elizabeth Garrett Anderson to Charlotte Anderson, 15 June 1871. Anderson family papers.

219

immense activity of the Victorians, salves its conscience with the comforting reflection that, after all, they had plenty of servants. In fact Elizabeth ran 20 Upper Berkeley Street, on five floors, without electricity or central heating, both as a home and consulting rooms, with the help only of a cook and a housemaid. She planned the domestic routine; the maids burnished grates, lit coal fires and carried brass hot-water cans upstairs with admirable regularity and were happy enough to stay with her for years. She enforced a yearly ritual of spring cleaning, when the house was scrubbed, scraped and repainted after the embrowning winter fog of London. Like many brides she found it testing to provide a manly breakfast every morning, but took the trouble to write to Aberdeen for recipes of Skelton's favourite fishballs and other breakfast dishes.[1] Bills were settled 'minus discount', as she noted firmly, by return of post. The lack of a garden was a deprivation to her until she had the inspiration of making a roof garden on the leads. 'The leads are outside the consulting room window, a French casement, and as this is always wide open the flowers form part of my constant still-life society. I am like an anxious mother over the plants, enjoy looking at them, and think they can't get on without me.' She gave dinner parties, at which the food was good, and an occasional reception, known as a 'big drum', which made her as nervous as any normal hostess. 'Seeing one's friends is anxious work, it is so terrible if they are dull! Dinners I am not afraid of, but long evenings with nothing to do are terribly risky.' Her parties were good, and she was also a popular guest, having the gift of enjoyment. 'I certainly do very much like meeting my fellow creatures, especially when I know them,' she said. 'I begin to think it is one mark of a good heart to like to go to evening parties.'

20 Upper Berkeley Street was the social centre of a large and lively family circle. To Skelton's sisters Elizabeth was a warmly affectionate friend. An elder sister, Mary Marshall, had been

[1] Elizabeth Garrett Anderson to Charlotte Anderson, 29 June 1871. Anderson family papers.

widowed after a few months of marriage and lost a posthumous
son at birth. Elizabeth helped her to study medicine in Paris.
When the School Board was meeting three hours daily she found
time to choose a dress as a present for an unmarried sister
Charlotte and to debate at length by post the merits of scarlet or
blue brocade, square necks and Brussels lace.[1] Ford Anderson
she knew well and loved; she understood the loneliness behind
his bachelor reticence. She thought he needed a wife; he made her
think, she told Charlotte, of 'Miranda's state of mind, when, as
Coleridge remarks somewhere, if Ferdinand hadn't come she
would certainly have married Caliban.'[2] In return for her affection towards his family Skelton welcomed the lively Garrett
sisters, advised Agnes when she came to London to train as an
interior decorator[3] and kept close ties with Millicent and Henry
Fawcett. He also did his best to establish good relations with his
father-in-law, sending him four dozen bottles of champagne on
his birthday, together with a letter in cautious but conciliatory
terms.

From their early married days the Andersons created a pattern
of companionship natural enough today, but revolutionary in
their generation. At work they lived separate and independent
lives; at home they shared leisure and pleasure. Both loved books,
the theatre, good music, good conversation, the countryside. On
their first regular holiday together in April 1871 they tramped
over the hills around Braemar, carrying only a flask of whisky and
some sandwiches: when they were tired, they rested in the woods,
watching the blue hills in the distance.

Marriage, far from withdrawing Elizabeth Garrett Anderson
from public life, gave her new poise and confidence. In the year
of her marriage she did more public work than ever before. The

[1] Elizabeth Garrett Anderson to Charlotte Anderson, 3 and 9 July and
20 Oct. 1871. Anderson family papers.
[2] Elizabeth Garrett Anderson to Charlotte Anderson, 4 Jan. 1872. Anderson family papers.
[3] Newson Garrett intended to put her in the malting business, but Edmund objected to the scandal this would cause.

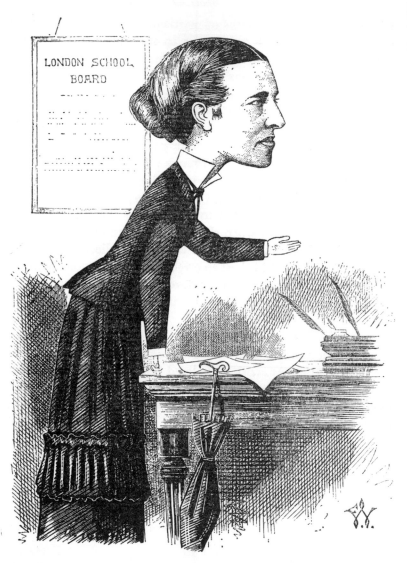

A caricature in 1872 shows Elizabeth Garrett Anderson as a member
of the London School Board

demands of the School Board were heavy. London education had been haphazard; gangs of street arabs haunted the courts and alleys, mudlarks roamed the river. Now, teachers, buildings, books, the very habit of going to school, must be built up in the face of the two enemies called by T. H. Huxley 'skinflint economy and stultifying sectarianism'. The School Board met every Wednesday afternoon at the Guildhall among a welter of papers and plans which had to be digested week by week. Elizabeth, elegant in black silk with cherry-red bows and a gold locket on a chain, took her place at the conference table among the morning coats of the gentlemen.[1]

In July 1871 she was elected to the Statistical, Law and Parliamentary Committee. This body was to collect returns, draw up a census and maps and estimate London's social and educational needs.[2] In two years its members produced a report of over three hundred pages, providing for the first time a census of all the children and schools in London. Elizabeth also served, *ex officio*, on the School Management Committee, where Huxley, with his genius for lobbying and string-pulling, found her an ally worth having. He called several time at Upper Berkeley Street during the summer of 1871, to plan the strategy of forthcoming meetings.

On 21 June Elizabeth voted in support of the regulation that only females should teach infants and senior girls, a decision which opened a professional career to hundreds of young women from relatively humble homes.[3] A week later she proposed herself, and saw carried, a motion 'that in the Senior Schools *Domestic Economy* should be added to the discretionary subjects'.[4] Her own taste would have been for the independence of the village schoolmistress's country cottage and garden. She encouraged the refounding of Bishop Otter College at Chichester in 1872 to train needy middle-class girls, or 'reduced ladies' as certificated

[1] Group portrait by J. W. Walton at County Hall, London, S.E.1.

[2] *Minutes of the London School Board*, Vol. I, p. 206. L.C.C. County Record Office, County Hall, London, S.E.1.

[3] ibid. p. 164.

[4] ibid. p. 169.

teachers. Elizabeth insisted that children need light and air, water closets and washrooms and space to play. She returned to these needs more than once during October 1871, while the other members of the Board were locked in controversy over religious teaching. She would have liked to see a special sanitary committee to safeguard conditions in the schools, but agreed not to press for this if she and Huxley could be present when the works committee dealt with health questions.[1]

She also played her part on the House Committee of the Women's College which proposed to move the students from Hitchin and to build on a site at Girton, two miles from Cambridge. Elizabeth agreed to speak at the first appeal meeting at St James's Hall, Piccadilly, on 15 May 1871. It was not easy to raise public enthusiasm for educating girls. The gathering was heavily weighted with bishops and members of Parliament to guarantee respectability, but Mrs Anderson was the speaker everyone wanted to hear. She admitted that the idea of collegiate life for women was revolutionary, but claimed they needed education, not merely as a preparation for the professions, but as wives and mothers. She made her invariable point. 'Women are not harmed by regular and steady work; on the contrary many of the most miserable cases of nervous weakness in women are due to the want of it.' Hers was the speech of the afternoon, and when she sat down she was loudly cheered.[2]

Money began to come in, and Elizabeth suggested that Skelton with his city experience, would be a valuable member of the Committee. Emily Davies privately doubted whether Skelton, a man of principle, would be willing to accept the necessary compromises. In less than six months she was proved right. Skelton could not accept Emily Davies's insistence that the college should reassure the public by providing religious instruction and services 'in accordance with the Principles of the Church of England as by law established'. 'It seems to me a building of the Tombs of

[1] ibid. pp. 299 and 330.
[2] Stephen, B., *Emily Davies and Girton College*, pp. 257–8.

the Prophets,' he said bluntly. Other members gave way, but he preferred to resign from the committee. Elizabeth was torn between her husband and her oldest friend, but she refused to let an emotional situation develop. Keeping principles apart from personalities, she considered the point on its own merits.

Not that I think the point a small one actually [she wrote to Skelton], but that it is so in comparison with the great ends that we hope the College will further. It seems to me that women want that which the College will give them so very, very much that those who can help them to it ought not to allow *any* minor disagreements to take from the duties of allies. Of course you do not quite share this feeling, to help women is not the passion of your life as it is of mine and Miss Davies's, and if you really think it is more important to help Liberalism, this argument goes for nothing.[1]

James Skelton Anderson did think Liberalism more important. He resigned, while at Girton the towering red-brick pile of Waterhouse Gothic buildings rose on the heath. Parties of undergraduates tipped the foreman to let them lay signed bricks at sixpence a time and even senior members of the University climbed ladders to look in at the windows. Elizabeth and Emily Davies remained friends, but inevitably saw less of one another.

In May 1872 Elizabeth began to give courses of lectures for women on anatomy and physiology. She charged a substantial fee, and was determined to make the lectures vivid and practical, although it was illegal to procure anatomical specimens for private use. 'We could manage a baby or an arm or a leg but no more away from a School,'[2] she wrote with professional sang froid.

---

[1] Probably Emily Davies was the more prudent in this case. A clergyman, passing the college at Hitchin in the train, looked out and was heard to remark, 'There go the infidel ladies!' It was necessary to live down such prejudices.

[2] Elizabeth Garrett Anderson to Mrs Webster, 22 April 1872. Fawcett Library.

All these activities, School Board, Girton and lecturing, remained side-lines. The core of Elizabeth Garrett Anderson's
working life was always her patients and her Dispensary. Before
long she had to give up the pleasure of a brisk walk between visits
as unsuitable to her consultant status. Reluctantly, 'for the good
of the practice', she drove everywhere in her carriage. The charity
patients at the dispensary were now more than she could handle
alone. In the first five years of the dispensary 40,000 attendances at a penny a time were recorded, and raising the consultation fee to sixpence had not reduced the number.[1] Fortunately
Frances Morgan, who had attended clinics as a student, had now
taken her M.D. at Zürich, and returned in March 1871 as the
first assistant member of the staff.[2] Each held three clinics of
two hours each during the week, and took emergency calls in
rotation.

The nature of the dispensary's work had changed. At first the
patients had been the women and children of the Lisson Grove
slums, suffering from a variety of general complaints. By 1871
they were increasingly women from all over London who wished
to be treated solely by women for gynaecological conditions.
Elizabeth was distressed by the plight of those too ill to travel
long distances and wait their turn as out-patients without considerable suffering and she was forced to turn away many urgent
surgical cases. With Skelton's support, she now made an important decision. She determined to open a new hospital for women,
equipped to treat serious medical and surgical cases as in-patients.
Its distinctive feature would be that the working medical staff
should consist entirely of women.

She would begin with ten beds above the dispensary premises
in Seymour Place. The house was small, dark and inconvenient,
but fresh paint-work, running water, ventilation and drainage

[1] Prospectus of the New Hospital for Women. Elizabeth Garrett Anderson
Hospital.
[2] She married in 1873 George Hoggan, a Fellow of the Obstetrical Society,
who had lectured to the women students at Edinburgh, and with whom she
published several scientific papers.

could be installed for about £300, and it would do for a start. James Skelton Anderson and James Smith both advised on finance and Elizabeth wrote to Mr Nixon, Secretary of the London Hospital, for advice on the constitution. As her mind moved forward in enthusiastic leaps, she added.

We wish to find a woman competent to act as our permanent paid secretary . . . thoroughly familiar with the organization of a good hospital, with the method of keeping its accounts and with the usual devices for raising money. It has occurred to me that if you have daughters you might, better than almost any-one in London, train one for such a post as this and that a sensible well-trained young woman might find the work both interesting and suitable. Pray pardon me for making this suggestion.[1]

Mr Nixon failed to provide a suitably well-trained daughter, but a young woman named Mary Parnall was found to fill the post. The New Hospital for Women, as it was finally named, was an entirely private venture and had to find at least £600 a year by its own efforts to cover expenses.

The hospital was opened in February 1872 by the Earl of Shaftesbury, who praised the venture as a new way in which educated women might minister to other women without the stigma of pauperization, while increasing their own skill. Women worked at the New Hospital as doctors, nurses, dispensers, caterers, secretaries and unpaid social workers. The in-patients, for the most part, were seriously ill women; the responsibility for caring for them was heavy, but the satisfaction great.[2] On

[1] Elizabeth Garrett Anderson to Mr Nixon, 3 Dec. 1871. Elizabeth Garrett Anderson Hospital.
[2] Within a year 103 in-patients were admitted to the hospital for periods varying from a few days to ten weeks. The out-patients' department received 10,704 visits, the greater part of them gynaecological cases. By 1873 the number of in-patients had risen to 119 and by 1874 to 133, of whom eleven were re-admitted, making a total of 144. Of these 81 were suffering from gynaecological complaints. New Hospital for Women *Annual Report*, 1873.

14 December 1871 Elizabeth Garrett Anderson ventured for the first time to report two interesting cases to the *British Medical Journal*.

One was of unilateral chorea in a girl of eighteen. The second was of clot in the heart and cerebral embolism. They had admitted a woman of fifty suffering from ovarian dropsy, and after consultation Frances Morgan decided to tap the tumour, with Elizabeth assisting. The operation went smoothly until the trochar had been withdrawn and the wound closed. While they were fastening the bandage the patient suddenly sprang up in bed saying she could not breathe. Suddenly she became livid, with lips and finger-tips of the deepest blue. To all appearances she was at the very point of death. The situation was made worse by the fact that Frances Morgan, an unregistered practitioner because of her foreign degree, had performed the operation. For over an hour they worked, applying hot flannel fomentations to the chest and back, mustard over the heart, ammonia to the nostrils and vigorous rubbing to the feet and hands. They had almost lost hope when, after an hour and a half, to their intense relief the blueness and lividity diminished, the dyspnoea was relieved and the patient slid into a comfortable sleep. 'It is I think impossible to doubt', concluded Elizabeth Garrett Anderson, 'that the symptoms in this case were due to an obstruction in the right side of the heart or in the pulmonary artery and that it was caused by a fibrinous clot.'[1]

For Elizabeth surgery represented a new and heavy burden. She was still the only active woman doctor on the Medical Register, and remained for twenty years the only member of the staff who could undertake major surgical work. In the year of her qualification, Lister's first experiments in antisepsis had begun to transform the practice and scope of surgery. For nearly ten years many surgeons stubbornly resisted his conclusions, but Elizabeth, young and enthusiastic, accepted them as 'one of the greatest glories' of science in her time. She scrubbed, boiled

[1] *British Medical Journal*, 14 Dec. 1871.

instruments and soaked dressings in carbolic, with good results. 'To be thoroughly aseptic as a surgeon requires the drilling of years,' she told her staff. 'It cannot be picked up after habitual disregard of the infinitely little.' Antiseptic technique added to the resources of the surgeon, yet the death rate from shock and haemorrhage remained high. Frances Hoggan, fearful of the responsibility, fell from grace by suggesting that a man should be called in for abdominal surgery. Elizabeth's reply was terse: 'No men or no hospital.'[1] Her courage as a surgeon was severely tested by her first case of ovariotomy. This operation had been performed by McDowell in Virginia as early as 1816, but the mortality rate was so high that it had fallen into disrepute, and was actually prohibited in several London teaching hospitals. When Elizabeth decided that it offered one patient's only hope of survival, Mrs Hoggan resigned in protest and the management committee refused to allow the operation to take place in the hospital. Elizabeth therefore rented a room in a private house, had it scrubbed, whitewashed and disinfected, then installed patient and nurse. Thomas Smith of St Bartholomew's, once apprentice and now assistant to Sir James Paget, volunteered to be present at the operation, which Elizabeth successfully performed. Skelton met all the expenses out of his own pocket, remarking cheerfully when the patient was well on the way to recovery, 'If Elizabeth's surgical practice increases we shall be in the bankruptcy court.' The next case remained in the hospital, and these two were almost certainly the first ovariotomies ever performed by a woman surgeon. Thereafter, when Elizabeth felt that in the interests of the patient a surgeon of greater experience should be present, she knew she could ask for help from the leaders of her profession. Sir James Paget, Sir Spencer Wells and Mr Knowlsley Thornton all assisted and tutored her when she performed major operations for the first time.

It was only many years later that Elizabeth Garrett Anderson revealed how much she had suffered before each major operation.

[1] Anderson, L. G., *Elizabeth Garrett Anderson*, p. 244.

Elizabeth Garrett Anderson

To see a skilled surgeon do his work [she said] is a very different
thing from doing it oneself. . . . In surgery the *nerve* has to be
trained and that is only done by actual work of your own. I
believe it is impossible for any but those who have gone
through it to realize what a tremendous tax upon one's nerve it
is to attempt a great operation, especially of the kind where
exact previous knowledge of the difficulties cannot possibly
be had. I speak of this with feeling because I know what it
is.[1]

By sheer determination she became a competent general surgeon
of excellent judgment and won the respect of her colleagues. A
hostile critic who had watched her operate could only say, 'I
admire your pluck.'

In 1873 Elizabeth Garrett Anderson operated in a variety of
gynaecological conditions, fibroid of uterus, prolapsus, cancer,
imperforated vagina, mammary abscess, ovarian tumour and
fistula.[2] She did not slacken either medical or surgical work during the year, although, at the age of thirty-seven, she was expecting
her first child. She wrote, lectured, attended cases and operated
within a few days of her confinement, revealing to middle-class
women a new attitude towards child-bearing. The only circumstance which disturbed her serenity of mind during the
summer of 1873 was the news that Sophia Jex-Blake intended to
open a medical school for women in London.

For the last four years the success and fulfilment of Elizabeth's
life had moved in ironic counterpoint to Sophia's struggles and
disasters. In 1869, on the day of Elizabeth's first triumphs in
Paris in the M.D. exam., Sophia had written in her journal
'Monday March 15th to Edinbro'. How I dreaded the journey and
sequence!'[3] She prepared to attack the University of Edinburgh

---

[1] Elizabeth Garrett Anderson, MS. draft for a speech, Royal Free Hospital
School of Medicine.
[2] New Hospital for Women *Annual Report*, 1875. See Appendix V.
[3] Todd, M., *The Life of Sophia Jex-Blake*, p. 226.

and take it by storm. In the autumn of 1869 she led the seven young women who settled down to the separate classes which the medical faculty of Edinburgh agreed to provide, while Elizabeth collected a scholarship fund for them. By the time Elizabeth completed her Paris M.D. and received her hospital appointment, hostility to the seven was building up. On 18 November 1870, while Elizabeth was campaigning successfully for the School Board election, Sophia and her six companions were facing the jeers and shouts, the cabbage stalks and rotten eggs of the Surgeons' Hall riot. Sophia Jex-Blake, reckless as she was brave, accused a member of the university staff of leading the riot, and in May 1871, during the early months of Elizabeth's happy marriage, had to fight an action for libel. Her opponent was awarded a farthing damages, but she was left with a bill of nearly a thousand pounds costs to pay.[1] In 1872, while Elizabeth was founding her own hospital, Sophia was battling day and night on behalf of her fellow-students for entrance to the Edinburgh Infirmary and professional examination. In October 1872 when the results of her own first examination came out, she had failed and, in one of her most calamitous indiscretions, claimed that she had been unfairly marked. In 1873 the hard-won right of entry to the Infirmary and examinations was withdrawn by the Court of Appeal. The case of the Septem contra Edinam, as they were called in the lawsuit, was at an end at last. Four years of toil and distress had apparently achieved nothing, and Sophia Jex-Blake returned to London to take up the struggle there.

Elizabeth had been disturbed by the situation at Edinburgh, the four years of battle, lawsuit, and riot, and the emotional atmosphere which now surrounded a question of principle. It seemed to her that all she had achieved by quiet persistence was being thrown away by a display of public histrionics, which personally she found intensely distasteful. Both she and Elizabeth Blackwell disapproved of using subscribed funds to fight a legal action, and were embarrassed when Sophia Jex-Blake turned an

[1] Todd, M., *The Life of Sophia Jex-Blake*, pp. 356–7.

231

Elizabeth Garrett Anderson

explanatory lecture at St George's Hall into a public fighting speech. People who had suffered the rough side of Sophia's tongue held her responsible for the failure at Edinburgh, and Elizabeth was tempted to agree. She admired Sophia's generosity and intelligence, which were great, but recoiled from the stormy, passionate nature, which would not be governed even in everyday social life. She was not the woman to gloss over an unfavourable opinion. 'Your want of judgment and temper have done great harm,' she bluntly said.[1] Moreover, she had always opposed the idea of a separate 'Female Medical College' on the grounds that it could only offer an inferior education and produce an inferior race of doctor.

Sophia had understandably not thought of turning to her for advice, and was therefore very annoyed to see a letter of two full columns in *The Times* signed Elizabeth Garrett Anderson M.D.[2] The time, it said, was not ripe for the medical education of women in Great Britain, as the Court of Appeal's decision in the Edinburgh case had shown. 'The real solution of the difficulty will, I believe, be found in Englishwomen seeking abroad that which is at present denied them in their own country.' She praised the hospitals, the teaching and the searching examinations of Paris and maintained 'in no way could women better serve the cause we desire to promote than by going to Paris to study medicine and returning here as soon as might be to practise it'. A foreign degree of course would not entitle them to registration, but in practice colleagues would accept a woman with a good foreign degree. Nor should such women fail to observe the etiquette of medicine. 'Nothing succeeds like success and if we could point to a considerable number of medical women quietly making for themselves the reputation of being trustworthy and valuable members of the profession, the various forms which present opposition now takes would insensibly disappear. . . .' A change in the law of registration would inevitably follow.

[1] ibid. p. 423.
[2] *The Times,* 5 Aug. 1873.

232

'Never was there a case in which the truth of the adage "Solvitur ambulando" was more likely to make itself felt.'

Sophia Jex-Blake's very natural reaction after all the indignity and disappointment she had suffered was to write back[1] to *The Times* 'protesting as strongly as lies in my power against this idea of sending abroad every Englishwoman who wishes to study medicine'. The idea of practising without legal recognition was utterly unpractical, and as for foreign degrees, wrote Sophia bitterly, let 'those who covet such ornamental honours go through the examinations requisite to obtain them'. She urged would-be women doctors to be 'like myself thoroughly resolved to fight it out on the line and not be driven out of our own country for education.'

It is easy from the vantage point of a hundred years' experience to see that here Sophia was right in principle. Her judgment, generally speaking, was less keen than Elizabeth's, but she had more imagination. She could foresee the future woman student, not fluent in foreign languages with no influential friends or rich father like Newson Garrett to smooth her path to expensive private teaching or foreign examinations. She could also see that the Edinburgh struggle, with all its humiliations, had forced the cause upon the public's notice at last. She accused Elizabeth Garrett Anderson of being inconsistent since, after all, to 'fight it out on the line' was what she had done herself ten years before.

On her side Elizabeth simply could not understand the underlying causes of the Edinburgh disaster. Sex antagonism had no part in her nature. Her hospital owed much to men, to Skelton's loyal support, to the generosity of honoraries and the trust of her patients' husbands and fathers. She had persuaded the public to accept her as a doctor. She feared the loss of good will to the whole movement if Sophia Jex-Blake precipitated a battle. For the first time there was division in the ranks of the medical women. The truth was, both women were needed, the fiery trail-blazer no less than the skilled, stubborn tactician. It was a

[1] Todd, M., op. cit., Appendix E.

personal tragedy for them both that they were forced to work together. Both were to suffer increasingly under it as they grew older.

Exactly one week before the publication of her *Times* letter, on 28 July 1873, Elizabeth's first child was born. To her joy it was a daughter. The baby was christened Louisa Garrett Anderson, and Elizabeth entered on a new rôle, as exacting as any she had played in her life. 'She hated noise', Louisa wrote later of her mother, 'and she could not enter readily into a child's mind or play with children, but love overcame these difficulties. She tolerated a baby banging two spoons together as she wrote and she was a devoted wife and wise mother.'[1] One decision which a professional woman now has to make was, of course, spared her. The unquestioned custom of her class and time was a nursery life for children in the care of a nanny. No one suggested that a lady, however leisured, should take sole charge of her own children. The top floor but one of the house in Upper Berkeley Street was converted to nurseries, where Elizabeth installed, as was still not uncommon, a wet nurse and a nanny. The latter, Helen Lorimer, was a little dark bird-like woman, quick and intelligent. She was still young when she left her father's farm in Banffshire for the first time to come to the Andersons. She stayed to see their children away to school, and returned to look after their grandchildren for the rest of her life.

Elizabeth did not use the nursery convention to exclude her child from everyday life. As well as their playtime together every evening, Louie rode about with her in the carriage, peeping out of the window at the back and holding out her small hand to catch the raindrops. As soon as she was old enough she went visiting, a little figure with a fringe and an immense blue sash who kissed her hand on parting in a most bewitching manner. She even went to the New Hospital and romped about on the beds of a whole wardful of patients.

The daily claims of nursery and hospital meant that Elizabeth

[1] Anderson, L. G., op. cit. p. 192.

must cut down her other work. In January 1872 she had already asked for her name to be withdrawn from the Statistical Committee of the School Board, since she no longer had time to attend its meetings. In the autumn of 1873 she decided not to stand for the triennial election to the Board, but to serve out her time and retire.[1] It need be no loss to the women's cause, for her sister Alice Cowell, home from India with her children, agreed to stand for the Board in her place. On 12 November 1873 Elizabeth attended her last School Board meeting. It was harder to take the next step, and to resign her honorary appointment at the Shadwell Children's Hospital. If Nathaniel Heckford had been alive she might have continued there, since his charm was so hard to resist, but he had died of tuberculosis at the tragically early age of twenty-eight. Elizabeth had never found it easy to work with Sarah Heckford's other-worldly temperament. 'We are not so made as to be capable of much active friendship,' she had told Skelton in the early days. In October 1873 she resigned her honorary post, hoping that one of the Paris or Zürich women graduates would be appointed in her place. Perhaps Mrs Heckford had had enough of medical women; the new consultant was a man, and Elizabeth did not hide her disappointment. She felt she was to blame. 'It was one of the greatest mistakes of my life,' she said candidly, but there was nothing she could do to retrieve it.[2]

By the new year of 1874, when Louisa was six months old, Elizabeth was again pregnant. Her superb health and vigour were undiminished, but the demands of professional life grew as fast as she could keep pace with them. She had achieved one ambition by her election to the British Medical Association. Ford Anderson applied to Dr Stewart, his chief at the Middlesex, who had always liked Elizabeth and who happened to be branch secretary. Dr Stewart searched the records, and reappeared at the hospital

---

[1] *Minutes of the London School Board*, Vol. II, pp. 34 and 48. L.C.C. County Record Office.

[2] Anderson, L. G., op. cit. p. 192. The next woman was not appointed until 1929.

delighted. The only proviso for election to the Association was that candidates should be registered medical practitioners; there was no mention of sex, so Mrs Garrett Anderson was certainly eligible. He himself signed her application to the Metropolitan branch, seconded by the senior physician of St Mary's, and she was elected.[1] The mills of the Association ground slowly in those days, and it was two years before the provincial members realized that a woman had been smuggled into their midst. With the Obstetrical Society, in the following spring, Elizabeth was less successful. In March 1874 she was proposed as a Fellow, but the Society's members ruled that no woman should be admitted. They were ironically congratulated by *The Scotsman* on 'deciding that no woman could ever be allowed to join in discussion concerning the treatment and relief of those sufferings which women alone have to endure'.[2]

In April and May 1874 Elizabeth Garrett Anderson's talent for putting a case was urgently called into play. Emily Davies and Miss Buss of the North London Collegiate School had been alarmed to read an article on 'Sex in Mind and Education' by the eminent neurologist, Dr Henry Maudsley.[3] Basing his remarks on a report published in Boston, he prophesied a gloomy future for the high school or college girl. It was true she might *appear* to enjoy her studies, but could a young girl 'bear, without injury an excessive mental drain as well as the natural physical drain which is so great at that time?' Nor was physical harm only to be feared. 'The consequences of an imperfectly developed reproductive system are not sexual only; they are also mental. Intellectually and morally there is a deficiency . . . the individual fails to reach the ideal of a complete and perfect womanhood.' In some cases 'nervous and even mental disorders declare themselves'.

Dr Maudsley's deserved fame as a physician made this opinion

[1] Anderson, J. F., *A Pioneer*. MS. Anderson family papers.
[2] In 1875 the Society's entire board of examiners resigned rather than examine Sophia Jex-Blake and two other women candidates for the diploma in midwifery.
[3] *The Fortnightly Review*, April 1874.

particularly damaging. It could not have come at a worse time, for the Girls' Public Day School Company which was to open twenty-eight High Schools for Girls during the next fifteen years, had just been founded. Parents could all too easily be frightened into thinking education meant exhaustion. For the next month, at Miss Buss's request, Elizabeth sacrificed her evenings to drafting a reply.

She attacked the fallacy that a good education must 'change women into men', since the masculine is not the only type of excellence, and went straight to the half-hinted crux of Maudsley's argument. Is menstruation really such an incapacitating affliction as he suggests? Working-class women must continue their daily work without intermission; domestic servants neither demand nor receive special consideration because of it. 'The assertion that, as a rule, girls are unable to go on with an ordinary amount of quiet exercise or mental work during these periods seems to us to be entirely contradicted by experience.' She goes on to point out that life at a good day-school, with time for fresh air and exercise, is healthier than sitting over the fire with a novel at home. She might well have quoted Sir James Paget, who used to say, when a delicate little girl was brought to him, 'Bring her up like a boy. Let her play cricket with her brothers.' The real danger to the health of middle-class girls, said Elizabeth firmly, was not education but dullness. Boredom and loneliness are potent causes of breakdown. 'There is no tonic in the pharmacopoeia to be compared with happiness, and happiness worth calling such is not known where the days drag along filled with make-believe occupations and dreary, sham amusements.'[1]

The last had not been heard of 'educational over-pressure'. Every attempt to broaden the syllabus in girls' schools for the next twenty years produced its crop of portentous threats. Elizabeth Garrett Anderson answered these in the press whenever she could. In this, as in other branches of health education, time has reduced her views to mere commonsense; comparison reveals

[1] *The Fortnightly Review*, May 1874.

that they were sometimes uncommon at the time of writing. She described overstrain at school as 'a risk which can be avoided by teachers and parents recognizing their divided and mutual responsibility in the matter'. On the same page of *The Times* Sophia Jex-Blake was urging government interference to reduce the curriculum in elementary schools. On ventilation Elizabeth Garrett Anderson advised a supply of fresh, *warmed* air equal to 1,200 cubic feet per hour per person. An enthusiastic hygienist in the same year, 1873, advised the British public to open all windows and sit in the drawing room with rugs and ulsters throughout the winter. On midwifery she wrote, 'There are not many callings in which ignorance and drink in combination are more likely to lead to disaster. . . . No one should be allowed to call herself a midwife until she has passed a qualifying examination in simple midwifery and maternity nursing.' When this apparently commonplace suggestion appeared in print Britain was the only country in Europe without its register of qualified midwives, a state of affairs which incidentally persisted until 1902.

Meanwhile the New Hospital for Women had grown until it was impossible to cram more beds into the old house at Seymour Street. The committee could not afford to build, but decided, in June 1874, to take fourteen-year leases of 222 and 224 Marylebone Road, unpretentious houses facing south, each with its strip of garden.[1] Six hundred pounds was spent on repairs and putting in baths, and a further hundred and eighty on new furniture. Servants and old patients joined to scrub the boards and sprinkle iodoform; friends gave linen, furniture, game, eggs, fruit, flowers and improving literature for the inmates. When the twenty-six beds were put up Elizabeth had the satisfaction of seeing her patients reasonably housed at last.

At the same time the Andersons themselves needed larger quarters. Elizabeth was reluctant for professional reasons to leave

[1] They later expanded to take in 220, having paid off their debts and the Seymour Place dilapidations by 1876. The whole terrace was demolished when the Grand Central Hotel was built.

Upper Berkeley Street, so in June 1874 they merely moved up the street to number 4, near the corner of Portman Square. This was one of a new block of six-storey mansions, massive in red brick and terracotta. Agnes Garrett and her cousin Rhoda, now London's first women interior decorators, advised on the furnishing. Their hall-mark was plainness and unpretentious comfort, well-polished oaken tables and Windsor chairs, plain drugget and oriental rugs, William Morris velvets and chintz and a prevailing wholesome smell of beeswax and turpentine polish.[1] 4 Upper Berkeley Street was a solid, hospitable house which was to become well known for good food and good conversation. Here on 9 September 1874 Elizabeth gave birth to Margaret Skelton, her second child.

[1] Garrett, R. and A., *House Decoration*, 1877.

CHAPTER FIFTEEN

A Women's Medical School
August 1874–December 1878

The years from 1874 to 1878 saw medical education for women secured at last. For Elizabeth Garrett Anderson the struggle was interwoven with the joys and sorrows of family life, and the leadership of the movement during these years passed into the hands of Sophia Jex-Blake. Sophia's vivid, tempestuous personality was a gift to journalists and their readers. In the public eye she became, and remained, the pioneer woman doctor. Elizabeth, fastidiously avoiding personal publicity herself, was content that it should be so.

Sophia throve on opposition and difficulties. By August 1874 she had collected a Council which met at the house of Dr Anstie of the Westminster Hospital to consider a new medical school solely for women. Elizabeth at first refused to be present; the whole idea filled her with misgivings. If the school issued its own diploma for women, she warned, 'they would at once be marked as a special class of practitioners, subordinate and inferior to the ordinary doctor'. The day before the first meeting she received a vehement letter, revealing in every line the hurt and resentment of Sophia at her criticism in *The Times* the previous summer. Sophia accused Elizabeth of listening to 'cock and bull stories' about Edinburgh and blaming her unjustly for the failure there.

> I never said it did not signify whether you joined the Council [the letter ended angrily], though I did say that I believed the

School was already tolerably certain of ultimate success. I think it is of very great importance, both for *your* credit and ours, that there should be no appearance of split in the camp, and I should greatly prefer that your name should appear on the Council.[1]

Elizabeth had one night to think over this discouraging invitation. Every instinct warned her to withdraw, but she knew that the enemies of women in medicine would seize joyfully upon her absence from the Council. If the school was inevitable, she decided, the only possible course was to make it a success. Next morning she attended the meeting and joined its unanimous vote 'that a school be founded in London with a view of educating women in medicine and enabling them to pass such examinations as would place their names on the Medical Register'. Once she had taken the decision, she did not look back. She joined the permanent Council and accepted the post of Lecturer, with Dr King Chambers of St Mary's, in the Practice of Medicine. The lectures covered 'the causes of diseases, also the application of general principles of pathology and treatment to the special morbid states enumerated'. She continued to work for the London School of Medicine for Women[2] to the end of her life.

On 11 October 1874 fourteen young women had walked into a small, tree-shaded house and garden in Henrietta Street, Brunswick Square. Without a formal opening ceremony they began their medical studies. In the same house their Executive held weekly and exhausting meetings. At these Sophia was not present, for with great self-denial she had decided the committee should consist of registered practitioners only, and she had not yet passed her qualifying examinations. Nor was Dr Anstie, who had died suddenly and tragically of a virulent throat infection, caught in the course of his work. A. T. Norton, a consultant surgeon at St Mary's, volunteered to take his place as Dean of the newborn

[1] Anderson, L. G., *Elizabeth Garrett Anderson*, pp. 214–5.
[2] Now the Royal Free Hospital School of Medicine.

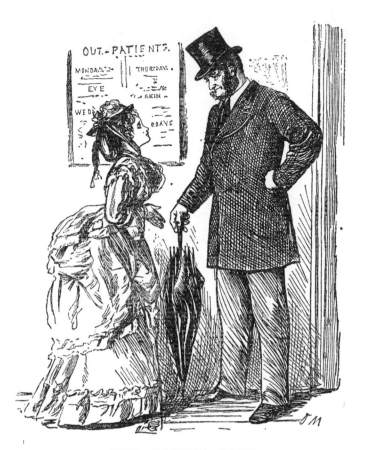

THE COMING RACE.

Doctor Evangeline. "BY THE BYE, MR. SAWYER, ARE YOU ENGAGED TO-MORROW AFTERNOON? I HAVE RATHER A TICKLISH OPERATION TO PERFORM—AN AMPUTATION, YOU KNOW."

Mr. Sawyer. "I SHALL BE VERY HAPPY TO DO IT FOR YOU."

Dr. Evangeline. "O, NO, NOT *THAT*! BUT WILL YOU KINDLY COME AND ADMINISTER THE CHLOROFORM FOR ME?"

A cartoon in 1872 salutes the Lady Surgeon

and struggling institution, a step which exposed him to abuse and ridicule by other doctors. Before the month of October was out a 'grand battle' raged in the Medical School Committee of St Mary's over the lecturers who also taught at the School of Medicine for Women. 'We were asked to reconsider our connection with it,' wrote William Broadbent stoutly. 'Of course we shall not abandon it.' Elizabeth Blackwell accepted the Chair of Gynaecology, but was soon forced by ill health to retire. The lease of the house had swallowed up the school's funds, the nineteen London examining bodies promptly refused to recognize it, and the staff had no hospital beds for clinical teaching. The students were full of enthusiasm; their numbers increased in one session to twenty-three; and it was plain that they needed a general hospital of at least a hundred beds for clinical practice. Elizabeth welcomed them as clerks and dressers, but the New Hospital could offer them only twenty-six beds and those solely for women and children.[1] The failure of the school in its early stages would be damaging beyond words to the cause and throughout 1875 Elizabeth worried over its future.

By contrast the New Hospital for Women flourished in its new quarters and began to attract favourable notice in the press. Already the comic possibilities of the woman surgeon in hospital had inspired *Punch* to a friendly cartoon. Now a correspondent of *The Queen* visited the ward and reported:

> Our visit was made in the early morning while the visiting physician was still on her rounds and the house surgeon busy with her work, while the dispenser was waiting in her workshop for patients. Although our visit was paid at so early an hour we were impressed with the orderliness which everywhere prevailed and with the feminine element pervading the place. We were told an operation was to take place that morning and saw the patient lying down for some necessary examination. As we looked at the patient and her surroundings, the thought

[1] New Hospital for Women *Annual Report*, 1875.

could not but come before us, if we had something similar to
undergo, how the suffering would be lightened by the fact that
only women were present.[1]

This was precisely the argument to win over the hesitant middle-
class reader of women's magazines; perhaps Elizabeth, while
making her rounds and preparing to operate, found time to im-
plant it in the journalist's mind. On a professional level, Elizabeth
continued to report interesting cases to the *British Medical Journal*.
One which gave her particular satisfaction was the recovery of
a woman of forty, in very poor general health, who had suffered
a pleural effusion. Since the other lung appeared sound, Elizabeth
performed a thoracentesis and the patient was discharged fit.[2] Her
report in March 1875 on a case of paralysis shows that she had
read the first series of Charcot's classic papers on nervous diseases,
which had appeared in Paris two years earlier. The number of
beds had been more than doubled by the move to Marylebone
Road; but the waiting list for in-patients was already so long that
Elizabeth persuaded her committee to buy the lease of an adjoining
house into which the hospital could expand when necessary. Mrs
Louisa Atkins, who had qualified in Switzerland, joined the staff,
an intelligent and kindly student from the London School of
Medicine for Women came into residence as a dresser, and by
March 1875 Elizabeth felt free to take her first holiday since the
hospital opened.

It was also the first time she had been parted from Skelton and
the little girls. 'I wish you were with me,' she wrote in the train
on the way to Dover. 'I shall never elope in real earnest. I don't
like leaving you and the bairns tho' I do most thoroughly enjoy
the sense of holiday.'[3] She was on her way to spend Easter in
Italy with Millicent. Neither was a good sailor, but Newson's

[1] *The Queen*, 31 July 1875.
[2] *British Medical Journal*, 24 April 1875.
[3] Elizabeth Garrett Anderson to Skelton Anderson, 18 March 1875.
Anderson family papers.

upbringing had taught them to endure discomforts cheerfully, and once in Italy the foreignness of everything filled them with childlike pleasure. They wrote home every day, ticked off the sights in their *Baedeker*, brewed tumblers of tea in their hotel bedroom and tramped round Rome until they were exhausted. Elizabeth insisted on having an audience of Pope Pius IX, not on her own account, but in order to have her old cook's rosary blessed.[1] The highlight of their holiday was a visit to Garibaldi at his villa. They tried earnestly to persuade him to say something in support of the women's cause, but the Lion of Caprera, well versed in the ways of English ladies, merely pointed to some photographs of himself and said, 'You would like me to sign them'? In spite of this disappointment Garibaldi remained their hero; to have been in his presence and actually touched his hand was a memory they both treasured. Elizabeth took her signed picture home; it still hung in her bedroom when she was an old woman.[2]

In August 1875 she again left home for a few days to read a paper at the B.M.A. conference in Edinburgh. She had always enjoyed her branch meetings and was quite unprepared for the storm which now burst about her ears. The president of the conference proved to be Sophia Jex-Blake's arch enemy, Professor Christison, who was heard to say in awful tones that 'a liberty' had been taken in admitting a woman member, still more in permitting her actually to address a section of his association. The fact that she was unquestionably on the Medical Register only added to the outrage. Elizabeth sat through this 'horribly dull and long medico-political' address, but was warned by the friendly editor of the *British Medical Journal* that a motion against the admission of women might be proposed. In some consternation she wrote home to Skelton.

I wish your wise counsels, beloved, were within reach. I should like to know what you would advise. I don't want to fail as

[1] Fawcett, M. G., *What I remember*, p. 106.
[2] Personal information, Sir Colin Anderson.

a leader even of a forlorn hope, but it grates against my taste making anything of a self-defensive speech to such a body. . . . Don't think I am unhappy, dearest. Someone must do it and with all my inner joys, you and the dear babies and my work, I can stand it better than most people could.[1]

She spent a whole morning walking alone on Arthur's Seat while she tried to compose a speech, only to be told that the question had been discussed in her absence and she would not be allowed to give her paper. By now, Elizabeth was really angry. She went straight to the head of the Obstetrical Section and said, 'If you can say that any one of your number has read my paper and thought it not worth producing, I acquiesce, but it ought not to be stopped in deference to prejudice.'[2] In the afternoon a message came, inviting her to speak that evening.

The hall was crammed to hear her read the paper she had prepared on Dysmenorrhoea. In discussing treatment she was critical of early surgical intervention, maintaining that 'various constitutional causes frequently gave rise to obstructive dysmenorrhoea, which could often be removed by constitutional measures'. The surgeons, not surprisingly, attacked this, but they were silenced by elderly Dr Keiller who stood up to express his hearty approval and admiration of the paper. 'It was just what I would have expected from my old pupil,' he said.[3] The meeting ended in cheers and handshakings, but Elizabeth was thankful to get home.

The children were at their most fascinating, Louie a high-spirited two-year-old, and Margaret flaxen-haired as a doll in white muslin and coral necklace. Elizabeth took them riding with her in the brougham, played with them on the nursery floor after tea and delighted in the sight of their two small figures walking hand-in-hand. They were so well that their parents stole a week together

[1] Elizabeth Garrett Anderson to Skelton Anderson, 4 Aug. 1875. Fawcett Library.
[2] Elizabeth Garrett Anderson to Skelton Anderson, 6 Aug. 1875. Fawcett Library.
[3] *British Medical Journal*, 8 Aug. 1875.

in September 1875 to go walking in the Yorkshire dales, map in hand and baggage slung over a moorland pony's back. They were utterly happy and it was as well, for this was the last happiness they were to know for some time.

On 9 October, when Skelton was in Glasgow at the shipyards, Elizabeth wrote to him in alarm. Margaret had been ailing for a few days and she had worried until she received the family doctor's time-honoured reassurance that 'it is simply a reflex irritation from the teeth'. But Margaret had a convulsion in the night lasting twenty minutes and in the morning she was drowsy and languid. Elizabeth clung to every hopeful sign; the baby was conscious, she recognized Louie and asked for her doll. Yet two days later the fever still kept up and the nights were very restless.

> She is now very ill poor pet [wrote Elizabeth to Skelton], and my chief reason for half asking you to come home was feeling that it was possible I might knock up before she was quite well. I don't think I shall but if I did I should like you to be here to look after her. It is hard work physically carrying her about and pacing the room hour after hour . . . I am not going out and am seeing scarcely anyone even here.[1]

Skelton hurried home to find Margaret worse and Elizabeth weary and anxious. The professional skill which had brought her success was quite powerless to help her own child. Ford Anderson, hearing the continuous high-pitched cry which rang through the house, tried to warn her gently of meningitis, but Elizabeth insisted obstinately that the evidence was entirely against what she called 'any brain mischief'. During November two very senior and distinguished physicians were called. Both said that the child might die, but offered no diagnosis. After they drove away Ford went up to the night nursery alone. Bending over Margaret's cot he swept the edge of his forefinger round the child's forehead in the form of a sickle and watched for the white track which

[1] Elizabeth Garrett Anderson to Skelton Anderson, 9 Oct. 1875. Anderson family papers.

followed, the classic 'tâches meningitiques' which then heralded certain death. All he wanted was to arrive at the truth; intent on his examination, he did not hear Elizabeth come softly into the nursery behind him, and was quite unprepared for the torrent of anger and tears which she poured upon him. She understood only too well what her brother-in-law was looking for. How dared he suggest, she cried, that her precious Margaret was dying of meningitis? Ford said nothing but went away.

December came and the baby grew rapidly worse. Towards the end Elizabeth and the nurse, completely exhausted, had to rest. Skelton took their place and for a whole night paced up and down the nursery floor, soothing the dying child with firm, gentle hands. At dawn on 15 December Margaret died with her head resting against her father's cheek. On the day of her burial Elizabeth sought out Ford. 'You were right and I was wrong. I have come to say how sorry I am that I spoke to you as I did.' The reticent Ford was deeply touched; he drove home reflecting that his sister-in-law had the quality of greatness, since even in the deepest personal grief she acknowledged her own mistakes.[1]

In the new year of 1876 Elizabeth prepared to take up her hospital work again after more than two months' break.

> I feel it is a great blessing [she wrote to Skelton's father] not to be one of those poor mothers who have nothing to do but to think of what they have lost, but on the other hand one would not like to hustle out of sight, as it were, all the tender memories of a grief, or to hide them too soon in commonplace cares.[2]

She found it hard to bear the sight of Louie, searching the house and asking anxiously, 'Babee? Babee?' She and Skelton, drawn even closer together in grief, were both heart-broken and puzzled by the cause of their loss. Margaret had been fed according to the best medical opinion of the day on 'milk from one cow', and it

---

[1] Anderson, J. F., *A Pioneer*. MS. Anderson family papers.
[2] Elizabeth Garrett Anderson to the Rev. A. Anderson, 2 Jan. 1876. Anderson family papers.

now seems likely that bovine tuberculosis from an untested cow was the source of the infection. Elizabeth, however, in common with all her contemporaries, believed tuberculosis to be a hereditary disease, which would probably attack her other children. Margaret's death left a legacy of fear and distress which was to haunt her for years to come. A photograph taken with Louie soon after Margaret's death, shows Elizabeth with both arms clasped round the rather frail little girl in a gesture of passionate protectiveness, while her face, sad in repose, looked at last as old as her forty years.

By the summer of 1876 Elizabeth was again pregnant. She tried not to wish too hard for another girl, especially as Skelton would enjoy a son, but confessed, 'My heart goes out so much more spontaneously to women than to men that I take more interest in having them and doing the best I can to give them a good start.'[1] In any case, she said, she would try to steel herself against loving the new baby too much; it would hurt her less if once again she had to lose it.[2] Fortunately she had little time to dwell on her fears, for the London School of Medicine for Women was now facing a life-and-death crisis.

From the first the school had faced two overwhelming difficulties: to find a body which would examine women, and to find a hospital which would give them clinical teaching. After nearly two years they were no further forward. By January 1876 the executive had been driven to report gloomily: 'Several students have already left the school in consequence of its inability to afford them qualifying hospital practice and they have reason to fear a still further decrease of numbers for the same cause.'[3] After further unsuccessful attempts they added that 'they cannot conceal their conviction that this point is of capital importance, that on it must eventually turn the usefulness – more, the very existence – of the

[1] Elizabeth Garrett Anderson to the Rev. A. Anderson, 19 Dec. 1876. Anderson family papers.
[2] Anderson, L. G., op. cit. p. 202.
[3] Moberly Bell, E., *Storming the Citadel*, p. 101.

School'. Three months after Elizabeth's return to work, in March 1876, she went on a deputation from the school to the Privy Council to explain the two-fold difficulty of examinations and clinical teaching. In her speech she asked the government to legislate. Women were not asking for special privileges, she said, but merely for the removal of special disabilities. Nothing followed, and the School was at its darkest hour. A year later, against all expectations, the whole scene had changed.

The examination problem was the first to be resolved. Help came from Elizabeth's old friend Russell Gurney, M.P. His health was failing and he was, in fact, within two years of his death, when in the summer of 1876 he steered through Parliament an act enabling all medical corporations to examine women, notwithstanding any restrictions to be found in their charters. At first it seemed doubtful whether any examining bodies would be willing to use their new powers, but in October, after inspecting the work done at the school, the King and Queen's College of Physicians, Dublin, agreed to do so. Five of the Edinburgh students, including Sophia Jex-Blake, at once presented themselves for examination, to be followed by two holders of the Zürich M.D. All seven were successful and all joined the British Medical Register, four in London, the others in Leeds, Birmingham and Edinburgh.

Their success was cheering, but it did not help the seventeen girls at the school who still could not present themselves as candidates for lack of clinical practice. In June 1876 Elizabeth suggested approaching the London Hospital asking for certain teaching wards to be set aside for women. She knew well that the vast building in the Whitechapel Road contained nearly 800 beds and that male students visited only a fraction of them. The House Committee was willing; for a month there was jubilation at the school until in July the medical and surgical staff of the London gave notice that they 'declined to entertain such a proposal'.[1] Elizabeth had no further plans to offer, and it was the Honorary

[1] New Hospital for Women *Annual Report*, 1877.

Treasurer of the school, J. B. Stansfeld,[1] who took the next step. The Royal Free Hospital stood nearby in the Gray's Inn Road. Its founder, the compassionate surgeon William Marsden, had died without realizing his dream of adding a medical school to his wards. The hospital doctors had already refused to consider women students, but Stansfeld now fell in on holiday with the lay chairman of the governing body who, he noted with some surprise, 'did not appear to be in awe of the staff'. Slowly over the winter of 1876–7 Stansfeld felt his way with this possible ally, reporting each step to Sophia Jex-Blake. Negotiations with the governing body and staff of the Royal Free went on throughout February 1877, but Elizabeth took no part in them, for she was fully engaged elsewhere.

On 2 March 1877 she organized a large charity concert at Grosvenor House for the benefit of the New Hospital. Clara Schumann played for her, and although the artists' fees came to a hundred pounds, Elizabeth, who had personally sold over four hundred pounds worth of tickets, cleared six hundred pounds profit. Her accounts were made up just in time. On 9 March she gave birth to a son.

The sight of the baby dispelled Elizabeth's fears for his health and her resolutions not to love him too much.

> His father's nose exactly [she wrote to Charlotte Anderson], very shapely even now, large, well formed mouth, good sized eyes and a broad placid brow, rather more after me than his father. I only see any likeness to myself above the eyes and as this is my most respectable part he has certainly chosen wisely. He has J.G.S.'s long shapely limbs and large hands. He is not *fat*, but also not disreputably lean.[2]

To her mother's great pleasure Louie, at three and a half, received

[1] J. B. Stansfeld, M.P., was member for Halifax from 1859 to 1895. He led the movement in the House of Commons for repeal of the Contagious Diseases Acts.

[2] Elizabeth Garrett Anderson to Charlotte Anderson, 13 March 1877. Anderson family papers.

the fable that this important figure had arrived in the doctor's bag with considerable scepticism. The only problem was his name. Elizabeth refused to start him off with a 'brand new Brummagem name utterly bare of association' and the handsome, sturdy boy was eventually christened Alan Garrett Anderson.

His mother's lying-in was as brief as usual. One day after he was born a telegram from J. B. Stansfeld to Sophia at the school announced 'Royal Free Hospital have unanimously accepted my proposal'. The hospital governors had driven a hard bargain. They were to receive guaranteed fees of £400 from the students and a further subsidy of £300, in case the admission of women students should cause a withdrawal of outraged subscribers. To Elizabeth this seemed a small price to pay for overcoming a mountainous difficulty. She wanted to go to the school and join in the cheer which was given to Stansfeld when he announced the agreement to the students, but had to content herself with writing from her bed. 'We all owe more to you than to anyone. I do not imagine there will be any difficulty about the £700 a year for five years, and I shall hope to be able to contribute £50 a year as my share.' J. G. S. Anderson agreed to act as one of three guarantors of the annual payment. The school was now in a position to appeal to the public for funds, and on 25 June 1877 held a large meeting at St George's Hall, with the Earl of Shaftesbury in the chair. Elizabeth's duty, as usual, was to win over the doubters.

> In the matter of health [she said] the medical education of women is less trying than the life of a fashionable lady. As to morals, the study of medicine is of an elevating character; and as to good manners I think the habit of dealing with people of different tempers can be of the utmost value to women and afford an exceedingly wholesome discipline.[1]

Her own feminine charm and the presence of her husband gave point to these words. The public response was good.

[1] New Hospital for Women *Annual Report*, 1878.

The Executive Committee members were shortly faced with a new, more personal crisis. For the past three years Sophia Jex-Blake, unasked and unpaid, had shouldered the donkey-work of organizing secretary. Members of the governing body had not found her easy to work with, but she had achieved miracles each term by sheer drive and determination. She had been away from London a good deal visiting her invalid mother and taking her M.D. in Berne and Dublin. Now she was qualified, there were governors who looked forward with sinking hearts to the time when she would return and really hold the reins. In early spring 1877 the Executive met to appoint an official organizing secretary, the post Sophia longed for and confidently expected.

She was away, but Elizabeth Garrett Anderson, who was there, heard Stansfeld in the chair speak of the qualities the new secretary would need, in particular 'the tact and judgment to enable the . . . working of the school and its students to go on smoothly with the Hospital'. The school's agreement with the Royal Free was still provisional, he reminded them; one tactless outburst could wreck it for ever. The committee members took this hint; when one proposed Miss Jex-Blake, another countered with Mrs Anderson. Elizabeth was appalled. She foresaw an emotional situation of the kind she most disliked. She genuinely did not want the post since she was very busy with practice and hospital and her son was only a few months old. She knew Sophia's gifts and past services deserved the appointment. On the other hand she knew as well as anyone present the calamitous possibilities of Sophia's temper and temperament. She hedged: 'I do not wish to take unfair advantage over a colleague, but if it were to be for the good of the school – ?' She suggested that the election should be postponed until the next meeting.[1]

The thought of Elizabeth as secretary was more than Sophia could endure. The crack in the wall, so carefully papered over in 1874, was now about to break through again, to the embarrassment of all beholders. To avert an open quarrel, Isabel Thorne,

[1] Todd, M., *The Life of Sophia Jex-Blake*, p. 446.

one of the original Edinburgh students, sacrificed her own career in medicine which she loved, to serve at the committee's request as secretary. Elizabeth was intensely relieved and Sophia accepted the bitter disappointment with fine generosity. 'About the best possible with her perfect temper and excellent sense, so much better than I,' she wrote of Mrs Thorne in her diary.[1] Nevertheless her hurt was deep. She could not bear to stay in London and see the school in other hands. Apparently without seeing Elizabeth again, she left to make a practice and found her own women's hospital in Edinburgh.

On 1 October 1877 the London School of Medicine for Women opened for the winter session with its future assured. The committee had bought an excellent private museum for use in teaching and was beginning to build up a library of which Elizabeth was honorary librarian. Elizabeth 'looking well in black with a large fichu of cream-coloured muslin' gave the inaugural speech to the students. She wasted no time in congratulations but warned them that they had four years' hard work ahead. They would be tested, she said, far more severely at the bedside of suffering patients than by any board of examiners. Women would understand disease in proportion to their knowledge and intelligence and not through any occult or mysterious sympathy with its subject. They should, however, understand better than men the conditions of life which underlay much chronic disease or disability among women. Finally Elizabeth begged the thirty-four assembled young women to remember how much depended on the judgment, moderation and good taste of the earliest supporters of a cause, and how necessary it was, especially in England, that they should carry the feeling of the community with them. 'From this day forth you are not merely women who desire to help other women', she ended. 'You are members of a noble profession. Seek in all things to promote its highest aims and add to its honour.'[2]

The school's only remaining legal disability was that its students

[1] Todd, M., *The Life of Sophia Jex-Blake*, p. 448.
[2] *The Standard*, 2 Oct. 1877.

254

were not yet admitted to the University of London's examinations. The Senate was willing but the medical faculty had protested in Convocation. One member, Sir William Jenner, declared 'he would rather follow his dear daughter to the grave than see her subjected to such questions as could not be omitted from a proper examination for a surgical degree'.[1] The Senate therefore laid before Convocation a new charter admitting women to *all* degrees of London University. Elizabeth, remembering too well how this very proposal had been defeated in 1862 by Lord Granville's casting vote, invited him to call on her, in hopes of winning him over. Lord Granville was famed for courtesy, but too experienced to commit himself. As he rose at the end of their interview his attitude was still uncertain. At this moment, from behind a sofa, the daughter of the house, aged four, appeared with some dignity, holding up a battered doll. 'You may kiss him', she said. The charter admitting women to London University degrees was carried by a substantial majority, and her parents agreed that Louie's intervention must have been decisive.[2] The Commissioners drafting the charter gave credit to the mother rather than the daughter. In deciding it was 'only fair and reasonable that women should be admitted to examinations on the same terms as men', they had been much influenced, they said, by 'the moderation with which the views of women have been laid before us by Mrs Garrett Anderson'.

This problem was no sooner settled than another arose. A new Medical Bill before Parliament made it essential, rightly, for all practitioners to hold qualifications both in medicine and in surgery. The General Medical Council proposed to admit women to a separate examination and a supplementary register. This was precisely the danger that Elizabeth had foreseen when the school was founded. Sophia Jex-Blake, pocketing her pride for the sake of the cause, wrote asking Elizabeth to protest. In a long, well-

[1] *The Standard*, 16 Jan. 1878. Not surprisingly, Miss Jenner became a militant suffragette.
[2] Anderson, L. G., op. cit. p. 228

argued letter to *The Times*, Elizabeth agreed the necessity for a compulsory triple qualification in medicine, surgery and midwifery, but proposed a conjoint board of the various examining bodies, with a uniform standard for all candidates, men and women. She foresaw the danger of different medical registers for the sexes, implying a separate and inferior race of women doctors.

> What women ask [she stressed] is that they should be *required* to know as much as men do. . . . Whether women should write their papers at the same table with the male candidates [she added caustically], or at another table in the same room, or in the next room, whether there should be one door, or two or none, or whether they should even be in separate houses and different streets, are matters which could probably be settled without the intervention of Parliament. Provided that the examination papers are the same, provided the standard for marking and conditions are identical, no one would care about these trifles.[1]

The point was of cardinal importance for her young students, and eventually she carried it. Meanwhile the Bill, in its proposed form, was dropped.

In the same year, 1878, Elizabeth completed a short medical textbook, *The Student's Pocket Index*, a modest aid to cramming for students of the L.S.M. Knowing the bugbear Latin was to many girls, she had asked the Royal College of Physicians for permission to reprint the English column of their *Nomenclature of Diseases*, but this was refused.[2] The little volume is the shape and size of a laundry book to slide easily into a petticoat pocket; each left-hand page contains a list of diseases or morbid conditions, under general headings such as 'Diseases of the Nervous System, of the Respiratory System, of the Female Organs of Generation' and so on. The right hand page is ruled into columns to be completed by the student: 'Seen. Lecture. Museum. P.M. Seen. Noted

[1] *The Times*, 8 May 1878.
[2] Elizabeth Garrett Anderson to the Secretary, the Royal College of Physicians, 20 Aug. 1877. The Royal College of Physicians.

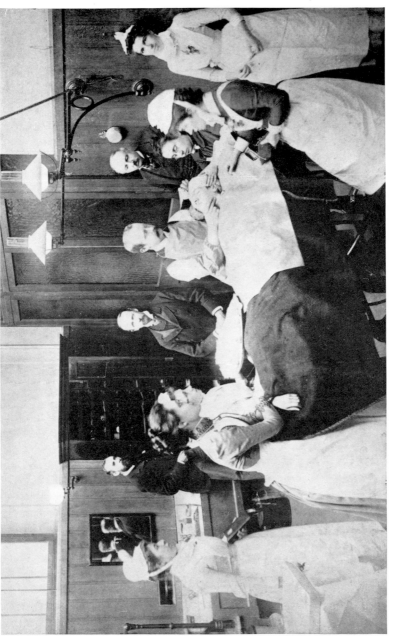

9. Women students in an operating theatre at the Royal Free Hospital

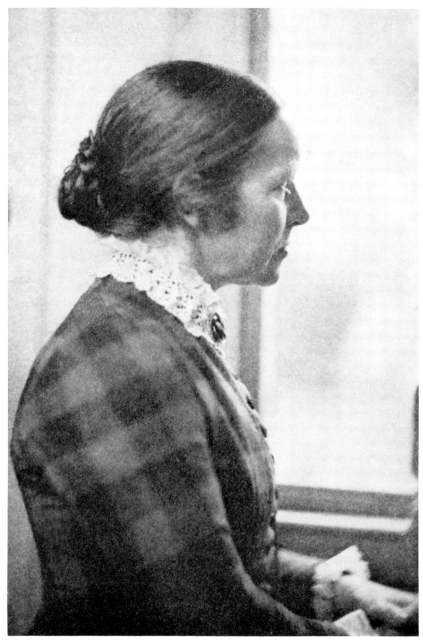

10. Elizabeth Garrett Anderson in middle life

in casebook p. —. Books Read', with spare pages at the end for bibliography and notes. The binding includes a slot for the owner's pencil. By means of this workmanlike arrangement the student could register all her clinical work for later reference.

Elizabeth never published her lectures, although she worked hard to revise them and keep them up to date. However Louisa Aldrich-Blake as a student attended Mrs Garrett Anderson's lectures on medicine, and kept detailed notes of the entire course.[1] To judge from these, Elizabeth's lectures were vivid, concrete and practical. She constantly urged the students to *observe*, to look in the patient's face, to notice, for example, the lips, very dry in fever, pale in anaemia, or a dull, dark blue in cardiac cases. She observed the full ritual of the tongue: '*Look* – How patient can put it out, size, form, surface, outline of edge, colour and whether *clean* (i.e. state of epithelium)' and gave a precise description of its appearance in different diseases. On treatment her recommendations were cautious but exact. '*In haemorrhage* from stomach, general treatment, rest and cold applications. Turpentine in mucilage. Ergot subcutaneously,' or '*In pregnancy* the worst thing to do is to get very fat. Best without any alcohol.' She believed that a good doctor should be able to give advice on home nursing. Her lectures on fevers recall sharply the almost vanished dangers of the Victorian nursery. '*Scarlet fever* if have to nurse at home. Ventilate well. Take up carpets. Disinfect. *Treatment*: Fresh air, cooling applications. In coma – pour cold water over nape of neck while holding child over a bath – put child into cold pack. *Prognosis* unfavourable in severe or irregular cases.' The approach she advised towards the patient was firm and forthright. 'For a person who has had gallstones order open air exercise, careful diet, especially avoid *fats*, *sugars* and *alcohols*.' She was firm with the students also and made no attempt to gloss over the difficulties of the subject, though in practice she helped them by a systematic arrangement of their work. Sometimes she set them to memorize, for instance, Celsus' classic definition of inflammation as 'calor,

[1] Now in the Wellcome Historical Medical Library.

dolor, tumor, rubor'. Sometimes she provided charts or diagrams. Nothing pleased her more than the intelligent response of an interested student. One such student of the 1890s, Louisa Martindale, still remembers Mrs Anderson's small, commanding figure, her un-academic approach and the dreaded moment when her eyes would swivel round the lecture room to settle on the vague or inattentive listener. 'Now what about the young lady in green, at the back? We haven't heard her views yet?'

Everywhere Elizabeth could see the results of her work consolidating. At the New Hospital for Women, Frances Hoggan, who had never been happy about the abdominal surgery, resigned, but another qualified woman, Mrs Bovell Sturge, living nearby in Wimpole Street, was ready to take her place. The old head nurse, kindly but uneducated, died, and Elizabeth was able to bring in the overdue reform of nursing. She found a matron trained in the Nightingale School, and with three years experience as ward sister at St Thomas's. Under her, two young nurses formed the nucleus of the New Hospital's own training school. The results of the change were immediate; the wards became gleamingly clean, bright with flowers, and 'a saving of about £20 per annum has been effected upon alcohol'.[1]

In the summer of 1878 Elizabeth had once again to brave a meeting of the British Medical Association. During the last three years, which had been so eventful in the Andersons' lives, the B.M.A. had laboriously circularized its members on the admission of women. About four thousand of the six thousand members replied, and of these about three to one had voted against women.[2] Sir William Jenner even threatened to resign, provoking a jibe from Elizabeth's old ally, *Punch*. 'What can the Council do to please Sir W. Jenner? Only turn the young Women out of their Society? The British Medical Association will always contain a certain number of irremovable old Women.'[3] Elizabeth could not

[1] New Hospital for Women *Annual Report*, 1878.
[2] Moberly Bell, E., op. cit. p. 137.
[3] *Punch*, 9 March 1878.

let the vote pass unchallenged. Remembering how roughly she had been handled at Edinburgh, Skelton would not let her go alone and she gratefully accepted his company to Bath, though he could not of course attend the meeting. 'That I must face alone as he is not a member,' wrote Elizabeth to her father-in-law. 'Happily my courage always rises to emergencies, so though I feel just now in a ghastly funk at having to speak before this unsympathetic audience, I dare say I shan't mind it so much when the time comes.'[1] The President moved that a clause should be added to the Constitution 'That no female shall be eligible as a member of the Association.' It was a forlorn hope when Elizabeth rose to speak against the motion.

Her speech was a triumph of self-control in one naturally hot-tempered. 'Mr President and Gentlemen, I shall treat this question from an entirely impersonal point of view', she began, and she was as good as her word. She pointed out that circumstances had changed since the last meeting; medical women were now recognized by law, they had a flourishing medical school and the practice of a large general hospital for their exclusive training. 'Eight Englishwomen are now on the Medical Register and every year will see their numbers considerably increase.' That being so, would either the interests of the profession or of medical science be served by cutting off a growing body of doctors from even the most limited amount of fellowship? Patiently she dealt with the old bogey of indelicacy. 'Considering how much of the practice of every doctor concerns women', she said, 'it is incredible to find that they find it impossible to speak upon medical topics in the presence of medical women.' She even ventured to tell the story of Charles Lamb, 'who had been heaping abuse on the head of someone when his friend said: "Lamb, how can you say that? How can you hate so heartily a man you do not know?" The answer was "My dear fellow, of course I do not know him. How could I hate him at all if I did?" '[2]

[1] Elizabeth Garrett Anderson to the Rev. A. Anderson, 7 Aug. 1878. Anderson family papers.   [2] *British Medical Journal*, 4 Aug. 1878.

There was general laughter mixed with the cheers of Elizabeth's supporters, but the voting was a foregone conclusion. The members protested that they were charmed by their lady colleague personally, but nevertheless they must act upon principle in excluding all future women members by a show of hands. In consideration of Mrs Anderson's standing in the profession and her personal popularity the motion was not made retrospective. By this singularly back-handed compliment Elizabeth became the only woman member of the B.M.A. She attended meetings, spoke in discussions and went to receptions in face of icy hostility. The thought of a forthcoming meeting was enough to give her a sleepless night. 'If I had known what it meant I could not have undertaken it,' she once told Ford Anderson. Nevertheless she refused to be driven away and continued for nineteen years to be the solitary woman member, reflecting that this was a minor irritation compared with what had been achieved. As she drafted her hospital's annual report in 1878, Elizabeth summed up the situation.

Parliament had expressed a decided opinion in favour of allowing women to practise medicine; the highest medical examining body in the United Kingdom has declared its willingness to confer its degrees upon them; a complete medical school, with a large hospital, a museum and a library has been organized for the use of female students; and we believe that when these facts are fairly considered the change must be accepted as accomplished, and that women must, from this time forth, be left to make the best mark they can for themselves in the practice of the medical profession.[1]

[1] New Hospital for Women *Annual Report*, 1878.

CHAPTER SIXTEEN

The Two Lives
January 1879 – December 1885

❄

'The fact is,' Elizabeth Garrett Anderson once remarked, 'a doctor leads two lives, the professional and the private, and the boundaries between the two are never traversed.' Because she was a woman, public opinion watched her for the least sign of failure or confusion, and to keep the two lives disentangled needed all her skill in planning.

By 1880, after fifteen years in practice, her professional as well as her family life was fully formed. In the opinion of Ford Anderson she possessed 'sound judgment as well as natural wit, aimed chiefly at the maintenance of health and research into the causation of disease'.[1] In an age often morbidly obsessed with the trappings of invalidism, this approach was unusual and opinions about Mrs Anderson varied greatly; but, as a colleague noticed, those who knew her best respected and loved her most.[2] No one could have been further removed from the conventional idea of a ministering angel. She had no interest in imaginary ailments and no inclination to imitate the fashionable physician of whom it was said 'most of the hypochondriacs in London spoke of him as their dearest friend'. Her bedside manner was her natural manner, dry, witty and often brusque. Her will was indomitable and she had never suffered fools gladly. It is true that her early rebuff at the Middlesex Hospital had taught her the dangers of an unguarded

[1] Anderson, J. F., *A Pioneer*. MS. Anderson family papers.
[2] Scharlieb, M., *Reminiscences*, p. 138.

manner, and during the years of struggle she had tried, on the whole successfully, to assume the ladylike demureness recommended by Emily Davies. Now, however, in middle life, established and assured, she allowed her character to show itself. Her public manner remained tactful and discreet, but patients found her private candour devastating at times. Stories began to gather round her in London, as they had around Newson Garrett in Aldeburgh.

'Dear Mrs Anderson,' said a would-be grateful patient, 'you must have had a great love for the sick to adopt such an arduous profession.' 'Not at all,' said Elizabeth shortly, 'I became a doctor because I detest sickness.'[1] A man who wrote asking 'if gout were in her line of practise' received the reply: 'Dear Sir, Gout is very much in my line; gentlemen are not. I advise you to consult Dr —. Yrs truly.' Totally unselfconscious, Elizabeth as she grew older tended to think aloud. On learning that a patient's husband had been offered a seat in Gladstone's cabinet, she remarked, 'Dear me! I had no idea things were as bad as that!' Another patient, whom Elizabeth had studied long and earnestly, was startled to hear her exclaim, with the satisfaction of one making a scientific discovery, 'It is true; you *do* paint your eyelashes!' Some people she offended mortally, but many more forgave her because she was unaffected and uncommonly good company. Where she detected self-pity she could be remarkably sharp. Was it true that she had carefully removed the flowers from a vase and poured the water over a hysterical patient? This story has enjoyed great currency.[2] It seems unlikely, less because Elizabeth had any great sympathy with hypochondria than because she was careful to set younger medical women an example of professional etiquette. The fact that irreverent nieces and students repeated it with such relish, however, is surely significant.

By contrast, when faced with real pain or distress, Elizabeth was kind beyond the bounds of mere professional duty. She

[1] ibid. p. 139.
[2] Mitchison, N., in *Revaluations*, p. 185, and elsewhere.

could also show unexpected imagination. Edith Simcox, the spinster radical, author of *The Autobiography of a Shirtmaker*, adored George Eliot and was prostrated by the death of 'my darling and my God'. Much to her surprise, Elizabeth came unasked to visit her. 'Dec. 26th, 1880,' wrote Edith Simcox in her diary: 'Mrs Anderson came to see me this morning – was very kind – spoke of people having spoken of Westminster Abbey; she seemed to understand about the dear one – thought she must have had Bright's disease and would have suffered more if she had lived.' Elizabeth stood beside Edith Simcox at George Eliot's grave on a bitter winter's day.[1] Also through George Eliot, she gained as patient Emma Paterson, the pioneer of women's trades unions, a born fighter, to whom she gave the plain and honest verdict 'You are dying'. Even when there was no hope, medically speaking, for a patient, Elizabeth offered the comfort of her presence. 'She told me how good you had been to her all through this sad year,' wrote Charlotte of a relative dying of a long and painful illness. 'She said she had felt your loving sympathy and all your visits very deeply. She wept, speaking of you.'[2] Courage, under physical or mental distress, was a passport to Elizabeth's affection. One of her patients, the writer Trelawny's niece, braved the Italian customs officials with his ashes in an urn to get them buried beside Shelley's in Rome. 'His daughter refused to carry out his will in these particulars, so the niece, who is one of the timid brave women with nerves of a mouse and heart of a lion did it all herself,' Elizabeth told Skelton admiringly. Her understanding extended to mental as well as physical illness. In this she was perhaps in advance of her time. She was consulted by the family of an elderly man who had suffered a breakdown.

A man of his fine type I can imagine never being able to get over the sense of personal humiliation involved in such an

[1] McKenzie, K. A., *Edith Simcox and George Eliot*, p. 112.
[2] Charlotte Clarke to Elizabeth Garrett Anderson, 20 Aug. 1893. Anderson family papers.

attack [she wrote]. It is however the kind of thing that may happen to the best balanced mind towards the decline of life and it ought not really to be thought of essentially as a malady of the mind when occurring at his age. . . . If as I suspect the fault lies in the arteries, and in their beginning to wear out, the disturbance may pass away with rest and the establishment of collateral circulation.[1]

Her insight perceived the suffering of a favourite butt of humour, the 'elderly, ugly daughter' imprisoned in the fortress of the middle-class home. The marriage market for such girls was early sold out, their lives were lonely and, she shrewdly pointed out, 'income derived entirely from their parents is not certain to last'. She advised them to train for some work and earn their own living; 'young women living away from their parents enjoy life much more and are more respected if they have a profession from which part at least of their income is derived'. With regained self-respect, ailing spinsters might find themselves happy and well. This bold advice led to some battles in country rectory or suburban drawing room, but many women who followed it found it good.

Elizabeth Garrett Anderson's reputation as a physician spread by personal recommendation from one family to another. 'I know many women', wrote a correspondent, 'who have for years taken the advice of Dr Garrett Anderson, and would never dream of employing a medical man after discovering the comfort which it brought them.'[2] One of the nearest, certainly one of the dearest, of Elizabeth's patients was her brother-in-law, Henry Fawcett. He had always been a chivalrous supporter of women's rights. When he became Postmaster General in Gladstone's 1880 government he created, as well as postal orders and the parcel post, a new field of employment for women as post-office clerks. To Elizabeth's lasting gratitude he appointed for these women

[1] Elizabeth Garrett Anderson to the Rev. A. Anderson, 21 Dec. 1876. Anderson family papers.
[2] *The Gentlewoman*, 19 July 1890.

clerks a woman medical officer at a salary of £350 a year, the first public appointment to be held by a woman doctor. In December 1882, at the height of his career as a minister, he had a severe attack of diphtheria and after a week of illness suffered a massive haemorrhage from the mouth. Elizabeth left home in the middle of dinner and hurried to him, collecting a surgeon on the way. They found Ford Anderson already there, attempting to control the bleeding by ice-packs. Harry's life hung upon a thread. Elizabeth and Ford, to the neglect of their own practices, took turns on duty until he was out of danger; even when he was recovering Elizabeth continued to visit him, sometimes three times a day.[1] 'I only feel that you make too much of the small service I was able to give,' she wrote in reply to his thanks. 'It was in strictest truth a service of affection, and you rewarded us all quite enough by getting well at the end of it.'[2]

In the administration of her practice, Elizabeth was prompt and efficient. She met many of the leading physicians and surgeons of the day in consultation and was courteously received by them. Some, like Sir James Paget, Sir William Broadbent and Sir Thomas Smith, became friends as well as colleagues. She kept open house to all women doctors, British and foreign. She made appointments, kept records and answered letters without the help of a secretary, able at short notice and in her own hand to provide full details of a patient on whom she had operated sixteen years previously.[3] Her own health was excellent, and the worst thing she ever complained of was 'a severe afternoon and evening over the bills'.

The relationship between doctor and patient is elusive and it is not easy at a distance of nearly a hundred years to form an estimate of Elizabeth Garrett Anderson's qualities as a physician. Naomi

[1] Elizabeth Garrett Anderson to Mrs Garrett, 2, 4, 11, and 14 Dec. 1882. Anderson family papers.
[2] Strachey, R., *Millicent Garrett Fawcett*, p. 95.
[3] Elizabeth Garrett Anderson to Dr Dobbs, 4 July 1894. Wellcome Historical Medical Library.

Elizabeth Garrett Anderson

Mitchison, attempting a revaluation of her by the standards of the 1920s, came to the conclusion that she was neither a brilliant nor a born doctor. It is true, of course, that any newly qualified house surgeon of the twentieth century could probably surpass her and her contemporaries in technique. She made no outstanding contribution to medical science; although she read widely, her temperament was not suited to laboratory work and she had neither time nor ambition to undertake original research. If one regards medicine as a pure science, her claims to distinction are not high. If one regards it as a skilled exercise in personal relationships, one must rate her very high indeed. It was as a general practitioner that she excelled, with all the qualities of character which that calling demands – courage, sense of duty, good judgment and warm humanity. By these she disarmed a hostile profession and won the trust of a whole generation of women patients.

As well as conducting hospital and private practice, Elizabeth continued to teach at the London School of Medicine for Women. In 1880 or slightly earlier she received a caller who was to play an important part in her life and the history of the medical women's movement. Mary Scharlieb was the wife of a barrister at the Indian bar and the mother of two children. Moved by the terrible sufferings of purdah women from lack of any medical care in illness and childbirth, she had trained at Madras for the Indian Medical Practitioners Certificate and now proposed, while her sons were at school in England, to study for the M.B., B.S., of London University. Elizabeth received her characteristically. Looking at the tall, slender young woman, hollow-eyed and pale from the heat of Madras, she said bluntly, 'I had hoped to see a much stronger person. With such health as you appear to possess you will do little as a medical student. Of course you shall join the School and of course I will do everything I can to help you.' Fortunately Mary Scharlieb was not offended. She saw in Elizabeth 'a little woman whose bearing was distinguished by alertness, determination and sincerity. . . . Mrs Anderson was one of those indomitable persons who are always willing and able to make the very best of circumstances. Like Napoleon she did not believe in the word *impossible*.'¹

Mary Scharlieb entered the London School of Medicine for Women and worked hard at Henrietta Street for the next two years. In the bitter winter of 1880-1, the pipes froze throughout the house. There was no water for the long anatomy room off the verandah; the students filled their kettles with snow from the garden and boiled up water over the open fire to scrub after dissecting. Elizabeth soon perceived in Mrs Scharlieb what she herself had never claimed, brilliant natural gifts as a surgeon. It was an intense pleasure to her when Mary Scharlieb took Honours all round, with a Gold Medal and Scholarship in Obstetrics. 'To think', lamented the examiner, 'that I have lived to give the Scholarship in my own subject to a woman! But there, it was an excellent paper and it can't be helped!'² Mary Scharlieb was out-standing, but all the early students did well, and by 1883 the school was so well established that A. T. Norton, who had acted as Dean for nine years, felt justified in resigning. He had seen the school through its early difficulties and felt it was time for a woman to succeed him. She would be the first woman Dean of a recognized medical school in the whole of British history, a figure on whom all eyes would be fixed.

The Council met in the spring of 1883 to discuss the appoint-ment and Sophia Jex-Blake made one of her rare journeys from Edinburgh to be present. 'There is only one Dean possible for the London School of Medicine for Women,' declared Dr Cheadle of St Mary's, a friend of the retiring Dean. 'She is, of course, Mrs Anderson.'³ There was a general murmur of agreement, sud-denly interrupted by Sophia's voice. Tension gathered in the orderly meeting like a rising electrical storm. Sophia had never forgiven Elizabeth for advising against the foundation of the school. She still suspected, not quite justly, that Elizabeth had

¹ Scharlieb, M., op. cit. pp. 44, 51.
² ibid. p. 77.
³ Anderson, J. F., *A Pioneer*. MS. Anderson family papers.

prevented her from becoming secretary. When Elizabeth had written to her, formally but kindly, on the death of her mother, as though nothing had happened between them, Sophia burned at having her feelings so easily dismissed. Now, while the members sat rigidly in embarrassment and apprehension, she spoke at the Council table. She wished, she said, to propose Miss Edith Pechey, one of the original Edinburgh students. There was a silence; no one spoke to second her proposal. Her suffering and distress were almost palpable to the beholders. Elizabeth would not withdraw. She was forty-seven, experienced, successful and mature. There was more steel in her composed manner than in all Sophia's outbursts, and she believed she was the right person for the appointment. She sat quietly and heard herself voted in as Dean, with only one dissentient vote. Sophia Jex-Blake went back to Edinburgh sore at heart. Her school, her child, had been handed over to a woman whom she neither liked nor trusted. She never attended a Council meeting again, although she wrote frequently to protest at decisions of which she disapproved.[1]

Elizabeth's first official duty as Dean was one she enjoyed. On the afternoon of 10 May 1883 she drove with Mary Scharlieb and Edith Shove to Burlington House. They were the first two women to gain medical degrees from London University, and it was Elizabeth's task to present them to Lord Granville the Chancellor for graduation. It seemed a long step from the day when her own petition to be examined by the University had been rejected by his vote. 'I think,' she wrote to her father, 'in memory of our efforts 21 years ago you should come up for it.'[2] Newson Garrett, burly in frock-coat with grizzled beard and eyebrows, took his place among the onlookers. The galleries were crowded to see the Chancellor, in full academic dress, hand scrolls recording their degrees to the two modest and graceful candidates, while artists from the picture papers recorded the scene for posterity.

[1] Moberley Bell, E., op. cit. pp. 109–10.
[2] Elizabeth Garrett Anderson to Mr Garrett, 6 May 1883. Fawcett Library.

Mary Scharlieb was due to return to Madras with her husband, but before she left she was summoned to Windsor to tell the Queen about 'her women subjects in India, the whole truth so far as I knew it'. After listening to Mary Scharlieb, Queen Victoria exclaimed indignantly, 'How can they tell me there is no need for medical women in India? Tell them how *deeply* their Queen sympathizes with them and how glad she is that they should have medical women to help them in their time of need.'[1] Only the previous year the Queen had let it be known that her patronage would be withdrawn from a medical congress if women were admitted. As Queen, she found the greatest satisfaction in political and administrative life, but for lesser women, she was convinced, home was the divinely appointed sphere. She had always resolutely opposed what she called 'this mad, wicked folly of Women's Rights'. Yet though she deplored the medical training of women at home, she now determined, with no sense of inconsistency, to send qualified women doctors to India.

Mary Scharlieb reported her interview with the Queen, and Elizabeth was astute enough to see at once that Victoria's interest could be turned to good advantage. Opposition to women was still stubborn and entrenched in certain sections of the medical profession, notably among gynaecologists and obstetricians, who had most to fear from their competition.[2] Royal approval would not remove these critics, but it would silence them, at least in public. Any shrewd observer could see the shift in public opinion which followed a royal lead. Many doctors had frowned on any attempt to relieve the pangs of childbirth until in 1853 Queen Victoria received chloroform at the birth of Prince Leopold, when apparently miraculous conversions occurred.[3] Even to please the Queen, Elizabeth would not allow the London School of Medicine to admit unmatriculated students or to teach what

[1] Scharlieb, M., op. cit. p. 92.
[2] The staff of the Hospital for Women, Soho Square, flatly refused to allow a woman doctor, though qualified and registered, to enter its doors.
[3] Frazer, W., *A History of English Public Health*, p. 336.

she called 'a little medicine to missionaries'. Instead, when the first two qualified women willing to practise in India were ready to leave for Bombay, she obtained permission to present them at Court. The Queen's interest was now firmly captured. At her request in 1885 the Viceroy's wife, Lady Dufferin, initiated a fund to bring women doctors to India. These doctors, as Elizabeth had foreseen, could only come from the London School of Medicine and the New Hospital for Women. Their training could not be separated in practice from the general medical education of women.

While her public and professional life grew in scope, the centre of Elizabeth's private life remained the Garrett and Anderson families. She felt strongly that emotional entanglements with patients or pupils were a mistake. 'Never make a friend of a patient', was always her rule. The friends of her young days, Emily Davies, Llewelyn Davies and his wife, Elizabeth Blackwell and the Gurneys remained the only close friends of her middle age. She followed the various building schemes at Girton and wrote warmly congratulating Emily Davies on the admission of women to the Cambridge Tripos.[1] When old Mrs Davies died, Emily moved to Marylebone and became a neighbour.

Elizabeth gave a considerable time and thought to her husband's business career, which during the 1880s was in the ascendent. Love of ships and the sea was in James Skelton Anderson's blood, inherited from 'old Tarrybreeks', a sea-captain ancestor. Shipping was more than commerce to him; it was a way of life. Moreover he was ambitious and extremely able. In 1878 his firm, Anderson, Anderson & Co., with F. Green & Co., conjointly founded the Orient Line, and thus made history in the shipping world.[2] His life was satisfying and he was remarkably free from petty possessiveness; he had not the slightest desire to interfere with his wife's career.

[1] Stephen, B., *Emily Davies and Girton College*, p. 236.
[2] Geddes, A. C., *The Forging of a Family*, pp. 266–9.

I take a decided line in this matter [he had written during their engagement]. I mean to be if I can a successful man of business neither interfering with your pursuits nor being interfered with by you (but having our confidences at off times and mutually advising and fortifying one another). I must let people know unmistakably not to come bothering me about your public affairs.[1]

It was a good resolution and he kept to it; at least half the credit for the success of their marriage must go to him.

As the richest member of his family, Skelton assumed responsibilities which his wife shared. With nine brothers and sisters on one side of the family and ten on the other, they were assured of a good supply of nieces and nephews. For the new year of 1879 and again in 1880, Elizabeth had 'Mabel and Mary Gavin, Murray and Bertha and the three Smiths – all v. energetic sightseers' to stay for ten days. 'After two or three days of not superfluous rest we shall begin again with five big girls.' Her comments on their characters were uncomfortably penetrating, but her kindness in amusing them was endless. She took them to the Tower of London and the theatre, organized charades and gave parties. She lined up her 'Ugly Ducklings', among them young 'Beau' Haldane, the future Lord Chancellor, and taught them to dance in the drawing room at Upper Berkeley Street. She remembered their birthdays and sent them presents. Among the young people, Uncle Jamie[2] and Aunt Elizabeth, though both distinctly alarming, were considered the good angels of the family.

Almost exactly two years after Henry Fawcett's first illness he was suddenly struck down at Cambridge by an attack of pneumonia. Millicent telegraphed to Elizabeth who went instantly, taking Sir Andrew Clark with her. When she saw Harry she telegraphed home that she would stay the night. That evening, 6 November 1884, he died, at the age of fifty-one. 'Our dearest Harry is gone,' wrote Elizabeth. 'It is a terrible calamity, a fine

[1] Anderson, L. G., op. cit. quoted p. 182.
[2] Elizabeth herself adopted his own family's pet name for James.

loving heart and a face set towards good in everything.'[1] From a relationship which might have been constrained, they had built a fruitful friendship. For Millicent it was an end and a beginning. From the time of her marriage she had acted as a secretary and reader to her husband. Society had regarded the blind man's helpmeet with sentimental 'approval, but an apprenticeship to blue books had developed in Millicent a considerable political intelligence. At the age of twenty-two she had spoken at the first public suffrage meeting held in London, when her youth and sincerity proved deeply appealing. Her mind, like her voice, was unemotional and very clear. Wearing the pretty clothes upon which Harry insisted, 'green silk with amber beads' or 'the beautiful pink-lined cloak', she had become increasingly in demand as a speaker on women's suffrage questions. Now, as a widow, she came to London to live for the rest of her life with Agnes in Gower Street. She refused the position of Mistress of Girton, because she knew her life's work lay in politics. When the National Union of Women's Suffrage Societies was formed, she was the obvious choice as its first president. Through all her years of public work, Millicent Fawcett used her great personal influence for good. She wanted votes for women, but refused to declare war between the sexes to get them. 'For my part', she maintained, 'I think that the spirit of generosity in men and of enterprise in women, is the spirit that brings progress.'

Elizabeth was always closely in touch with her own family, especially with her two sisters at Gower Street. Sometimes she went with them to the fisherman's cottage at Rustington in Sussex which Agnes had lovingly restored as a holiday home. There the Garretts were observed by young Ethel Smythe, gardening and swimming, or striding along the deserted shore in self-contained companionship. She found their reserve baffling, and their intense family loyalty exclusive towards the outsider.[2]

[1] Elizabeth Garrett Anderson to Skelton Anderson, 5 and 6 Nov. 1884. Anderson family papers.
[2] Smythe, E., *Impressions that Remained*, Vol. II, p. 54.

Elizabeth had never lost her love of the sea, and as her children grew out of babyhood determined to give them some of the health and freedom of her own childhood. Littlehampton and Bournemouth had both been tried, and found 'the dullest and dreariest of places', when, about 1880, Elizabeth received the gift of a house at Aldeburgh.

Newson Garrett had never willingly surrendered his daughters in marriage and was always looking for ways of gathering his grandchildren about him. During the 1870s a private company had bought thirty-five acres of land on the crest of the hill above Aldeburgh, planted ten thousand trees and planned to spend £5,000 on gentlemen's residences. The estate was to be called New Town and its success, according to the Aldeburgh Magazine, was certain. Success however was slow in coming, and while the company languished Newson stepped in and acquired the land.[1] He proceeded to lay it out as a private estate for his sons and daughters, with large houses and gardens surrounding the Alde House grounds, the whole designed in a strain of fantasy peculiarly his own. His country carts collected odd pieces of masonry or carving, a stone owl, a Corinthian capital or half a tombstone, which he embedded at will in the brickwork. Sam Garrett's house was named Gower House because it incorporated two truckloads of granite paving-stones which his father had commandeered from a demolition gang as he strode along Gower Street to visit Agnes.[2]

Elizabeth received West Hill, a large red-brick villa with lop-sided gables. It looked westward to the river, winding among its green marshes, and to the sunset in which the whole landscape of the Alde streams with translucent rays. Elizabeth loved West Hill. She spent holidays gardening with fierce energy in tweed suits and felt hats of singularly uncompromising design. She enjoyed being, for once, an ordinary housewife. 'A country house

---

[1] *East Anglian Daily Times*, 6 May 1893.

[2] Sam Garrett had become a highly successful lawyer, President of the Law Society and the first solicitor to accept women pupils in his office.

without servants and full of visitors is not exactly a rest for the mistress.' In a crisis she could always appeal to Skelton. 'Harry and Milly come here to stay tomorrow, so I particularly want you to arrive by the 6.30 train and to bring with you a very good rolled tongue, *not* a tinned one. It shd. be about 7/6. Be careful to get it from a trustworthy place, so that it is really good.'[1] Skelton cheerfully accepted such commissions, since he enjoyed Aldeburgh. His Scots eye had detected the possibilities of the open commons behind the town, where he founded a golf club.

At West Hill Elizabeth made for her children a home which reflected her own childhood. They could run by secret paths through the Alde House plantations to the beach to bathe. They could ride their pony Taffy, feed baby rabbits in the hutch, or swing on the home-made swing in the garden. 'It makes us feel sea-sick, it is so nice!' wrote Louie. They could catch roach in the garden pond and invite the cousins to fry it in Pig's Paradise, a children's cottage of two rooms with its own real stove and chimney.[2] Elizabeth was conscious of her own short-comings when compared with more home-keeping mothers. 'I never really know how to play with my own children,' she once said regretfully to an old friend.[3] She had insight enough to know she would quickly have become bored with unrelieved nursery routine. Yet her attitude had certain advantages from the children's point of view. She loved them, not as extensions of herself, but as people in their own right, entitled to their own opinions and interests. She and Skelton were both formidable personalities, but family letters make it plain that their children did not find them unapproachable. Skelton, a lion in the boardroom, allowed himself to be called 'dearest Poodle', a title of which the feminine was 'Moodle'. Even in London, Elizabeth went on bus

---

[1] Elizabeth Garrett Anderson to Skelton Anderson, 6 Sept. 1883. Anderson family papers.

[2] It still stands, very dilapidated, in an overgrown corner of a garden at Aldeburgh.

[3] Margaret Morison to Louisa Garrett Anderson.

and underground excursions with them to exercise their collie dogs, Col and Don of the strident bark. They romped on her bed in the early mornings, she never forgot to reward courage at the dentist with 'tooth money', and on foggy winter afternoons she staved off boredom with exciting games of Old Maid.[1] Above all, she talked to them as equals and listened to what they had to say in reply. She told them of a baby cousin born posthumously. Louie, aged eleven, said, 'Why, I thought babies could not come without fathers,' upon which Alan said, 'Well, I suppose God had started making this one to their pattern and he would not like to poison the poor little thing, would he Moodle?' Louie, 'No, and as it was being made specially *for them*, he could not send it to anyone else, I suppose,'[2] All this, with an account of their daily doings, Elizabeth recorded in letters to Skelton whenever business or a shipbuilding at Glasgow took him away from home.

In the autumn of 1884 Elizabeth's two lives, the private and the professional, were running so smoothly that she felt able to take another holiday abroad with Millicent, this time accompanied by sixteen-year-old Philippa Fawcett. Elizabeth equipped herself with studded boots and a curious little Boy Scout knife and fork for her idea of perfect pleasure, eight hours' hard walking and sightseeing every day. 'This sort of life is as blessed for the mind as Aldeburgh and the grey pony to the body,' she wrote in one of her daily letters home, 'no late lying in bed in the morning, no late starts, no grandeur!'[3] At Dresden she enjoyed the picture gallery, the china works and the opera equally. The Rhineland reminded her of her girlhood and her steady unfolding from that 'chrysalis stage'. 'When I was last here', she told Skelton, 'I was about Philippa's age. Life has gone very well with me since

[1] Elizabeth Garrett Anderson to Skelton Anderson, 19 Jan–10 March. Ten letters. Anderson family papers.

[2] Elizabeth Garrett Anderson to Skelton Anderson, 19 July 1884. Anderson family papers.

[3] Elizabeth Garrett Anderson to Skelton Anderson, 7 Sept. 1884. Anderson family papers.

then.'[1] Elizabeth returned from her holiday in high spirits to celebrate in October 1884 the tenth anniversary of the founding of the London School of Medicine. The founder would not be present; Sophia Jex-Blake could not bring herself to face a scene with such poignant associations. They must, however, have a party, 'and if I give a party,' said the Dean firmly to the students, 'it is a good one.' The Council voted ten pounds from the funds, and the students ran a 'Medical Dogs' Show' to raise money for hiring an awning. The beautiful little Adam House in Henrietta Street, where George IV had long ago visited Mrs Fitzherbert, was opened for an evening conversazione. Guests admired the panelled rooms, the long verandah, the garden overhung by a graceful weeping ash. They went away happy, and no one enjoyed the evening more than Elizabeth.

She was at this peak of confidence and happiness when suddenly, out of a clear sky, a series of misfortunes and sorrows struck her family. There was the illness of Henry Fawcett, already recorded, which led to Millicent's widowhood. In the same week Skelton Anderson was called to Aberdeen to the deathbed of his father. While he stayed on for the funeral and Elizabeth was alone in London, to her horror Louisa fell suddenly and seriously ill, apparently from a kidney infection. She was just eleven and a half, 'a bright, skipping little creature, full of character and intelligence'. Elizabeth nursed her in woollen blankets, fed her on sips of milk and water, and read aloud to her by the hour from *Robinson Crusoe*. She was haunted by the memory of nursing Margaret, nine years before, and at forty-eight she was less resilient than she had been then.

> I have been waiting in my heart all night and day [she wrote to Skelton], trying to put thought away while my duty lay elsewhere. . . . It will be too late to telegraph after [Sir Andrew] Clark leaves in the evening, but I will write then and telegraph

[1] Elizabeth Garrett Anderson to Skelton Anderson, 5 Sept. 1884. Anderson family papers.

early tomorrow. All I can feel is that we must try to be brave, or rather try to do what is right and to have self-command enough not to neglect any chance. But oh it *is* hard – that sweet darling the very centre of our heart's love. In spite of her delicacy, I had always thought of her as securely ours for years.[1]

The crisis of Louie's illness passed, but organic renal disease was suspected. 'Bed life', as Elizabeth feared, proved 'most un-wholesome to the nerves', and the poor child grew fretful and depressed. Elizabeth decided to abandon everything else and take her on a sea voyage.

Early in 1885 the Andersons, with both their children, sailed in one of the Orient Line's ships for a six-months' journey to Australia. It was the first time Elizabeth had taken a really long holiday since she began the study of medicine, twenty-five years before, and it had needed Louisa's dangerous illness to persuade her. She left her three colleagues in charge of the medical wards at the hospital[2] and enjoyed her freedom with immense gusto. 'I have scarcely had a day more full of physical pleasure than to-day,' she wrote home to Aldeburgh. Thankfully she rested her hard-worked body, read, wrote, worked a tapestry chair-back and watched her children gain strength from sunshine and sea air.

Australia, when they arrived, provided an unexpected en-counter. Elizabeth's eldest brother Newson Garrett, who had opposed her career when she was a girl, had himself gone into the army. After leaving the service and holding a variety of short-lived jobs, he had been sent in traditional black-sheep fashion to try his luck in a brickfield in New South Wales. Apparently this had not been a success, for suddenly one day he appeared at their hotel in Melbourne and asked for a loan. Skelton would have

[1] Elizabeth Garrett Anderson to Skelton Anderson, 29 Oct. 1884. Two letters. Anderson family papers.

[2] Louisa Garrett Anderson says that Mary Scharlieb took charge of the surgery, but she did not return to England until 1887. In 1885 it must have been left to some other member of the staff or to the male consultants.

given him money, but Elizabeth steadily refused. The vein of iron she had early shown in her dealings with her mother had never vanished where moral standards were concerned. She would go out of her way to help comparative strangers if they fulfilled her demands of courage and integrity, but had always disliked her brother's social pretensions, his contemptuous attitude to the Indians when serving in that country, and his shiftlessness about money. Not even family loyalty could overcome her rejection of all he stood for. She sent him away, though in her will she left him an annuity and she continued to welcome his wife and daughters in London.[1] This meeting was the only cloud on her pleasure in Australia.

On the homeward journey they called at Tristan da Cunha, where an islander's wife had just given birth to a son. Greatly struck by the sight of a woman doctor, the mother said to Elizabeth, 'I shall call my baby after you.' 'But Elizabeth is not a boy's name!' Elizabeth objected. The woman looked crestfallen. 'I know,' said Elizabeth, 'call him after my father; he is a very fine old gentleman.' The mother agreed and the small islander was christened Newson Garrett.[2]

By July 1885 the Andersons were back in Upper Berkeley Street, and Elizabeth returned to her life as a doctor. It had made a deep impression on popular opinion that Mrs Anderson, so successful in public and professional affairs, had been willing to put aside her career when her child's health was at stake. Elizabeth disliked any reference to this, which she regarded as an intrusion on her privacy; the mention of it in a newspaper more than twenty years later she considered 'complimentary and quite hateful'. Nevertheless it was important to public opinion which, in the 1880s, still wavered between accepting and rejecting the professional woman. Elizabeth Garrett Anderson's greatest service to the women's cause was her normality. Florence Nightingale had become the heroine of a nation and achieved incom-

[1] Mitchison, N., op. cit. pp. 189–90.
[2] Dr Ford Anderson to Louisa Garrett Anderson. Undated.

parable work by shattering her health and spending the rest of her life upon a couch, free from ordinary claims or duties. No one could suggest that as a pattern for the new woman's life. Elizabeth Garrett Anderson, by contrast, a 'thoroughly ordinary' woman with 'no particular genius' as she claimed, lived happily as wife and mother of young children, enjoyed the good things of life and yet did a man's work more than usually well. 'The woman question will never be solved in any complete way', she had written, 'so long as marriage is thought to be incompatible with freedom and an independent career.' She set herself to live 'two lives, the professional and the private'. Any woman since, who has attempted to do the same, must admire her.

CHAPTER SEVENTEEN

Building a Hospital
1886–1892

Each morning Elizabeth Garrett Anderson went to her hospital to make ward rounds. As she passed from bed to bed the members of her retinue, house surgeon, dressers and students from the school, learnt that in these crowded, poky rooms their chief insisted on standards of work worthy of a great teaching hospital. On diagnosis her teaching was: 'Get away from the bondage of theories and hypotheses; be able to question and cross-question facts until their full meaning becomes plain.' If she detected carelessness or inaccuracy, she could be scathing. 'There is absolutely no demand for an increased supply of mediocre doctors of either sex.' Visitors to 220–2 Marylebone Road marvelled at the quality of work that was done in the two little houses.

The main problem during the 1880s was to make staff and funds keep up with the number of patients. Skelton's sister Mary Marshall had qualified and joined the medical staff, bringing its number to four, all married women. By common agreement their policy was to have no masculine member of staff 'not even a tom cat!' This was not unreasoning prejudice on their part; hostile critics would have given credit for the success of their hospital to any man who happened to be on the premises.

In an average year Elizabeth reckoned to spend about £2,000, all raised by gifts and subscriptions.[1] She, the medical staff and the consultants all served without payment. In her case, since she

[1] New Hospital for Women *Annual Report*, 1881.

gave so much time to the hospital, this represented a very considerable loss of income, which fortunately she could afford. The patients contributed what they could, an average of one pound each for the whole length of their stay, or sixpence for a first visit as out-patients.

Patients came in steadily increasing numbers.[1] The mere fact of their presence was proof of their trust in a woman doctor. When Elizabeth asked, 'Have you been here before?' a common reply was 'No, but a friend of mine has', or 'A fellow-workman told my husband his wife had been here'. Elizabeth cherished a letter from a hearty Londoner who wrote, 'The lady doctors for me! I shall send all my friends here when they are ill.' Patients came from Wales and Scotland; one even made the journey from America to be operated on by Elizabeth.[2] In 1886 she performed a rare and dangerous operation. 'My patient is doing excellently,' she wrote to Skelton who was in America on business. 'It turned out to be a very uncommon case and I have offered the tumour to the Museum of the College of Surgeons as [Sir Spencer] Wells says they have only one like it.' This was a tactful and unanswerable reminder to the surgeons of their women colleagues' existence. Two years later Elizabeth wrote, 'I have had an operation which I had never done before or seen done and which is more often than not fatal.' Later she added, 'Both the cases at 222 have done well, which as I was entirely without outside help is a great comfort. I shall leave them tomorrow practically convalescent.'[3] At fifty she was still in the position, which she had filled for nearly twenty years, of being the only staff member of the New Hospital for Women who undertook major surgery.

She was privately looking for a successor when, in 1887, Mary Scharlieb was driven by increasing exhaustion to leave the

[1] Two thousand five hundred out-patients in 1880 had become more than four thousand by 1885, more than five thousand by 1887, and a total of 15,488 attendances was recorded in 1888.

[2] Elizabeth Garrett Anderson, MS. draft for a speech, Royal Free Hospital School of Medicine.

[3] Quoted in Anderson, L. G., *Elizabeth Garrett Anderson*, pp. 245–6.

humidity of Madras and begin her career over again in London. Elizabeth at once went to call at her lodgings. 'Don't worry,' she said, 'I can put plenty of work in your hands.' 'But what should I charge,' asked Mary Scharlieb diffidently, 'for an ordinary consultation at my own house?' 'Oh, I should think one guinea,' said Elizabeth, looking round the shabby room. 'Yes, one; you are certainly not smart enough for two.' She appointed Mary Scharlieb as assistant lecturer at the school, and shortly after went abroad for a holiday with Skelton, leaving her in charge of all the surgical beds. Generously she insisted that any new private patients should remain with her locum.[1] The hospital committee protested, but as usual Elizabeth had her way. When she returned she demanded a detailed account of the cases and, armed with this, went to her committee demanding that Mary Scharlieb should be appointed her clinical assistant. In February 1888 the appointment was made, and though Elizabeth still operated, the surgical ward was put under her assistant's care.[2]

The change was overdue, for Elizabeth, as the leading woman doctor in London, had endless calls on her time. She repaid a debt of gratitude by serving with Emily and Llewelyn Davies on a committee for the admission of women to Cambridge degrees as well as degree examinations. The Council of the Senate by eight to seven declined to consider the matter. In 1890, when a proposal to admit women to the M.B. degree threw Oxford into a furore, it fell to her to write to *The Times*: 'I am unable to believe that if the statute is passed Oxford is threatened with moral cataclysm.'[3] The proposal was defeated, but only by four votes.

Elizabeth was always on the alert for any circumstance that could be turned to the advantage of her hospital staff or her students at the school. When in 1886–7 all nineteen of her candidates passed their finals, she made sure that this hundred per cent success was known in the medical world. When women practitioners were

[1] Scharlieb, M., *Reminiscences*, p. 128.
[2] ibid. p. 146.
[3] *The Times*, 18 Nov. 1890.

admitted to post-graduate lectures at Charing Cross Hospital,[1] this made a good springboard for a tactful approach to the Harveian Society. Could she 'be admitted to some dark obscure corner to hear the lectures on lupus? The good Charing X people are admitting women to their post-graduate course, so it wd. not be quite novel if the Harveian Soc. were disposed to be gracious. Do not trouble to answer unless you find you can say "Yes".'[2]

Tactful in what she asked for, Elizabeth was equally tactful in what she avoided. She seldom made the same mistake twice, and having burnt her fingers over the Contagious Diseases Acts, she was careful not to involve medical women in any controversy likely to lose them support. During the 1870s and '80s the growing tolerance of public opinion in matters of politics and religion was balanced by an intensified intolerance of everything connected with sex. Elizabeth Blackwell, who was not in active practice, lectured on sex education and sexual hygiene; women doctors, she told the students of the school, 'must be the moral guides of society'. Elizabeth Garrett Anderson, by contrast, took care not to move too far in advance of public opinion, especially on sexual questions. In 1885, when W.T. Stead began his campaign in the *Pall Mall Gazette* against juvenile prostitution, she refused to be drawn in. She did not dispute the facts, but she thought Stead's sensational journalism harmful to the women's cause. She wrote, 'I myself believe such things are done on some scale or other, having seen children on the streets, or creatures dressed up to represent children. But I cannot accept Stead's methods.'[3]

She was equally cautious on the subject of birth control. By many people contraception, from whatever motives, was regarded as evidence of immorality. In 1876, after the prosecution of Bradlaugh and Mrs Besant for circulating a pamphlet said to

[1] London School of Medicine *Annual Reports*, 1887 and 1888.
[2] Elizabeth Garrett Anderson to Mr Hutchinson, 25 Nov. 1887. Royal College of Physicians.
[3] Strachey, R., *Millicent Garrett Fawcett*, p. 111.

contain indecent physiological detail, the latter lost the custody of her daughter, and the little girl, shrieking and struggling, was forcibly removed from her. As late as 1887 a doctor was struck off the Medical Register for issuing a 'Wife's Handbook' at sixpence a copy. Yet no one knew better than a woman doctor in hospital practice how desperate was the need for contraception among the really poor. Freedom and equality were meaningless words while the wives of working men still bore the crushing burden of almost continuous pregnancies. A select committee in 1890 found that 'there is a very considerable number of infants in this country who are starved to death each year, often to cash in on insurance policies'. Baby-farming, infanticide and criminal abortion were on the increase, a fact which must have been well known to Elizabeth Garrett Anderson, since it formed the subject of a campaign by a personal friend, E. A. Hart, editor of the *British Medical Journal*. Yet she chose to remain silent in public on the subject of family planning. Contraception, by whatever means, was never mentioned in the courses at the London School of Medicine for Women, and its graduates were perplexed if in general practice they were asked for advice on this point. A young woman doctor, being interviewed for her first assistant-ship, was asked for her views on birth control. She replied tentatively that she had always thought large families rather jolly, and was relieved when this appeared to be the right answer.[1]

The entry of new students to the London School of Medicine in 1885 and 1886 had been the largest ever. Elizabeth as Dean pointed out that 'Rooms and tables to accommodate twenty or thirty will not do for double that number, and the students are suffering from the overcrowding.' The Governors recognized that they would have to rebuild eventually, but meanwhile she insisted, in spite of the protests of the neighbours, on a temporary 'Iron Room' in the garden. In a manner with which any member of an educational body will be only too familiar, the temporary Iron Room became a permanency. Here for thirteen years chemis-

[1] Personal information Miss Louisa Martindale, F.R.C.O.G.

try and anatomy classes grilled or froze according to the season, while the sound of rain on the roof competed with the demonstrator's voice. By 1888 the school was again overcrowded, and during this summer recess Elizabeth and the executive spent £500 of capital on alterations. This drew down upon her the anger of Sophia Jex-Blake, who had now founded her own medical school for women in Edinburgh. She wrote protesting at the use of capital, and claiming that in Edinburgh she achieved 'complete professional efficiency on a much smaller outlay'. 'I trust', she ended, 'that my very great interest in the welfare of the school for which I am perhaps more directly responsible than any other will be my excuse for this long letter.'[1] Not dismayed by this, nor by the dirt and dilapidation of years, Elizabeth took possession of the house next door and by autumn 1889 had it ready to receive the overflow of students. A boarding house was also opened in Mecklenburgh Square for student clerks and dressers on call day and night.

At the hospital no such temporizing measures were possible. The lease of the houses in Marylebone Road was running out, and the owner, Lord Portman, refused to renew it. A crowd of poor women and their babies, waiting outside the hospital every afternoon for the out-patients' clinic to open, was not an advantage to property-holders in the neighbourhood. Elizabeth soon learnt that Lord Portman was not alone in his objection to her patients. During 1888 she wasted hours looking at large houses in Marylebone and Bloomsbury suitable for conversion.

If we were free to choose a house as private people would, I could have found excellent quarters over and over again [she reported]. But everywhere the landlord objected to a hospital and the only houses we could have bought were wretched tumbledown places in the most squalid districts.[2]

[1] London School of Medicine, *Governor's Minutes*, 18 July 1888. MS., Royal Free Hospital School of Medicine.
[2] Elizabeth Garrett Anderson. MS. draft for a speech, Royal Free Hospital School of Medicine.

After long consultation the committee decided to buy a site and build a hospital of forty beds, nearer the London School of Medicine for Women. Before the year was out, they had bought a seventy-years' lease of 144 Euston Road for £3,000.[1]

Elizabeth Garrett Anderson assumed responsibility for the financial as well as the medical, surgical and administrative work of the hospital. She planned a campaign which should be of value not only in raising money but in educating public opinion about the work of women doctors. It opened on 6 July 1888 with a meeting at the Mansion House, chaired by the Lord Mayor and shrewdly buttressed with snob appeal. Elizabeth's trump card was a letter from Florence Nightingale. She sent a donation of fifty pounds, thereby becoming a life governor of the hospital, and a letter which was read aloud to the crowded audience.

> You want efficient doctors for India most of all [she wrote] whose native women are now our sisters, our charge. There are at least 40 millions who will only have women doctors, and who have none. But for England too you want them. What woman of us has not known many, many poor women who would rather go through any suffering than undergo the necessary examination before men students at a general hospital? To the Women's Hospital, women by preference would go. . . . We want to press the whole of women's faculties, the scientific, the executive, as well as the sympathetic and the more contemplative into the service of the sick, which is the highest service of the noblest love. Good speed to the Women's hospital is the earnest prayer of – Florence Nightingale.[2]

Elizabeth was able to announce that plans for the new hospital, drawn up by J. H. Brydon, were being submitted to Miss Nightingale for approval – a tactical triumph on her part.

The staff of the hospital were whirled along on the tide of

[1] See Appendix VI.
[2] Florence Nightingale to the Governors, 6 July 1888. Elizabeth Garrett Anderson Hospital.

their chief's determination. 'Mrs Anderson was not the woman to let the grass grow under her feet,' wrote Mary Scharlieb with rueful admiration, 'nor was she one to consider unduly the effects of overwork or fatigue on herself and her colleagues. She was a persistent, shameless and highly successful beggar.' One day she appeared at the building committee and said,

> I wrote to some friends in the country asking them to contribute liberally; they sent £100, but I returned it immediately with a note saying 'If old friends and rich people like you send me £100, what can I expect from the general public? I quite thought you would send me £1,000!

She laid a cheque on the table. 'The £1,000 came by return of post!'[1]

To carry out the educational side of her campaign Elizabeth had to overcome her dislike of personal publicity. She was photographed working at her table, a woman in the early fifties, in bustle suit and striped gilet, with austere chignon, beautifully kept hands and strong face. She gave a speech with which she took great pains, drafting and re-drafting it upon any scraps of paper that came to hand, old letters, fly-leaves, discarded reports. In it she told with modesty and considerable humour the story of her own early struggles and the founding of the hospital and the school. 'Now', she said, 'we pursue exactly and strictly the same education as the men, pay the same fees, pass the same exam. side by side with the men and get the same diplomas – or sometimes we don't get them, also like the men!' The one disadvantage women doctors suffered, she said, was lack of practical experience after registration, since no general hospital would offer them house jobs. As physicians and surgeons they needed this training. 'If we want to learn a new step in dancing, we have to do it in order to learn, a new stitch in needle work, a fresh knot, a trick with cards, anything which requires a complete command of hand and eye in an unfamiliar way, has to be practised – *to be done*, not

[1] Scharlieb, M., op. cit. p. 155.

merely *to be seen.'* No one needed this practice more than the young doctors who would go out year after year to work in India. Skilfully she played upon this theme of India, the vast, lonely field of work to which women doctors had been led by Providence. 'Our New Hospital must do its utmost to drill them in practical work before they start. To do this we must not cease to exist for want of a house.' With a good deal of effort and much crossing out, Elizabeth succeeded in ending on a personal note most unusual for her. 'I have had the honour of being a leader, and so far as my limited powers permitted, I have tried to *lead* . . . and while my day lasts, I want to see this work completed.'[1] The speech was so successful that she repeated it at thirty-seven different meetings, not only raising money but finding in all classes of the community an unexpected interest in her work.

By 7 May 1889 the site had been cleared for the Princess of Wales to lay the foundation stone of the new hospital. It was the first gesture of royal recognition towards the hospital and Elizabeth made the most of it. The day was dull, but she had provided a huge marquee, filled with palms, shrubs and flowers. The Artists Rifles, whose depot was nearby, provided a guard of honour and a band, Liza Lehmann sang and the Archbishop of Canterbury led the prayers. Elizabeth made a brief speech. The contractors, Messrs. Higgs and Hill in person, were presented. The Princess tapped with her silver trowel, while press reporters fervently described the graceful figure in green velvet dress and bonnet with diamond stars. They also mentioned, as Elizabeth intended they should, the novelty of a woman's hospital staffed entirely by women. A very large crowd gathered in the street to cheer the royal party as it drove away. The publicity was all that Elizabeth could have hoped.[2]

Florence Nightingale was not so easy to manipulate for

[1] Elizabeth Garrett Anderson, MS. draft for a speech, Royal Free Hospital School of Medicine.
[2] *The Times, The Pall Mall Gazette, The Daily Telegraph, The Standard,* 8 May 1889.

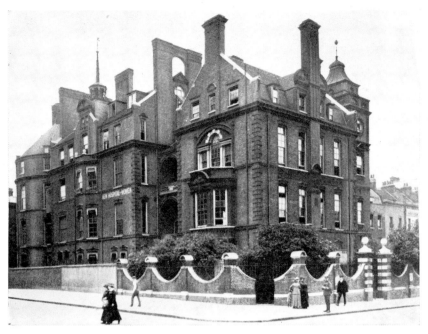

11a. The New Hospital for Women.
It had started its work in a house like those on the right of the picture

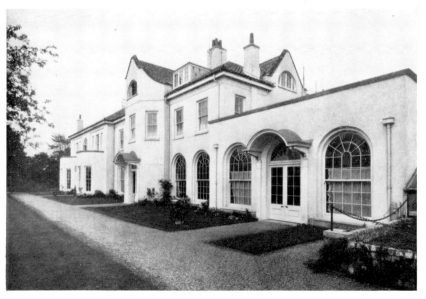

11b Alde House showing the additions built by Elizabeth Garrett Anderson

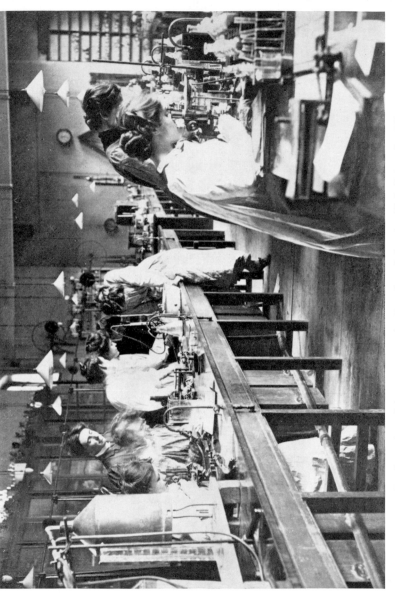

12. Students in a laboratory at the London School of Medicine for Women

publicity purposes. She returned the plans with a characteristic note.

The first thing for a hospital is that it should do the patient no harm. In the women's hospital there will always be a large number of the cases most sensitive to hospital harm, that is not only to foul air, but want of fresh air, or light of sun, of cubic space, to whom any crowding is *fatal overcrowding*.

There followed detailed and severe criticisms of the plans by herself and Sir Douglas Galton, chairman of the Sanitary Institute. How Elizabeth received these is not revealed, but work on the building went forward without any apparent alteration. By 25 March 1890 the hospital was ready for the patients to move in. When the time came to leave the 'Old New', the committee wished to change its name to The Elizabeth Garrett Anderson Hospital but its founder would have none of this. The change of name they desired had to wait until after her death.

The new hospital was built of bright red brick diversified with terracotta decorations and a variety of gables, soon to receive a bloom of Euston soot. Indoors, narrow passages, sharp turns and unexpected flights of stairs complicate its work to this day.[1] Yet the interior had character, a homeliness that flowed from Elizabeth's warm feeling for her sick women. The wards were comfortable, with polished parquet floors, bookcases, bedspreads of scarlet Turkey twill, old brown milk-jugs full of flowers and, as well as central heating, small open fires 'just to look at'. Here, before the patients arrived, Elizabeth organized a three-day bazaar to cover moving expenses. She herself presided with gusto over the hat stall. The main feature of the sale was an Indian temple where Hindu ladies in saris sold Benares brass,

[1] J. M. Brydon, who had worked in Norman Shaw's offices, was a partner in the firm where Alice Garrett trained, and like her, an 'unashamed Queen Annist'. His works include St Peter's Hospital Covent Garden, Chelsea Public Library and the pump room extension at Bath. He described his style as 'Georgian type English Renaissance', but the modern reader will recognize it more readily under the title 'Pont Street Dutch'.

embroideries and lacquer trays. Elizabeth was determined to identify her hospital with the work in India which had such strong public appeal. She was right. 'There can be no doubt,' wrote an intelligent and sympathetic journalist, 'that the imperative demand for medical women in India has had a great moral effect in disarming opposition to the education of women as physicians and surgeons'.[1] Privately, Elizabeth remarked that young women doctors come back from India 'a shadow of their former selves' and she would rather see them practise in England and earn good incomes.[2]

By the middle of May 1890 the forty-two beds of the new hospital were filled with patients. Twice as many could be treated, and for the first time the public could see medical women at work in a real hospital building. Elizabeth opened a room on the ground floor as a medical women's institute, where she began to build up a library of medical journals and transactions for the last twenty years, as well as important modern works on obstetrics and gynaecology from England, France, Germany and America.[3] Young medical women could at last hope for house posts; Elizabeth usually appointed her medical and surgical residents, anaesthetist and clinical assistants from among the graduates of the London School of Medicine for Women. The out-patient department, operating theatre and wards were open to students of the school; there was room to hold lectures and case discussions in the hospital building. It was possible at last to open a Maternity Department, where in the first year eighty-two women entered their names, and it is hard to say whether they or the students appreciated the service more.[4] In the rigid social hierarchy of British Medicine, immense prestige and influence attaches to a teaching hospital. Women now had one of their own, and it had taken precisely Elizabeth's combination of idealism with worldly wisdom to bring it about. Within the social framework of England in the 1880s, intelligence and devotion were not by themselves

[1] *The Queen*, 5 July 1890.   [2] Anderson, L. G., op. cit. p. 234.
[3] *British Medical Journal*, 21 Feb. 1891.
[4] London School of Medicine *Annual Report*, 1891.

likely to achieve material results. When allied to wealth, social position, influential friendships and an extremely hard head for business they could, and at the New Hospital did, work wonders.

The improved status of women doctors began to show itself. The British Medical Association, always a sensitive barometer, held its summer meeting in July 1892 at Nottingham, where Dr J. H. Galton proposed to expunge the twenty-year-old resolution barring women members. Elizabeth, called on to second, did not make a fighting speech. Instead she said. 'You are all disciples of Darwin and his great theory of evolution. Here before our eyes is the great evolution of women out of one stage into another. If you are all really good Darwinians, you will help this evolution.' Only three or four hands out of three hundred were raised against the motion.[1]

The years around 1890 were a high-water mark in the family fortunes of the Garrett family. Since young Mr Garrett went to London to make his fortune, England had absorbed in turn the Oxford movement, the rationalism of the Darwinians, imperialism, international socialism, the feminist movement and a vast increase in population. The country had peopled parts of three continents with hungry emigrants from its villages and towns. In the 1880s it had led the scramble for overseas possessions. It had enfranchised the labourer, though not his wife. It was even being dragged, kicking and struggling, to face the problem of Ireland. The Garrett family, like England itself, had observed change with steady, plain self-confidence. Newson Garrett, fighting old age as stoutly as he had fought his worst enemies in the Borough, stood for election under the reformed constitution of Aldeburgh and was elected first mayor under the new charter, wearing a chain of office presented by his children. In 1889 he was elected first county councillor and alderman for Aldeburgh. 'Ought you now to be addressed as *Alderman* Newson G.?' wrote Elizabeth, congratulating him. Affectionately she urged the old gentleman to have 'lunch and a rest before the meeting, then

[1] *British Medical Journal,* 30 July 1892.

dinner and a little good wine before starting home'.[1] Newson's vigour seemed undiminished. From his chair at a dinner for Queen Victoria's Golden Jubilee he promised 'a room worthy of the town'. He built at his own expense the Jubilee Hall, familiar to patrons of the present-day Aldeburgh Festival. When Newson Garrett's fellow townsmen elected him, at the age of seventy-eight, to a third term of office as mayor, his emotions remained as volatile as ever. 'Did Grandpa cry much?' asked Louie with interest after the ceremony. Nor would he submit to being looked after. When old age reduced him to a pony-drawn bath chair, he still insisted on driving himself and by speeding contrived to overturn even this sedate vehicle.

In June 1890 he went to Cambridge for a great family occasion. Among shouting, cheering and clapping in the Senate House, the name of Millicent's daughter Philippa Fawcett was read out as being 'above the Senior Wrangler' in the Mathematical Tripos. She was in fact 400 marks ahead of the Senior. Her mother and her aunts felt too keenly to dare to be present, but old Newson, though 'a good bit upset', heard the proceedings out.[2] Two years later another of his grandchildren, Alice's son Philip Cowell, was also placed Senior Wrangler; Newson was immensely proud of them both.

A few weeks after Philippa's triumph, Elizabeth's son Alan Garrett Anderson, who had done extremely well at his preparatory school at Elstree, won a scholarship to Eton. 'I can fancy all the kissings!' wrote his sister from school. As well as being intelligent and affectionate, Alan was in every way a boylike boy, devoted to dogs, pet rabbits, ponies, swimming, skating, sailing paper boats and reading *Ally Sloper*. He was companionable to his father, with whom he tramped round the Aldeburgh golf course,

[1] Elizabeth Garrett Anderson to Mr Garrett, 2 Feb. 1889. Anderson family papers.
[2] The undergraduates at Newnham, celebrating with fireworks in the garden, were joined by some young men from a neighbouring college. The head parlourmaid of Newnham, with the personality of a female butler, sent a message to the Principal: 'Do not be alarmed. I am here.'

and it seems to have been agreed at an early age that he should go into the family firm. Louie worked hard at school, wrote amusing letters home and was a devoted daughter. Everything their mother touched appeared to prosper. 'Mrs Garrett Anderson', remarked a much younger woman doctor, 'embodied those factors to success which the modern woman demands, skill in her profession, good social position, wealth, happy married life, absence of sentimentality. She understood her world, demanded much from it and obtained much.'[1]

Reality is seldom quite as simple as appearance. The woman who by her very presence could transfuse confidence to others, was prey to a secret, gnawing anxiety. The object of her fears was her daughter Louie, now entering upon adolescence. On Louie was concentrated all the love for young, growing feminine creatures, dammed up by the deaths of Elizabeth's adored sister and her baby girl. During Louie's childhood Elizabeth had been intensely happy. The shock when in 1884 Louie too was touched for a moment by death's finger remained to haunt her mother for a decade. She still believed, in common with her contemporaries, that the tubercular infection which had killed Margaret was hereditary. Perhaps at a deeper level she suffered an unconscious need to punish herself for the happy and successful career she had not given up when Louie was born. Her fears might have been eased if she had discussed them openly, but her rigid reserve in all personal matters forbade this. Only in letters to Skelton does anxiety for Louie's health form a pitiful, repetitive refrain.

A year after her illness Louie was well enough to go to school again. There were a number of girls' high schools now open in London, but for the sake of bracing air she was sent away in the autumn of 1886 to St Leonard's School.[2] For a sheltered thirteen-year-old, Louie met the change with detachment. 'It was one of the most delightfully unhappy days I have ever had, I think, for

[1] Martindale, L., *The Woman Doctor*, pp. 60–1.
[2] Founded at St Andrews by Louisa Lumsden, one of the first graduates of Girton.

I cried on and off, nearly the whole day.' She had pluck and intelligence; soon she was doing well in class, acting in amateur theatricals and helping to edit the school magazine. Her cousin Mona Geddes was at school with her and her Aberdeen aunts within reach; the sharp, frosty climate appeared to suit her and some colour came back into her cheeks. Nevertheless Elizabeth could not shake off her dread of illness. Years later she was still writing to Skelton, 'I am not happy about her. She eats so very little, especially of food of any value.'[1] 'L. is better. I have stolen all the serious books she brought with her, after speaking seriously to her and saying I really wished her to take complete rest.'[2] Louie was continually exhorted to wear warm clothes, take rest, a change of air, or, above all, more food. 'L. quiet and not looking well, but already I think looking a little better. I wish she were more satisfactory in mind and body. . . . We must hope balance will come before she kills herself from wanting it.'[3] Heat and cold alike were objects of dread to the anxious mother. 'She is provoking about her dress, *will* not put on an outside garment, though the wind is often cutting and she looks blue with cold.' On holiday the meals of this understandably rebellious adolescent were the subject of almost daily report. 'L. would eat nothing but bread and cheese for lunch and looked tired and white. Even then nothing would induce her to ride (instead of walking). I think she ought to know we are anxious, but she considers she is *quite well* and we are fussy.' Louie's creditable determination to lead a normal life in spite of being delicate met with no understanding. 'I think if she realized how her white face grieves me she would be more docile and manage herself better.'[4]

[1] Elizabeth Garrett Anderson to Skelton Anderson, 20 Sept. 1891. Anderson family papers.
[2] Elizabeth Garrett Anderson to Skelton Anderson, 8 April 1893. Anderson family papers.
[3] Elizabeth Garrett Anderson to Skelton Anderson, 7 Aug. 1893. Anderson family papers.
[4] Elizabeth Garrett Anderson to Skelton Anderson, 18 Aug. 1893. Anderson family papers.

Louie had inherited Elizabeth's independence of spirit, and though she loved her mother intensely, this anxious tutelage oppressed her. The death of a girl at the school threw Elizabeth into a panic.

> Perhaps I sent off a more excited letter than usual [wrote Louie in reply], but I don't think I have a mortal disease and I don't weigh the pros and cons of committing suicide. If I wrote to you in this frame of mind after having been impressed with Edith's peace and beauty, perhaps you will not misunderstand what I said, and think I meant something which I did not mean in the least.[1]

Next year Louie did in fact have a minor illness and Elizabeth wanted to rush to St Andrews.

> I must really expostulate against these sudden outbursts of excitement [wrote her daughter]. I do wish Miss Dove would not write to you about me. On Sunday I was a little wrong – not bad a bit – and since then my usual healthy appetite has not returned. . . . it's rather honest of me not to telegraph 'Not very ill but want Father to come'.[2]

When tension grew between these two, so devoted to each other and so dangerously allied in temperament, James Skelton Anderson held the balance between them. He had a rock-like character on which Elizabeth in times of weakness was glad to lean, and enough sense of humour to tease her out of obsessions. He was not an outwardly pious man, but his ethics were deeply engrained. 'Man is descended from the brutes,' he wrote to his sister Nellie; 'His present course is upwards and not downwards as held by the orthodox. . . . I think the substance of true religion is morality and so far as we are soundly moral we are "walking with God".' Elizabeth trusted his judgment and had experienced

---

[1] Louisa Garrett Anderson to Elizabeth Garrett Anderson, 20 July 1890. Anderson family papers.

[2] Louisa Garrett Anderson to Elizabeth Garrett Anderson, 7 March 1891. Anderson family papers.

the strength of his will. Only those very near to the family knew how much she relied on him.

At eighteen Louisa left St Leonard's. She had decided to read medicine, for she had an inherited interest in the subject, also perhaps a need to prove herself in the eyes of the mother whom, despite emotional friction, she so much admired. Before she entered the London School of Medicine, Elizabeth took her, Alan and a niece in September 1891 to Paris, where Louie was to spend a few weeks in a French family. Elizabeth's love had been for the Paris of the Second Empire. This was the Paris of the Third Republic; Boulanger had just fled with a charge of high treason hanging over his head and the name of Dreyfus was soon to ring around Europe. In the Place de la Concorde stood the crêpe-shrouded statue of Strasbourg. Yet the brilliance and rationality of French civilization still fascinated her. Together they travelled by river steamer along the *quais*, admired Versailles and the coloured fountains of the Trocadéro, and sat sleepily through an hour-long sermon at a French Protestant church. Even now Elizabeth's fears did not leave her. 'She ate next to nothing and had a bad headache. It is such a pity not to recognize that her spirit is in advance of her real strength. . . . She will turn into a sweet, delightful woman *if she lives*, but I should much like to see her stronger.'

Stress and anxiety were hidden from the world at large. Elizabeth Garrett Anderson's career was about to enter on a new phase. With her hospital rebuilt and continuing to cover its heavily increased expenses, her remaining task was to secure its future work. She decided, with whatever personal regrets, that paradoxically the only way to do this was to retire herself 'and give the younger women a chance'. To make the transfer smoothly would need skilful generalship of the Management Committee, which disliked change. Late in 1892 she announced that, though she would still act as a consultant, she had decided to retire from the staff of the New Hospital for Women. The committee, alarmed, implored her to remain, since in the eyes of the public she *was* the hospital.

296

At least, they begged, she must give them time to look for a successor. 'I have done better than that,' said Elizabeth firmly, 'I have provided a successor.' She reminded them that Mary Scharlieb had been in charge of her work during her long absences and that all had gone well. 'In my opinion you cannot do better than appoint her.'

She further told the committee that if they wanted the surgery of the New Hospital to be a credit to it they must put all the major surgery into the hands of one person. There were not enough cases in the wards to give good experience to more than one surgeon, she told them, and 'no one can operate well who is not operating constantly'. The committee had hardly taken this in when she went on to say they must give Mrs Scharlieb a regular first assistant, who by working continually with her could train as senior surgeon on her retirement.[1]

These proposals completely took away the breath of the committee, but Elizabeth had thought the matter out, and as founder and senior member of staff she was far too strong for them to fight. They made the appointment, and as their founder went off to her daily rounds they voted a resolution that 'to her indomitable energy and ability the hospital owes not only its foundation and its great and continued success, but that to her is owing the recognized and established position of medical women in England'.[2]

[1] Scharlieb, M., op. cit. pp. 134 ff.
[2] New Hospital for Women *Annual Report*, 1893.

CHAPTER EIGHTEEN

Portrait of a Dean
1893–1903

On 4 May 1893 Newson Garrett died at Aldeburgh. Two days earlier he had gone for a long carriage drive, and on the previous day had been in excellent humour. As he was getting into bed in the evening his heart suddenly ceased to beat; he left life swiftly enough even for his impatient spirit. He was buried in the family vault which he had built in Aldeburgh churchyard. Bunting flew at half-mast all along the beach; the mayor and corporation, the freemasons, the Volunteer Artillery, the lifeboat and coastguardmen followed him to his grave. Old Mrs Garrett survived her husband by ten years, continuing to pray for him serenely every day as she had in his lifetime. Her mind remained clear and her handwriting firm. She continued to order the affairs of Alde House and subscribe to her favourite charities, among them Elizabeth's hospital and the London School of Medicine for Women. She made her way to church on the bitterest winter Sundays and took a cold bath daily until her death. Steadily writing and receiving letters, she followed the careers of seventy-five children, grandchildren and great-grandchildren, recording every birth and death with appropriate moral sentiments. Elizabeth had once found her mother's pieties exasperating; now she regarded them with affection and respect.

For Elizabeth her father's death brought new responsibilities. She was his eldest child and he had made her, without respect of sex, heir of Alde House, its twelve acres of garden and the park lands adjoining, after her mother's death. The sons divided malt-ings, wharves and warehouses, while shares in the family firm were divided among his children.[1] In a career which might have formed a minor chapter of social history Newson Garrett had put together property to the value of £51,800.

Skelton Anderson was already an alderman of the Borough, a trustee of the lifeboat and the quay, and for the past five years a Justice of the Peace. Aldeburgh people, slow to accept strangers, had adopted this shrewd and kindly Scotsman as one of themselves. By general agreement he was invited to succeed his father-in-law as mayor. Elizabeth was both pleased and proud; she was determined that his year of office should be successful and threw herself ungrudgingly into the work it brought.[2]

In May 1896 Elizabeth, to her intense pleasure, was elected President of the East Anglian branch of the British Medical Association. She chose to give her first reception to the members in the grounds of Alde House. Newson was not there to see the triumph of the daughter in whom he had gloried; old Mrs Garrett wandered among the guests, welcoming the doctors in radiant forgetfulness of her horror thirty years before when Elizabeth had become one of them. Elizabeth gave a presidential address of some interest in its own right.[3] Its opening words might almost have been spoken by her father who had returned to make his fortune in the county of his birth.

My first duty [she said] is to thank you most heartily for the honour I am receiving at your hands. To be invited to preside over the senior branch of your Association would in any case be a great and valued distinction. The honour in my case is

[1] The exception, under the will, was his eldest son, Newson Dunnell. Skelton Anderson was one of three trustees appointed to hold his share 'in the residue of my estate as one of my nine surviving children', and to ad-minister it at their 'uncontrolled discretion'.
[2] Elizabeth Garrett Anderson to Skelton Anderson, 11 Oct. 1894. Ander-son family papers.
[3] See p. 320 below.

enhanced by the fact that it has been given by my own country-
men, by those among whom my family has lived for so many
years.

Her election was an encouragement to medical women everywhere, and she valued it for their sake as well as her own.

The 1890s were the years when as Dean she put her seal on the
development of the London School of Medicine for Women.
She had found it a jumble of small shabby houses, providing the
bare essentials of medical education. She was to leave it, through
wise administration, a college of London University. Members
of the executive committee found 'it was a treat to sit and listen
to Mrs Anderson's use of the English language'. Experience had
made her tactful and conciliatory, but she was still the same
woman who had roused the Board of the East London Children's
Hospital to fight a bad appointment. Her natural instinct was to
arrive at the root cause of any problem, and when occasion demanded she could denounce or condemn with scathing calm.[1]
She was bold but cautious. By 1892 she had convinced the committee that the school must eventually be rebuilt and was already
buying neighbouring houses to round off the site. In them she
contrived, at minimum cost, temporary laboratories, a pathology
museum and, for the first time, a common room.

Elizabeth took special care over relations with the Royal Free
Hospital. She spoke of the school as a bride, marrying the groom
of her choice. 'The alliance formed years ago has gone on very
comfortably and happily up to the present time and I hope there
is no reason to think it will ever end.'[2] In one year more than half
the honours in medicine at London University were taken by
students from the London School of Medicine for Women. The
connection was a credit to the hospital; the physicians and surgeons were now openly proud of their young women students.
The annual indemnity was a thing of the past; indeed the hospital

[1] Anderson, J. F., *A Pioneer*. MS. Anderson family papers.
[2] London School of Medicine *Annual Report*, 1894.

governors generously paid back to the school building fund a portion of the fees received for clinical teaching. The marriage had never been happier.

By June 1895 Elizabeth felt it was time to address to the Royal Colleges of Physicians and Surgeons a memorial asking for the admission of her students and other women candidates to the examination for the Conjoint Diploma in medicine and surgery. She pointed out that the two hundred women now on the Medical Register were generally accepted by their male colleagues, and their numbers were sure to increase. Yet they still had to face the fatigue and expense of a journey to Scotland or Ireland to obtain their Royal College Diplomas. The memorial presented on 8 July 1895 was signed by the lecturers of the School, by Paget, Spencer Wells, Broadbent, Treves, Hughlings Jackson and other leading doctors. It put the Royal Colleges in a position of some difficulty. The College of Physicians, with a caution proper to their calling, resolved to defer discussion to 'the close of October or the early part of November'. The Council of the College of Surgeons decided to submit the memorial to the annual meeting of Fellows and Members. There was something in the very idea of women doctors, as an observer had already remarked, 'which carries away a certain section of the profession and leads to the display of an antipathetic feeling unsurpassed in intensity by any which is called forth by any other professional topic'.[1] The annual meeting, representing the rank and file of the M.R.C.S., rejected the petition by 58 votes to 39. Meanwhile the Royal College of Physicians had also decided to refuse. After a long and apparently heated debate the Council of the College of Surgeons could only write to Elizabeth Garrett Anderson assuring her that 'had the matter rested solely with them the prayer of the memorialists would have been granted'.[2] This was at least something gained since 1861 when the college would 'in no way

[1] Rivington, W., *The Medical Profession*, 1st edn, p. 135.
[2] Royal College of Surgeons of England, Minutes of Council 1895–1897, pp. 19–21, 44, 75–8, 81. Royal College of Surgeons.

countenance' the entry of women to the profession. Elizabeth thanked them civilly and was prepared to wait. *The Lancet* remarked that 'so great has been the change of opinion in the profession on the general question'[1] that the present decision would probably be reversed; but women were not finally admitted to the Conjoint Diploma until 1910.

In the autumn of 1896 fifty new students entered the school, a record number since its foundation. A hundred and fifty-nine students were now crammed into the old houses and rebuilding could wait no longer. The executive committee took the decision to raise a loan and start rebuilding on the existing site, though in the process the charming, shady garden must be sacrificed.[2]

Elizabeth took considerable thought before appealing in the press. For one thing, rebuilding would almost certainly involve her in an open quarrel with Sophia Jex-Blake; for another, the whole idea of a women's college was less attractive to the charitable public than a hospital for women and children. The letter which she finally sent to *The Times* was drafted with some guile.

About thirty-five years ago a movement was initiated which had two objects in view. It aimed at enabling women to obtain, if they desired it, medical advice from qualified practitioners of their own sex, and at enabling such women as were able and willing to go through a long and severe professional training to earn their own living in a way not hitherto open to them. . . . The two things hung together; if medical women were welcomed they would be employed, and if employed a new and large field of professional work would be open to women.

The movement had succeeded, she claimed. The wards of the New Hospital were always full and there was a waiting list for admission; the school had aimed at quality rather than quantity in output and had always given first-class teaching.

[1] London School of Medicine *Annual Report*, 1896.
[2] London School of Medicine *Annual Report*, 1897. See Appendix VI.

These two bodies are *both* now in want of help. The New
Hospital has no endowment and this year it is behindhand with
the funds needed to pay Christmas bills. . . . The School has
for many years been carried on in small hired houses, and it is
now proposed to pull these down and build good laboratories,
library and lecture-rooms.

She invited any 'large hearted man or woman' to endow either
a bed at the hospital or a laboratory at the school, 'thus linking
his memory with the history of one of the most striking social
advances seen in the present generation'.[1]

This appeal called down upon Elizabeth, as she had feared, the
wrath of Sophia Jex-Blake. Relations between the two women
had followed their usual course ever since the storm over the
school's endowments in 1888. Sophia's friends had been anxious
over her Edinburgh School of Medicine for Women. 'It would in
my opinion', wrote the loyal Isabel Thorne, 'have been wiser to
have consolidated and developed the original school before starting another.' The Edinburgh School, like all Sophia's creations,
did excellent work which her passionate temperament then en-
dangered. In 1890 two of her students sued her for wrongful
dismissal, after she had accused them of 'mean and dishonourable
conduct'. They won their case and were awarded fifty pounds
damages with costs, which she had to meet.[2] That autumn a rival
women's medical school opened in Edinburgh. Sophia would
not, could not, conciliate. She refused to allow its students access,
with her own, to clinical teaching in the wards of Leith Infirmary.
At a large public meeting she was openly sneered and jeered at
by old adversaries of her Edinburgh student days. Elizabeth
could not work with Sophia Jex-Blake, but she would not allow
the accusation that the Edinburgh School 'exists for Miss Jex-
Blake's benefit'. Their quarrels had been honourable differences of
principle; she could not stand by and see Sophia suffer under this

[1] *The Times,* 11 Dec. 1896.
[2] *The North British Daily Mail,* 16 July 1890.

mean attack. 'Knowing what it costs in time, thought, labour and money to create and sustain even a small medical school,' she wrote to *The Times*, 'this statement seems to me one that ought not to have been made.' Instead, Sophia Jex-Blake should be publicly thanked for the 'immense services rendered by her in the last twenty years'.[1] It was bitterly humiliating to Sophia to receive support from this quarter. Still worse, students from the rival school, among them Elizabeth's niece Mona Geddes, were admitted to the Edinburgh Royal Infirmary, where she had so long battered in vain for admission. Their classes swelled as hers dwindled; in 1898 she was finally forced to admit defeat and give up.

It was therefore with deep resentment that Sophia Jex-Blake wrote on 27 January 1897 to protest against the rebuilding scheme at the London School. By her own request, her letter was printed and circulated to members of the Council. The increase in numbers, she said, was probably only temporary, and she accused the governors who had incorporated the school under the Companies Act of 'shifting on to the school a liability too great to be incurred by them personally'. Indignantly she questioned the need for 'this vast expenditure'. Elizabeth Garrett Anderson had expected this attack and was completely unshaken by it. 'The expense of altering the present premises would be considerable and the gains only temporary,' she said. The governors supported her, and the plans went forward. Sophia then wrote, 'As no attention was paid to my suggestion, I can but free myself from all responsibility in the matter. You will please report my resignation to the Executive Council.' This Elizabeth did on 26 May. Whatever she felt, relief, regret, sorrow for an old friendship, she did not allow it to appear. 'I know,' she said, 'that the governors will wish to record their appreciation of Doctor Sophia Jex-Blake's past services to the School. I feel sure that but for her energy and determination the School would never have been established in 1874, and that a deep debt of gratitude is owing to

[1] *The Times*, 2 March 1891.

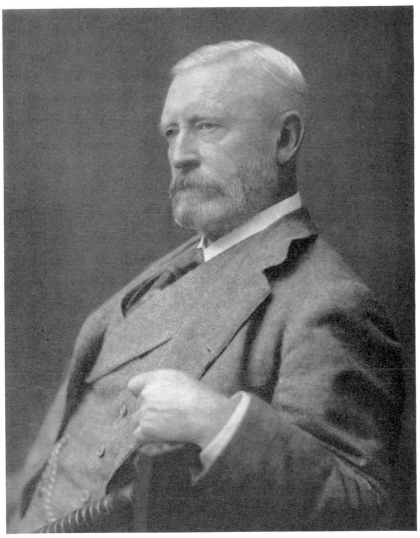

13. James Skelton Anderson during his Mayoralty at Aldeburgh

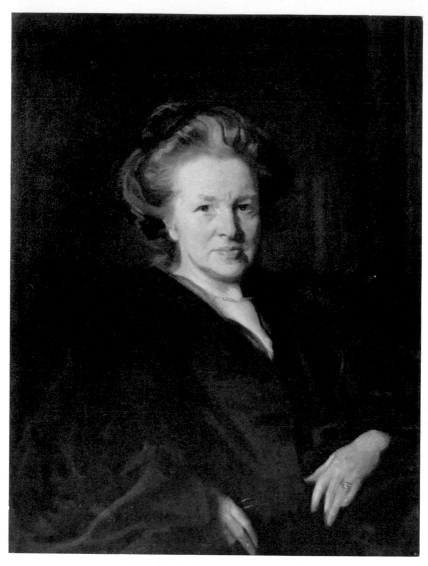

14. Elizabeth Garrett Anderson in 1901
painted by Sargent upon her retirement

her.'[1] This was generous and just; it formed a fitting end to a relationship, stormy but always sincere, which had lasted for thirty-five years. Sophia had broken the last link which bound her to the school and to Elizabeth.

In the long vacation of 1897 building work began on the new block at the end of the garden. It continued through the winter session and into the summer of 1898. Lawns were ravaged, disorder, dust and noise were continuous, but the Dean did not allow the work of the school to slacken. As the first building was completed, with physics, chemistry, anatomy and physiology laboratories, work began on a second right-angled wing which would link the new block with the old buildings. No sooner was this under way than a third wing was planned, giving a new library and a new entrance to the school, with a new address – Hunter Street – which it still retains.[2] Elizabeth was determined to get the work finished, restore order in the garden 'and give back to the students their lawn tennis court'. She resigned the post of Lecturer in Medicine, which she had held since the school opened in 1874, in order to concentrate on administration and keep a sharp eye on the builders.[3]

Meanwhile the hospital had already outgrown its new quarters. The wards were congested by teaching rounds from the school; there was nowhere to isolate infectious diseases, and no space to maintain vacant beds for casualties. Overcrowding in the out-patients' department was still worse. Doctors and nurses toiled their way through queues of waiting women, but Elizabeth would not allow them to hurry. 'It is of far more importance to the patients that they should be seen properly than that they should be dismissed with a word and a bottle of medicine, without careful enquiry into their case.'[4]

[1] London School of Medicine Council Minutes, 27 Jan., 3 Feb., 27 May 1897. MS., Royal Free Hospital School of Medicine.
[2] London School of Medicine *Annual Reports*, 1898 and 1899.
[3] London School of Medicine *Annual Report*, 1900.
[4] New Hospital for Women *Annual Report*, 1896.

She achieved one ambition for the hospital at a modest cost of £322. This was a room to serve as a pathological laboratory. She furnished and equipped it with gifts from friendly doctors, and encouraged her staff to work there. Women, as well as practising, should make some contribution to science and 'pathology is the basis of scientific medicine'. During the building operations at the school, the hospital received two large donations, and Elizabeth without hesitation began to build there as well. The outpatients' waiting hall was enlarged, to the relief of everyone concerned. A cancer ward was opened on the top floor and a new operating theatre built on the same floor as the surgical wards 'to avoid the labour involved in carrying the patients up and down stairs'. The staff themselves donated a new table, sterilizers and instruments. Sir Thomas Smith, who had assisted at Elizabeth's first ovariotomy operation, came some twenty-five times to watch major operations in the new theatre, and said in a public meeting how extremely good he thought the surgical work – 'indeed it could not be better'. His praise meant a great deal to her.

Throughout 1898 Elizabeth went to and fro between the Euston Road and Hunter Street sites, marshalling committees, balancing accounts and superintending building works. She had inherited Newson's knowledgeability and love for bricks and mortar; a dilatory plumber or careless bricklayer never knew when Mrs Garrett Anderson might appear at his elbow. Miraculously, to those with experience of large-scale public works, both buildings were finished in time. Brydon's style was better suited to college than to hospital building. The new laboratories were large and well lit, their fittings plain and solid. The roof of the south wing was low-pitched, so that the sun shone into the central courtyard. The sense of enclosure gave privacy for working and the inner rooms looked on to a paved garden. The Dean was photographed, a small but intensely dignified figure in academic dress, standing under the arches of the garden cloister.

11 July 1898 was fixed for the ceremonial opening of the new

school. Elizabeth, who had seen what royal approval could do for the hospital, secured the Prince and Princess of Wales for the occasion. The Prince agreed to visit the school beforehand, officially incognito. On the morning of his visit the Dean appeared carrying under her cape a small package, which she unwrapped in the privacy of her own office. It contained a bottle of excellent whisky, personally chosen. Refreshed from this, the Prince of Wales was taken upstairs by Elizabeth to the new chemistry and anatomy laboratories, where carefully selected students were at work. Whether they were chosen for scientific ability or feminine charm, the Prince was impressed. 'I can only say', he remarked, 'that I was very much struck by the assiduity of the students who were at work.'

The opening itself bore all the marks of a Garrett Anderson occasion. Elizabeth was up before anybody else to supervise the preparations. The devastated garden had been re-turfed and decorated with flags lent by the Orient Line, which flew gaily in the breeze. The students had arranged flowers in all the public rooms, and later served as ushers showing guests to their seats in the main hall. The staff in academic dress hovered over the tea-cups, ready to pour out for the royal visitors.[1] Outside the window a military band played vigorously in its tent, while in the street a regiment of policemen held back the crowd as swelling cheers in the distance announced the approach of the royal party. Among the 250 women doctors present was Elizabeth Blackwell, who never could understand the British adulation of royalty. She wrote home to America with refreshing tartness

. . . the Royal Party were arriving to occupy their gilded chairs: the fat Prince looking good-natured but silly, the ladylike Princess in a grey gauzy dress with a large boa of mauve-coloured ostrich feathers and a hat trimmed to match. Mrs

[1] *Le National*, 14 July 1898. 'Ce serait aller trop loin', noted the correspondent regretfully, 'que de prétendre que la coiffure academique anglaise est de nature à faire valoir les avantages d'une femme.'

Anderson, looking like a fat college don in her robe and
trencher (which is most unbecoming to her) read a long address, to which the Prince replied with fluent, amiable common-
places, patting the lady medicals on the back. Then a procession
of little tots presented small bags of money (occasionally
dropping one which the Prince picked up). Rev. Mr Paget made
appropriate prayer and finally all were invited to tea.[1]

Elizabeth Garrett Anderson understood her British public
better than Elizabeth Blackwell. The 'procession of little tots'
contributed some £4,000 to the building fund. More important,
the London School of Medicine for Women, like the New
Hospital for Women, was now assured of impregnable respectability. A month after the official opening, the school was granted
a Royal Charter of incorporation. With the willing consent of the
governors of the hospital it became the London (Royal Free
Hospital) School of Medicine for Women. What pleased Elizabeth
even more, the hospital committee unanimously decided to open
two of its resident posts to women. In 1902 the once struggling
school became a college of London University, with its lecturers
represented on the Faculty of Medicine.

The students gave a Christmas party in their new common
room, and the Dean, who believed in moving with the times,
contributed 'a cinematograph' for their entertainment. Her care
for them was serious and sincere. A good teacher does not build
in bricks and mortar, or even in institutions, but in people. Elizabeth Garrett Anderson taught generations of students her own
unemotional but deep devotion to the ethics of medicine. Medical
ethics were, for her, an aspect of religion. She seems to have felt,
as Huxley said, 'that a deep sense of religion was compatible with
the entire absence of theology'. She never lost her reverence
before the mysteries of birth and death. In a rare moment of self-
revelation, she spoke of 'that which is most precious in our life,
and surely one of the cornerstones of its foundation – Charity,

[1] Ross, I., *Child of Destiny*, p. 260.

that genuine care for others, which makes us ready to postpone our own interests, and even the interests of our children, when by doing so we can help'.[1] Elizabeth did not preach these virtues to the students, she lived them. 'What struck me more than anything', a student remembered, 'was her absolute honesty. I never met anyone who gave me such an impression of sincerity.'

The Dean could be stern, but she was fair and her students knew exactly what she demanded of them. Her demands began even before they were admitted. Candidates must have a good general education. To encourage this she herself served as a governor of the North London Collegiate School and Bedford College. After school they must not drift into a desultory home life where they would lose the habit of mental work. They should go, at eighteen, to university, where they could learn their preliminary science, and 'what women so much need, the value of self-guidance and government'. Her judgment of character was shrewd. She was not taken in by intellectual pretensions, nor did she under-value modesty. Indian students were particularly welcome at the school. The Dean was bold enough to say that purdah women and children needed women doctors of their own nationality, who would understand them as foreign missionaries never could. Once a student was accepted, Elizabeth demanded courage of body and mind. 'People who wish to be leaders', she said, '*must* lead.' She expected students to take responsibility for their own health. If they broke down, she told them, it would be from lack of food, lack of sleep and lack of proper holidays, not from 'overwork'. West Hill at Aldeburgh was filled in the vacations with students who could not otherwise afford the sea air and good food they needed.[2]

Sometimes a student near the beginning of her course was overwhelmed by the weight of work ahead. Elizabeth from her own experience encouraged such girls to look forward to the clinical part of their training, when the facts they had struggled to

[1] MS. draft for a speech: Royal Free Hospital School of Medicine.
[2] Scharlieb, M., *Reminiscences*, p. 139.

learn would gradually fall into place. 'No one dislikes dissecting, though everyone expects to do so,' she told Dr Rivington. 'The later subjects of study, medicine and surgery, are more attractive than the earlier ones, botany and materia medica; and surgery attracts more than medicine. Finally hospital practice is exceedingly popular.'[1]

For many women public examinations represented a terrifying ordeal. Elizabeth did not attempt to minimize this, nor to deny that some of them would fail, but she did ask them not to concentrate on examinations at the patients' expense. On the whole, women candidates met with courtesy from their examiners. She told of a woman who had emerged from her viva at Dublin, to find a crowd of men waiting outside. 'Did he *curse* at you?' they asked. 'Oh no,' said the young woman, surprised. 'He was very civil.' 'Civil to you, was he?' said the Dubliners. 'Well, he curses us!' On the other hand students might meet the rare bully, who does his best to shatter the nerve of the candidate, whether man or woman. In that case it was their duty, and their only hope, to put a bold face on it.

Once they were well qualified, she thought women particularly well suited to public health work and preventive medicine. She wanted to see her graduates as medical officers in workhouses, women's prisons, asylums and school boards, as well as in counties and boroughs. In 1899 Dr Barnardo appointed the first medical woman to supervise children boarded out in families by the Barnardo Homes, and the experiment was a notable success. At the New Hospital, Elizabeth opened a clinic for public vaccination, believing that women doctors would be able to overcome the mistrust of this procedure among working-class mothers. Former students served as medical officers to the L.C.C. and the Metropolitan Asylums Board. By 1900 the demand for graduates of the school in public health posts exceeded the supply.[2] This seemed to the Dean to justify her policy of 'quality rather than quantity'.

[1] Rivington, W., op. cit. 2nd edn, 1887, pp. 290–1.
[2] London School of Medicine *Annual Report*, 1900.

She was not concerned by the relatively small number of medical women in training. It was to be expected since parents had to meet the full cost from their own pockets. The real scope of her work did not show itself until after her death, when state-aided students in ever larger numbers enjoyed the rights she had won for the few.

Graduates from Hunter Street had been well schooled in professional etiquette. 'The first thing women must learn', said their Dean, 'is to behave like gentlemen.' Her standards of gentlemanly conduct covered every side of their working life. They must be courteous to their colleagues, the nurses, their patients, however poor and humble. She quoted Sir James Paget. 'Always do unto others as you would they should do unto you and your etiquette will be perfect.' They must resist the temptation to seek personal publicity. A notice in Elizabeth's largest and firmest handwriting hung in the common room; it drew students' attention to the resolution of the B.M.A. Ethical Committee that the publication of biographical details in the press, 'partaking more or less of the nature of advertisement is undesirable and improper'. She could not endure loud or hearty manners and her standards of dress were impeccable. 'Now put on your smartest evening gown, my dear, and come with me to a reception,' she commanded a harassed house surgeon. 'I want you to look pretty and be charming.' With whatever qualms, the young woman obeyed. The owner of a scalloped pink flannel coat like a bed-jacket, and the deplorable student who proposed to finish out an old evening frock in the dissecting room were left in no doubt of their Dean's disapproval. The students were frightened of the Dean, her sharp eye and sharper tongue, but they were proud of her as well. Her achievement fascinated them, and because, though pioneers, they were women of their time, so did her wealth and social position. 'It did a great deal for women doctors,' said a distinguished graduate of the London School of Medicine for Women, thoughtfully, 'that Mrs Anderson *dressed* so well.'[1]

[1] Personal information Miss Louisa Martindale, F.R.C.O.G.

Elizabeth intended the young women at the school to enjoy the pleasures of university life, which she had missed in her own single-handed struggle. She welcomed them to her own home; she wrote quite casually of 'a pretty large party, probably seventy or eighty, all to a sit-down supper'. Every Christmas she gave a dance at the school, with an entertainment. One year this was provided by the music-hall comedian Corney Grain who gave 'a take-off of two fashionable doctors', one of them the proverbial hypochondriac's friend, Andrew Clark. Sir Andrew was in the audience, but to Elizabeth's relief he 'enjoyed the fun as much as anyone present'. She believed in self-government through the students' representative council; she encouraged clubs for music, fencing and various outdoor games. She provided study-bed-rooms for renting, on the top floor of the building, and a students' refectory. In her view 'a bun and a cup of tea' was no meal for a working woman.

As Elizabeth Garrett Anderson passed her sixtieth year, she began to show one failing as Dean. She could not remember her students' names. Their faces passed her by, she confessed to Louisa, and as their numbers increased so did her difficulty. She became adroit in concealing her forgetfulness, and her manner was so full of warmth and goodwill to them all that they did not guess how hard she found it to put the right name even to the last gold medallist.[1] Nevertheless it was a sign that she could not go on working for ever. 'The cause', the women's movement to which she had given her life, was fast changing its character. Hundreds of young middle-class women had received the education at school and college won for them by the pioneers of twenty years before. Working-class girls, meagrely provided with a minimum of schooling by the Act of 1870, were hungry for opportunity. A whole new generation had come into the ranks. In 1905, at the first militant suffrage demonstration in the Free Trade Hall, Manchester, the new recruits were to show their strength. Meanwhile it was time for the pioneers to retire, before

[1] Anderson, L. G., op. cit. p. 230.

they were elbowed out of the way. In 1899 Sophia Jex-Blake left Edinburgh and settled to a contented old age in a house on the Sussex Downs, the storms of the past forgotten. Emily Davies resigned the Honorary Secretaryship of Girton, in deference to the wish of the college to be governed by its own Mistress and Fellows. Barbara Bodichon had died tragically in 1890, after a series of strokes which reduced her to a life of invalid frustration. In 1899 Millicent Fawcett received the Hon. LL.D. of St Andrews. Standing in the robing room, as she put on the heavy black gown with red buttons, she thought of the pioneers in every branch of woman's work and said, 'I am reaping in a field where many have sown.'[1] In January 1901 Queen Victoria died. Elizabeth had been born the year before Victoria's coronation, and had achieved a life's work in her reign; the Queen's death was the signal for her to depart in peace. That year she began to prepare for retirement.

Sargent painted her portrait. She sat to him in the famous studio at 31 Tite Street, Chelsea, where he had painted the Three Graces and the stylish Misses Wertheimer. Artist and sitter in this instance were not created to understand one another. Elizabeth wished to be painted in her M.D. gown. Sargent begged for some jewellery, so she added a pearl necklace costing sixpence. She was annoyed to find Sargent had painted her with affected, tapering hands. 'They are nothing like mine!' She spread her scrubbed, capable surgeon's fingers. Sargent hid one hand under the black silk gown, which by common consent he painted superbly, but the remaining hand is still his and not hers. A friend who came to the studio pronounced the portrait charming. 'Oh poor Mr Sargent,' said Elizabeth with a certain malice, 'you will have all the ugly old women in London asking you to paint them!' He had certainly captured her bright eyes, her crisp grey hair, and her air of easy mastery. The picture was shown at the New Gallery and on the whole admired, except by the *Magazine of Art*, which commented, 'The furioso method and temperament of the painter has shown the lady violently aggressive and totally

[1] Strachey, R., *Millicent Garrett Fawcett*, p. 82.

unsympathetic, which we well know must belie the charm of the sitter.'[1] Elizabeth Garrett Anderson, who had never sought personal publicity or favour, found herself even more of a popular figure, a part of the London scene.

In 1902 she retired from the office of Dean of the London School of Medicine, which she had held for nearly twenty years. The college owed a new building and full university status to her flair for administration. She had won for its graduates the right of entry to hospital appointments, public health services and medical societies. She had set the pace for the women doctors who followed her. There was no risk now that they would be content with inferior qualifications or with under-selling their male colleagues. Above all, she had left the impress of her character on hundreds of students who worked under her. Her courage, her independence of mind, her honesty and kindness were the touchstone for a new generation of medical women. In recognition of all this the council of the college created for her a new office, President of the Royal Free Hospital School of Medicine, 'one they think is now most fittingly conferred'.

[1] Downes, W. H., *John S. Sargent*, p. 194.

CHAPTER NINETEEN

Writing and Travelling
1893–1903

In *Who's Who* Elizabeth Garrett Anderson listed her recreations as travelling and gardening, a pair of pleasures not easy to combine. To these she added a long-standing interest in the history of medicine. From 1893 onwards, no longer tied by daily visits to the hospital, she indulged all three tastes. A day's digging, a week's research or a fortnight abroad gave her more satisfaction than months of desultory leisure could have brought, for these recreations were not chosen at random; each fulfilled a profound need in her nature. Reading and writing about medicine provided a continuing intellectual interest, gardening took her back to her own roots in the East Anglian soil, and travelling satisfied a need for adventure which had not grown less with the years.

As soon as she had resigned from the staff of the New Hospital she took a month's holiday in Switzerland with Louie, Alan, her brother Newson's daughter Ruby and thirteen assorted pieces of luggage. Thereafter she travelled every spring and autumn, either with her husband or with parties of young people. Often Skelton Anderson could not leave his office for more than a few days' golf at Aldeburgh. He saw no reason why this should deprive his hard-working wife of holidays she enjoyed, and he was totally indifferent to conventional opinion on the subject. If he stayed at home, Elizabeth marked down particularly interesting places for 'our next trip together'. She wrote to him almost every day, long letters full of affection and a childlike pleasure. She loved the Lake of Lucerne, deserted by tourists in the sharp spring sunshine. They climbed five thousand feet of the Rigi where eight hours on foot gave Alan a blistered heel, but left his mother quite unsubdued. Next morning she was up at a quarter past five to see the sun rise above the glittering mountain peaks and a few days later walked through deep snow up the zig-zag path to Andermatt, 'boots and petticoats as wet as could be', to sleep cheerfully in 'a dampish bed'.[1] The morning after her return she made her usual round of patients at the hospital, for although no longer on the staff, she was still a consultant.

The university vacations which allowed Elizabeth to travel also gave her time to write a series of papers on subjects connected with medicine. These were usually commissioned, either as lectures or as review articles, and were addressed to laymen interested in controversial topics. Her first, 'The History of a Movement', published in *The Westminster Review*,[2] was an account of the admission of women to the medical profession in Great Britain, covering the last forty years. In it she was scrupulous to pay tribute to Mary Putnam for winning entry to the Sorbonne, and to 'the energy and courage of Miss Jex-Blake'. She gave a brief account of the New Hospital and the London School of Medicine and mentioned the new development of mixed colleges for men and women in Ireland. 'It is pleasant to record that at Cork the movement last autumn [1892] in favour of removing all restriction in the way of women studying in the hospitals started from the men students.' She reviewed the present position of the 144 women on the Medical Register, who worked in private practice, under the Asylums Board, in workhouse infirmaries and in children's hospitals. Looking back, she hoped it would appear that women doctors 'have done good service to the community at large as well as to themselves'. She returned to this subject a few years later when she contributed a short intro-

[1] Elizabeth Garrett Anderson to Skelton Anderson, 20 March–10 April 1893. Ten letters. Anderson family papers.
[2] *The Westminster Review*, March 1893.

duction to a volume on careers for educated women. She told the intending doctor frankly that 'it is equally important to avoid being too ambitious or too modest in her estimate of her powers'.[1] A reasonable choice of schools and medical degrees was now open to well-educated women. Acceptance by the profession, she said, was largely but not wholly won. This was true. Opposition was in the last ditch, but remained firmly dug in there. Members of the Glasgow Royal Medico-Chirurgical Society collected a number of ballot papers admitting new members before discovering that apparently harmless initials represented feminine Christian names. An indignant objection was lodged, the papers were destroyed uncounted and no woman was elected to the Society until 1911.[2]

In 1899 Elizabeth Garrett Anderson contributed two articles to *The Edinburgh Review* on subjects of popular controversy. Vaccination, though bitterly opposed by some sanitarians, had been compulsory in Britain since 1853 and from 1890 to 1896 a Royal Commission on Vaccination had examined the evidence of thirty years. Smallpox, it found, formerly a lethal disease of childhood, had become mainly a disease of adults, suggesting that children were protected by vaccination. Doctors and nurses exposed to outbreaks were seldom infected; therefore re-vaccination protected adults. The old method of vaccinating children from arm to arm had carried a risk of accidental infection, but this was greatly reduced by the use of glycerinated calf lymph.[3] In spite of this evidence a vociferous anti-vaccination movement persisted and led to a change in the law. The Vaccination Act of 1898 allowed the rights of parents to conscientious objection. To Elizabeth Garrett Anderson this concession seemed weakness and folly. She served as honorary secretary to the Imperial Vaccination League, which conducted a campaign to tighten up the

[1] Osborn, C., Manuals of Employment for Educated Women, *Medicine*.
[2] Power, D'A., *British Medical Societies*.
[3] This method was evolved by Dr Monkton Copeman, a personal friend of Elizabeth Garrett Anderson.

administration of the law and to promote the re-vaccination of children at school age.[1] On 30 January 1899 she herself lectured to a crowded audience at St Luke's Rooms, Nutford Place, showing by carefully prepared diagrams that even the virulent smallpox epidemic of 1871–2 killed only half as many as any one of the thirty-two epidemics in the century which preceded vaccination. Three months later she was invited to put this lecture into permanent form.[2] In 'The History and Effects of Vaccination' she acknowledges that the subject has been a centre of controversy for the last half century, but insists that a historical approach will educate the public. Historically, smallpox was one of the great scourges of humanity. She quotes Ben Jonsons's epigram

> *Envious and foule disease, can there not be*
> *One beauty in an age and free from thee?*

supporting it from evidence of smallpox deaths in the yearly London bills of mortality since 1538. She describes the observations which led to Jenner's discovery of vaccination and gives figures of the fall in mortality which followed it. She admits that vaccination is not invariably or indefinitely effective; 'we have no reason to expect mathematical precision in what is fundamentally a vital process'. Re-vaccination increases efficiency; among post office staff, re-vaccinated upon appointment, 'there was not a single death from smallpox in the years 1870–80, although this included the great epidemic of 1871'. She admits the risks of infection, but ascribes them to faults in technique, largely overcome by the use of glycerinated lymph, and quotes in support of this the findings of the Royal Commission, now embodied in the Vaccination Act of 1898. She carries the war into the anti-vaccinators' camp, maintaining that they were believed only because the general public has forgotten what an attack of smallpox is like. Has anyone, she asks, ever met a doctor in a smallpox hospital who was an anti-

[1] Elizabeth Garrett Anderson to Mr Wellcome, 15 Dec. 1902. Wellcome Historical Medical Library.
[2] 'History and Effects of Vaccination': *The Edinburgh Review*, April 1899.

vaccinator? Have the antivaccinists seen the disease in action? 'Have they not seen it only with the eyes of their minds in the safe seclusion of the British Museum Reading Room? . . . As apostles of mischief and misery they have much to answer for.' Finally she reminds the authorities that 'every practical improvement in the administration of the Vaccination Act will tend enormously to remove opposition', and hopes than an enlightened public opinion will play its part. 'The History and Effects of Vaccination' is a good paper, partisan but just. Laborious research in the historical section has been assimilated with a deceptive air of ease; the style is clear and vigorous and the article is quoted as authoritative by the *Encyclopaedia Britannica*.

This contribution was so successful that Elizabeth Garrett Anderson was commissioned in the same year to write for *The Edinburgh Review* on the even more vexed subject of vivisection.[1] The ethics of vivisection had been a topic of more or less acrimonious discussion between scientists and the public since the Royal Commission of 1875 and the Cruelty to Animals Act of 1876.[2] In contributing to the discussion Elizabeth first attempts to define the terms Pain and Cruelty. 'The birth of every child causes the mother severe and prolonged pain but we do not think of it as cruelty. It is not useless or purposeless. Cruelty begins when pain is inflicted without adequate cause.' She is honest enough to admit that physiologists from lack of imagination may be careless, but this is a matter for education; 'if the operator sets himself to minimize suffering, he can reduce it in almost all cases to a point which is not out of proportion to the advantage to be gained'. She examines the provisions of the 1876 Act, sets out the categories of licence covering differing types of experiment, and gives figures from the inspectors' report of 1897 on licences issued by the Home Office. The treatment of this section is full and factual. Of the antivivisection campaign she remarks that 'the language cannot be said to have the lucidity

[1] 'The Ethics of Vivisection': *The Edinburgh Review*, July 1899.
[2] This Act is still in force and governs all experimental work with animals.

proper to writing that deals with scientific matters. Men who give up their lives to the difficult and often disappointing work of searching for truth . . . should not lightly be called "inhuman devils".' She illustrates pungently the illogicality of many anti-vivisectionists. 'A duke going to preside at a meeting against vivisection dines off animals which have been vivisected. The ladies with him wear fur, feathers and ospreys. He drives to the meeting behind vivisected horses.' All this is sanctioned by custom, but experimental vivisection is new, and therefore attacked, as in their day were anaesthesia and dissection. Finally and justly, she urges the need for humanity towards the vastly greater number of animals who suffer at man's hands in their daily work, in the slaughter-house or on the farm. 'The Ethics of Vivisection' is a temperate and factual contribution to a problem which still concerns the scientist and the general public.

The most interesting of Elizabeth Garrett Anderson's medical papers is 'On the Progress of Medicine since 1803',[1] expanded in 1903 from her presidential address to the East Anglian B.M.A., 'On the Progress of Medicine in the Victorian Era.'[2] The earlier version is of particular interest, since it records many developments which she had seen during her working life as a doctor, and reflects her own appreciation of them. The years of Elizabeth Garrett Anderson's early practice, during which Pasteur's researches were first applied to the treatment of wounds and disease, formed a watershed in the history of surgery. Those who could not accept them were forced to look always backward. Thus Elizabeth Blackwell writing in 1891 could speak of Pasteur pursuing 'a false method of research', of vivisection as 'a grave error' and bacteriology as 'a mischievous exaggeration'. Elizabeth Garrett Anderson, well grounded in science and open-minded, looked forward to a future of boundless possibilities. She contrasts the old art of medicine, based on observation and general

---

[1] 'On the Progress of Medicine since 1803': *The Edinburgh Review*, Jan. 1903.
[2] Reprinted as a pamphlet, Macmillan, 1897.

experience, with the precision which a physician of the 1890s could command.

> He looks into the eye, the larynx and other organs; he measures the heart, he listens to the sounds of the chest, observes the reflexes, tests the nutritional condition of nerves and muscles, examines excretions and records the temperature. By these means he forms a precise diagnosis and demands from the pharmacologist precise remedies.

How and when did this change of method in the study of medicine begin? Elizabeth personally dates it from Jenner's observations on immunity, though the explanation of them was not at first fully understood. The next step, in her judgment, was the discovery of anaesthesia, which released the surgeon from the need for haste. 'He could, for the first time, take time enough to be careful and minutely painstaking.' From this fact sprang much medical research work and the whole new field of abdominal surgery. She adds the interesting personal observation that anaesthesia has made highly skilled nursing possible. 'While all surgery was torture scarcely less terrible to see than bear' very few educated women would become nurses.[1] The third great step forward in medicine was the rise and development of the antiseptic method 'which we owe to Lord Lister, and which I venture to think will for ever be accounted one of the greatest glories of the Victorian Era'. She recalls her own memories of the opposition Lister had met, recorded for incredulous future students in the literature of the medical societies from 1868 to 1876. By his discovery 'the range of the art of healing has been almost indefinitely widened, and with much greater safety goes an amazing diminution in suffering'. In describing the effects of antiseptics in midwifery, she is careful to mention 'a man to whom the honour that is due has not even yet been paid – Semmelweiss,

---

[1] This was borne out by Paget. His young wife, living within earshot of St Bartholomew's during the 1840's, used to look 'worse than the patient' on operation days.

whose name should for ever be held in honour'.[1] Coming to more recent times she describes the rise of bacteriology from about 1880. 'Step by step, with infinite labour and patience, the specific micro-organisms of tuberculosis, glanders, anthrax, tetanus, cholera, malaria, plague and influenza has been found and its life history studied.' Allied to bacteriology, and like it dependent on the microscope, is the study of the blood and the glandular secretions, which had thrown new light on myxoedema, diabetes and Addison's disease.

The conclusion of 'On the Progress of Medicine' is a passage of remarkable force and scope.

> I ask you now to turn your thoughts to the future and to consider where further progress is most wanted. . . . We want in medicine more of the knowledge that can only be gained through research. We want to know the real nature of malignant growths, the complete life history of the bacillus of diphtheria, of the parasite of malaria and how to produce immunity from them and from tuberculosis.

In 1896 Elizabeth Garrett Anderson dared to look forward to a world in which diphtheria, malaria, tuberculosis and cancer could all, through precise knowledge, be controlled as effectively as smallpox. She left her audience of country doctors with a thought which, she said, gave her particular satisfaction. 'The study of medicine is big enough and young enough to fill all our lives to their end. To have a profession of which the intellectual interest is certain not to flag is an enormous addition to the pleasure of life, and it is one which we all enjoy.'

This paper and the review articles were intended to be of general interest. For working scientists she contributed articles to the *Encyclopaedia Medica*,[2] whose general editor was a connection by marriage.[3] The Garrett Anderson contributions to the

[1] Ignaz Semmelweiss, as early as 1847, almost abolished puerperal fever in his wards at Vienna by antiseptic methods, but died without recognition.

[2] *Encyclopaedia Medica*, gen. editor D. Chalmers Watson, 1899–1910, 15 vols.

[3] Skelton's niece, Mona Geddes, became the first woman M.D. Edinburgh,

Encyclopaedia were on vaccination, puberty, the menopause and neurasthenia. Even to a lay reader the style reveals the writer's personal approach. Consistently she advises a way of life that is self-disciplined, sane and simple. She might be describing herself in this account of normal living:

> In health the nervous force is sufficient for all the ordinary demands made upon it. We work and get tired, we sleep and eat and are again as new beings ready for another day's work. After some months of continuous work we are tired in a different way; the night's rest and the weekly day of rest do not suffice; we want change of scene and a complete rest. With these we renew our force and are presently again ready to enjoy work.

This balance of nature, in her experience, need seldom be disturbed either by puberty or the menopause. Of the first, she says, 'No special rules are required at this age for either boys or girls. They both need a healthy, active life, with much open-air exercise, plenty of good food and plenty of occupation.'[1] She held the opinion, general now but unusual in her day, that wide variations of masculinity and femininity must be accepted as a normal fact. As an example she mentioned her friend Mrs Grote. 'We all remember Sydney Smith's inquiry "Who is the gentleman in white muslin on the sofa?" in reference to a well-known woman who strove through a long life to be like the sex she belonged to physiologically but not mentally.' Willingness to face this fact, she said, would remove much prejudice and individual hardship. Of the climacteric she wrote

> in a natural menopause there is a beneficent absence of haste. Nerves, blood vessels and tissues have time, day by day, to adjust themselves to the new order of things; physiological compensation is established and in many cases the woman is in

and on the day she received her degree she married Douglas Chalmers Watson, editor of the *Encyclopaedia Medica*. Together they published many important papers on nutrition.

[1] *Encyclopaedia Medica*, 'Puberty'.

better health after the menopause than she was before it. She has paid her tax to humanity and she is now free from calls of that kind on her strength and activity.

Elizabeth Garrett Anderson did not show the insensitiveness of which a certain type of woman doctor has stood accused. She pointed out the dangers of attributing every ill in middle-aged women to the menopause. 'The diagnosis "change of life" is a very refuge to the indolent and ignorant and as such it should be shunned by all honest practitioners.' The increased risk of cancer, rheumatoid arthritis and other diseases at this age should be recognized and treated seriously, while for the housewife in mental distress 'there is absolutely nothing so good, when she really wants it, as a real holiday away from her family, with no duties and no housekeeping'.[1]

The article on Neurasthenia urges the general practitioner to recognize the reality of nervous debility; in 1901 the advice was probably more necessary than now. 'Of the two broad causes of neurasthenia, heredity and stress, heredity stands first except in cases with a pronounced traumatic factor.' She points out the difficulty of defining undue stress; 'a task that would strain a pony is nothing to a cart horse'. She describes some of her own cases vividly and with sympathy, urging doctors not to label such people as freaks or 'err by dogmatically insisting on one programme for everyone, be he sound or unsound. . . . We are all neurasthenic when we are dead tired from want of sleep, undue exertion and the absence of food.'[2] Taken as a whole Elizabeth Garrett Anderson's medical writings cannot claim scientific originality, but they do display an intellect of considerable judgment, clarity and force. She was outstandingly free from prejudice. If she had wished she could have been a good historian. In writing on scientific subjects, she commanded a style swift, vigorous and humane, which has now almost vanished from that field of work.

[1] *Encyclopaedia Medica*, 'Menopause'.
[2] ibid. 'Neurasthenia'.

The intellectual stimulus of writing medical papers was heightened during the vacations by the pleasure of young company. Elizabeth kept open house to her children's friends and cousins. The young people had to understand that they were staying with a busy woman. 'There, my dears,' she would say at breakfast, handing a golden sovereign to each, 'you may go where you like and do what you like. Don't let me see you again until the evening. Dinner will be at seven and you must be at home in time to dress.'[1] The guests had to display intelligence, good manners and sheer physical stamina. Elizabeth's way of dealing with them was crisp; she remained slightly formidable, even to her own family. She helped one of Skelton's nieces to get her degree at Cambridge, but the niece remembered

my youthful affection for her was tempered with a good deal of awe, because of her clear cut mind and great efficiency. I remember that in my second year at Girton, about 1901, I had poisoned fingers on both hands, which would not yield to treatment and I turned to Aunt Elizabeth for advice and help. I was summoned to London, where she met me, took me straight to a surgeon, who removed the nail from one finger and lanced the other. I felt pretty unwell after that and was in great pain, but I sat up for most of the evening and it was Louisa who suggested that bed might be a good thing, not my aunt. Next day Spartan treatment continued and I was sent back to Cambridge with my two bandaged hands. A few days later I was rebuked quite firmly for leaving a small toilet article behind and reminded that it was the mark of a well-bred guest not to leave anything behind her! Later on she mellowed greatly and when I last saw her, which must have been ten or twelve years later, she had grown into a dear and gentle old lady and such a kind one. I was much attached to her.[2]

Frequently Elizabeth took parties of young people on holidays

[1] Anderson, L. G., *Elizabeth Garrett Anderson*, p. 269.
[2] Personal information, Miss Mary Clarke.

abroad. In August 1893 she went walking in Switzerland with a niece, Christina Cowell, Louisa, Alan and Millicent Fawcett. Idle for once, the sisters sat together on the balcony at Lauterbrunnen, watching 'the Jungfrau lit up before us with a wonderful after-glow. This comes later than I had expected in silver white, not red. The mountain was shining brightly with it long after we were in complete darkness.' The young people explored a glacier, and Alan, who was sixteen, longed to tackle the overnight climb up Titlis. Elizabeth would not permit this on her own authority; Alan had to wait for his climb until his father in London had been consulted and had telegraphed permission. Meanwhile his mother, with childlike pleasure, journeyed 3,000 feet by funicular up to Mürren. 'It is really like being in a *balloon*! The up and down trains balance each other, and the top one starts by being weighted with water which is let out at the bottom.' She cut her knee on a rock and could not walk, but sat in the sun alternately reading a novel by Dumas and looking at the mountains through a telescope. When she could walk again she was touched that Alan took her arm over steep places. 'It is a great opportunity of knitting hearts together, a little jaunt like this.'[1] The following spring, in April 1894, she visited Lake Como for the first time. Louie, in the middle of her medical course, could not spare time for a holiday, so Elizabeth's guests were her sister Alice, Alan and two nephews. Skelton again preferred to spend Easter on the links at Aldeburgh. 'I was sorry, dearest,' his wife wrote, 'to hear you were beaten before the last round, but you did so well that it was almost as good as a victory.' Como was beautiful, but overrun by English tourists: 'we are incog. no longer and so have to be aff.' reported Elizabeth in disgust. Half the charm of travel for her lay in escape from her official personality. She left the hotel and took a rowing-boat on the lake. 'The water was sapphire blue one way crossed with orange brown, such a mixture as one could never believe if seen in a picture. It is quite delicious – such colour and blue

[1] Elizabeth Garrett Anderson to Skelton Anderson 7–25 Aug. 1893. Twelve letters. Anderson family papers.

haze everywhere.'[1] Her enjoyment was not dependent on weather; to relax and to be free was pleasure in itself. In 1895, during an August of wild thunderstorms at Zell-am-See, she and Millicent entertained one another quite contentedly by taking turns to sew, while the other read aloud from Motley or Erasmus.[2]

Millicent Fawcett was now a recognized political leader. In 1897, when a Women's Suffrage Bill actually came to a second reading, she was elected President of the National Union of all the women's suffrage societies. Like Elizabeth she tempered her feminism with self-control, saying, 'We can't afford a good honest rage yet!' and under her rule the suffrage movement was constitutional and orderly. Two years later the Boer War broke out. Kitchener, the British Commander-in-Chief, brought Boer families into hutments, to which he gave the new name 'concentration camps'. Here an epidemic of measles followed by pneumonia killed children in their hundreds. Millicent Fawcett, with two women doctors, a woman inspector of factories and a Guy's Hospital sister, was sent to investigate conditions in the camps. They reported, 'Bully beef and bread are quite unsuitable food for young children' and some improvement followed.[3] Neither Millicent nor Elizabeth, however, was in the slightest degree pro-Boer.

Elizabeth could review her own happiness in 1896 from the vantage point of her silver wedding. The marriage, entered with such fears that she was failing in her duty as a leader of women, had proved a true working partnership. The Andersons were united yet independent, loyal and affectionate yet unpossessive in personal relationships. In the anguish of love and loss for her children Skelton's strength had been his wife's support, and she in return had respected his authority as a father. After twenty-

[1] Elizabeth Garrett Anderson to Skelton Anderson, 1 April 1894. Anderson family papers.
[2] Elizabeth Garrett Anderson to Skelton Anderson, 15 Aug. 1895. Anderson family papers.
[3] After the war ended Philippa Fawcett went out to set up public elementary education for the government of the Transvaal.

five years their minds still struck sparks from each other. Their letters are full of glancing references to international affairs, concerts, the books they happen to be reading and the current exhibition at Burlington House, along with the domestic minutiae of social engagements, frozen cisterns and clean shirts. When they disagreed, it was upon a foundation of mutual love.

> I am sure you know that I am not disloyal to you [wrote Elizabeth upon a controversial decision during his mayoralty of Aldeburgh]. I am only trying to keep you from making a mistake which you would regret afterwards. . . . I have worked hard to make your year of office a success and I think I have a claim to be listened to on this disputed point.

She ended with a quotation from their children's babyhood, which only he would recognize. 'But in any case you know "Bay's *heart* is good all the time" and I know the same about yours.'[1] To say this, after a quarter of a century, was to say much.

Louisa Garrett Anderson was at Clapham, doing her midwifery on the district with Dr Annie McCall, where Elizabeth sent her hampers of country food after every trip to Aldeburgh. She qualified in 1897. Alan was still in his last year as an undergraduate at Trinity College, Oxford, and his life seemed to his mother full of masculine mysteries. She visited him at Oxford, found him much occupied with a boat club supper, and took the chance to go to bed at nine o'clock at the Mitre and enjoy a long read at the last volume of Justin McCarthy's *History of Our Own Times* before falling asleep. The years it covered, from 1880 to the Diamond Jubilee, had been the busiest in her public life, but she had found time to be a faithful newspaper reader. She had followed the Boer rising, the defeat of the British at Majuba Hill and the death of her old acquaintance Empress Eugénie's only son in battle. She had read of the murder of General Gordon at

---

[1] Elizabeth Garrett Anderson, 11 Oct. 1894. Anderson family papers. The disputed point was an alteration to the exterior of the Moot Hall at Aldeburgh. It was not made.

Khartoum before a relief expedition could reach him, and the Phoenix Park murders in Dublin. She had followed the rise of Parnell, his ruin in the O'Shea divorce scandal and his death, 'a cold blast to wither the prospects of Home Rule cause'. She had seen the London School Board on which she had served taken over by the London County Council in 1888. She had read of the great dock strike, of the Jameson raid, of the deaths of Browning and Tennyson. It was satisfying to her orderly mind to gather together the threads of contemporary experience as she read McCarthy's new volume. 'It is entertaining,' she wrote to Skelton from her hotel bedroom 'and his style is as good as ever. . . . I shall be glad to see all he says about Parnell.'[1]

Louie was shortly to take up her first post as assistant medical officer at the Camberwell Infirmary. In April 1897 Elizabeth, her son and her daughter went for their last family holiday together, ten days walking on the coast roads of Brittany, and scrambling out to Mont St Michel, perfumed by the golden-brown wall-flowers which clung to every cranny. On this fresh ground Elizabeth could look at her two children and see them as independent adults. Louie was a rare person in mind and character, but she could no longer be protected; in any case she was 'eating famously and looking younger. Alan is quite nice, kind and aff., but I suspect he gets a lot of flattery,' wrote their mother frankly. He was good-looking and had considerable charm. 'I hope you will arrange to put him in an office not your own, where he will have to submit to discipline and work pretty hard.'[2] For the first time Elizabeth could speak of her children with some of the objectiveness she brought to her work, and the fact brought her a blessed peace of mind.

In the same year, 1897, she went for a second foreign journey, this time in the winter, to Ravenna and Florence, with yet another

[1] Elizabeth Garrett Anderson to Skelton Anderson, 5 June 1897. Anderson family papers.
[2] Elizabeth Garrett Anderson to Skelton Anderson, 23 and 26 April 1897. Anderson family papers.

niece. At sixty-one she was still a resilient traveller. 'We were over-turned in our voiture today,' she wrote casually on a postcard, 'but not at all hurt luckily. It was done so slowly we had time to step out.' Unaccountably, however, her mind kept turning to Alde-burgh and the gardens at Alde House. Her letters to Skelton were full of hedges, wind-breaks, flagged paths and lily ponds. In the clear golden light of Florence her eye was caught by 'a marble Madonna, a relief, rather high, an old one. I hope you will like it. I had the future dining-room in my mind, but if you liked better it could be let into the wall of the sunk garden among the sprays of roses.' Lying awake at night in her hotel, while the swollen Arno roared over its weir outside, she mentally planted a bank with plants that like sea air, and designed a dry stone wall to dis-play a Luca della Robbia plaque. She ordered a pair of wrought-iron gates and had them shipped home to form an entrance to the new garden.[1] The sights of Florence, the cloister and the cells of San Marco, the view from the terrace at Fiesole, reminded her of a visit with Skelton in the early days of their marriage. She went again to Italy in 1899, but increasingly she missed him. 'It seems so long since your last little note,' she wrote, 'but I hope it only means that you are busy all day and tired at night.'[2]

Early in 1900, Skelton Anderson was overtired and convalescent after a winter illness. For his sake Elizabeth was willing to take a much more leisurely holiday than usual and they went together to Cannes where Mary Marshall had a villa. The *Edinburgh Review* articles on vaccination and vivisection were finished, her con-tributions to the *Encyclopaedia Medica* half written, and the new buildings at the school would be complete by the autumn. She confessed to feeling a little tired herself.

[1] Elizabeth Garrett Anderson to Skelton Anderson, 22 Nov–5 Dec. 1897. Anderson family papers.
[2] Elizabeth Garrett Anderson to Skelton Anderson, 7 April 1899. Anderson family papers.

CHAPTER TWENTY

Return to Aldeburgh
1903 – 1917

In 1902, when she was sixty-five, Elizabeth and Skelton Anderson retired from work in London to West Hill, Aldeburgh. A year later, after the death of Mrs Garrett, they moved into Alde House. Louisa Garrett was ninety when she died. She had witnessed a revolution in the position of women and seen her own daughters play a leading part in it. In old age she had come to accept their work gladly. 'To have had such a radiant centre in our family life is an immense blessing,' wrote Elizabeth. 'It is not given to many people to get so near their fellow creatures' hearts as my *dear mother* did.'[1]

Retirement did not mean rest. Not even the trials of a journey by the Great Eastern Railway could keep Elizabeth away from council meetings at the School and the New Hospital. She continued to keep an eye on the finances of both. Thanks to her promptness, the Royal Free was the first medical school to receive aid from the Treasury[2] when Campbell-Bannerman's government instituted grants towards technical education. Bequests or savings were carefully invested.[3] At home she worked closely beside Skelton Anderson when he was re-elected mayor of Aldeburgh. Together they supported the Jubilee Hall, the Victoria Bridge at

[1] Elizabeth Garrett Anderson to Adelaide Anderson, 23 Jan. 1903. Anderson family papers.

[2] The first payment, in 1911, was of £169.

[3] Elizabeth Garrett Anderson to Mr A. G. Pollock, Chairman of the New Hospital for Women, 22 Feb. 1908. Elizabeth Garrett Anderson Hospital.

Thorpe[1] and the Church House. Skelton turned cheerfully from ocean-going liners to fishing smacks and yachts. He found jobs in Orient Line ships for many Aldeburgh boys, and on one occasion invited the entire crew of the lifeboat to visit a new Orient liner in the Albert Dock. As mayor he was troubled by the seasonal unemployment of a fishing and holiday town, and planned to develop some permanent industry on the banks of the Alde. Meanwhile he employed local labour on dredging at Slaughden Quay. Elizabeth tried to revive rural crafts among the fishermen's wives. The Andersons' service to Aldeburgh was generous; in return they were liked and respected.

Elizabeth's recreation and chief pleasure in her retirement was to work in her house and garden. She built an extension to Alde House, a long, white, garden front with an arched gable in the centre and tall Palladian windows through which sunlight streamed into the rooms. In one wing a winter-garden sheltered her rare plants; in the other an old barn made an open sun loggia, where she sat to read or work at her drawn-thread embroidery. The rooms at Alde House were calm and orderly; bowls of flowering plants stood everywhere. Music was played in the evenings. The house was fastidiously kept, the Chippendale furniture polished and scented with beeswax, the curtains of William Morris chintz freshly laundered. In the winter-garden sunlight filtered mysteriously through the ferns. Above the hall fireplace a portrait of Newson Garrett looked down on his descendants.

Elizabeth poured into gardening all the creative energy that had shaped her career. People still living who remember her garden at Alde House describe it simply as 'a dream'. She found beech avenues and fine lawns; she added walks and vistas, the Italian wrought-iron gates, a circular fountain, coloured lilies, rare shrubs. An exotic tree fern was persuaded by her determination to grow in the Aldeburgh air. She had been modest about her intellectual achievements, but now she openly boasted of having 'the best rock garden in East Anglia'. She built the rockery with

[1] Now demolished.

her own hands, around a little stream which flowed westward down the hill to the marshes of the Alde. Truckloads of natural limestone, specially quarried in Yorkshire, went into its making. She worked on her knees, in old clothes, her hair tied up in a handkerchief, firming down the little plants into the soil. She even won, rare triumph for an amateur, the grudging tribute of the professional. 'Mrs Anderson', said the head gardener, 'be a power of help to me about the place.'[1]

Constant visitors came to Alde House to enjoy the beauty of the garden, and to be terrorized by Toddy, Elizabeth's fierce mongrel, said to be the offspring of the union between an Irish terrier and a door mat. Toddy, enjoying his mistress's protection, was Nero among the dogs of Aldeburgh and he knew it. One cautious dinner guest wore leggings under his evening trousers to protect his ankles from the dark presence growling among the folds of the tablecloth. The hostess's conversation was as lively as ever, with a directness which somehow did not give offence. 'Do you really suppose God would *mind*?' she inquired with interest when a clergyman refused meat at her table on a Friday. She genuinely wished to know; human nature had lost none of its interest for her. The guests departed, after signing their names in the visitors' book, to which their hostess added comments of extreme frankness. 'Never want to see her again' appears against one name.[2] No doubt she never did.

Louisa Garrett Anderson had taken her M.D. in 1900 and to her mother's pleasure served as secretary to the Obstetrical Section of the B.M.A. meeting in 1905. Alan Garrett Anderson married in 1902, and the first of four grandchildren became, as Elizabeth wrote, 'the joy of our lives, the sweetest of children'. Alde House was open to grandchildren, and to a second generation of nieces, nephews and cousins, as it had been to their parents. Among them was a shy, solitary little girl, whose widower father was a cousin of James Skelton Anderson. Winifreda

[1] Personal information, Mrs M. L. Spring-Rice.
[2] Anderson, L. G., *Elizabeth Garrett Anderson*, p. 270.

333

Yuill had run wild on her father's estate in Australia; when she came to England at the age of ten she could hardly read or write, and English ladies alarmed her exceedingly. The one exception was Elizabeth Garrett Anderson, who welcomed her with warm and understanding affection. The child, a sensitive and perceptive observer, never forgot. 'She was in her sixties, but did not seem old; she was so alive. Everything about her was beautifully clean-looking, *scrubbed* – her hands, her clothes, her lovely curly grey hair.' Elizabeth created an atmosphere of peace and reassurance. 'She had wonderful, subtle taste; she was devoted to her family and to me she was a most delightful hostess.'[1]

Old friends left the circle one by one. Mrs Gurney, Mrs Llewelyn Davies and Lady Stanley were all dead. James Smith, the quiet brother-in-law who had given Elizabeth a home during her student years, soon followed. Sir William Broadbent and Sir Thomas Smith both died. Sir James Paget, who had accepted old age and infirmity as though it were part of his work, most of it rather dull, some of it interesting, some of it almost amusing, died at last and was buried in Westminster Abbey.

> It is grievous [wrote Elizabeth to a cousin] to see so many friends leaving us, but it is one of the penalties, and a heavy one, of getting old. Death is as much one of the beneficent laws of the Universe as birth is, and we ought not to think of it as an enemy. Especially is this true when people have had a life and have used it well.[2]

This philosophy was soon put to the test. In March 1907 Skelton Anderson had a stroke. His heart had been failing for some time. He was moved to London for a consultation and was in Louie's rooms at 114a Harley Street when he had a second stroke and died. Elizabeth, who was with him, took comfort from the memory of their work together. To friends who

[1] Personal information, Winifreda, Countess of Portarlington.
[2] Elizabeth Garrett Anderson to Adelaide Anderson, 29 Sept. 1905. Anderson family papers.

sympathized she said simply, 'He lived a very good life.' The Council wrote her a letter of condolence, to which she replied, 'My dear husband had the interests of Aldeburgh very much at heart, and I feel that the loss we have suffered is really shared by all who knew him here.'[1] This thought was deeply consoling to her. She decided her husband's memorial must be in accord with his character, and remembered how 'the impulse to help all who came to him in suffering or in need was very strong'. A service was held at the New Hospital, where she herself endowed and dedicated a bed in his name.[2] She aged noticeably after his death and, lacking his balance and humour, her judgment was perhaps less sure, but she had no intention of retiring from active life. She allowed herself to be photographed in widow's weeds, carefully posed in cap and shawl, her mittened old hands clasped in her lap. There is, though, a disconcerting sharpness in the sitter's eye, and this apparently struck her, for on the reverse side of the picture she wrote sardonically, 'A female Paul Pry!'

By Skelton Anderson's death the mayoralty of Aldeburgh fell vacant, and his term of office was served out by Elizabeth's youngest brother, George Garrett, maltster of Snape. During the year the Qualification of Women Act of 1907 opened county and borough councils to women, and Aldeburgh Corporation invited Elizabeth to stand for election. On 9 November 1907 'Mrs Elizabeth Anderson' joined the Council, her name being added in pencil to the minutes by a rather surprised clerk. A year later, 9 November 1908, she was proposed by the retiring mayor and seconded by his deputy as the new mayor of Aldeburgh. She did not hesitate to accept. Skelton would have wished it, and the challenge to pioneer was still irresistible. In her time she had been the first Englishwoman to qualify in medicine, the first woman M.D. in France, the first woman to be elected to a School Board, the founder of the first hospital staffed by women and the first

[1] Borough of Aldeburgh, *Council Minutes*, 24 April 1907. Borough Offices, Aldeburgh.
[2] New Hospital for Women *Annual Report*, 1908.

woman Dean of a medical school. Now, at seventy-one, she became Britain's first woman mayor. She was elected by the unanimous vote of the councillors, and her first official act was to send a telegram of congratulation to Edward VII on his birthday.[1]

Elizabeth Garrett Anderson was prepared to work as hard in Aldeburgh as she had done in London. The politics of the parish pump did not bore her, and she had always been strong on detail. She sat *ex officio* on every committee of the Council, so that no side of Aldeburgh life escaped her. The prosperity of the once-great sea-port now depended on its visitors and she took a realistic view of the amenities they would demand. In 1861 Edward Clodd, seeing the opening of the railway[2] as a turning point in Aldeburgh's history, had written: 'the streets must be paved, the lights better distributed, an effective system of drainage introduced and a water supply established'. Forty-eight years later Elizabeth Garrett Anderson was determined to carry out this programme in full. The Council *must* demolish the rusting old pier-head which disfigured the Crag Path, and plant waste open spaces with trees and shrubs. She urged them to make up the muddy roads on the estates where new houses had been built. She served notice on all owners of defective drains to connect their pipes with the common sewer. She insisted upon building public lavatories in time for the summer season, and appointed a sub-committee 'to consider the best method for efficiently removing the contents of dust bins'. The water tower was enlarged and rebuilt. The four-shilling rate which financed all these services also provided for such extras as the restoration of the sundial on the Moot Hall, and the purchase of tackle for hauling stranded animals out of dykes. Attempts to reduce the rate to 3*s*. 9*d*., Elizabeth considered, were unrealistic. During her second year of office, from November 1909 to November 1910, the decision was made to light the streets and pump water by electricity. In the bleak February weather of 1910 she compelled the Paving and Lighting Com-

[1] Borough of Aldeburgh, *Council Minutes*, 9 Nov. 1908.
[2] Now closed.

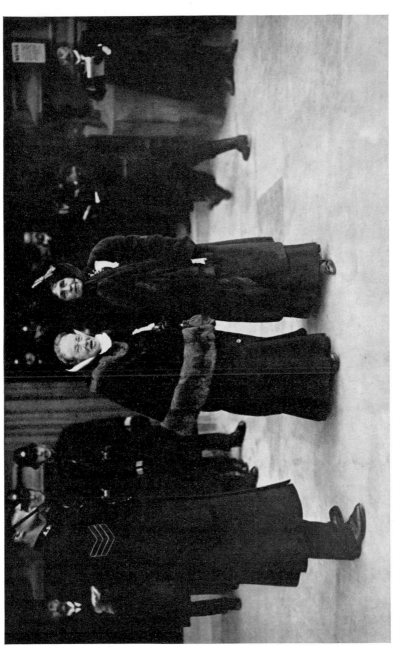

15. Elizabeth Garrett Anderson and Mrs Pankhurst present a suffrage petition to the House of Commons in 1910

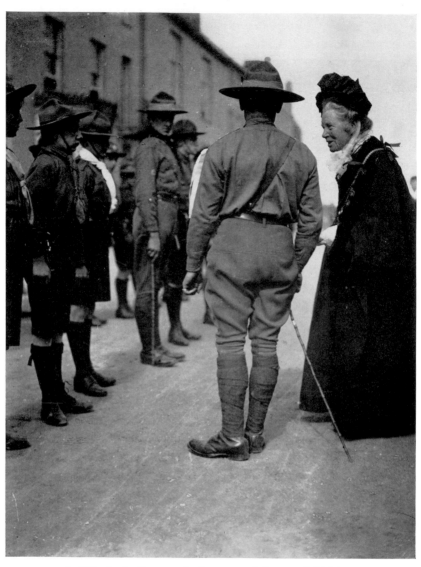

16. Elizabeth Garrett Anderson as Mayor of Aldeburgh
inspects the Boy Scouts in 1910

mittee to meet in the street and settle the exact position of the
new lamp standards. She walked the Leiston and Saxmundham
roads across open heathland with the Borough Surveyor to
satisfy herself that they needed making up. Thriftily, she obtained permission to hire a steam-roller for one or two days, when
a roller was within a short distance of the town. She urged house-
holders to re-lay any necessary drains or mains before the new
roads were made up, a piece of elementary common sense apparently beyond many municipal authorities to this day. Finally,
towards the end of her second year in office, she secured through
George Garrett, who was a county councillor, a grant of fifteen
hundred pounds from the County Road Board.[1]

The Borough conferred distinction upon itself by electing Mrs
Garrett Anderson mayor, but the Council quickly learnt that
they would have to accept her upon her own terms. She chose to
let Alde House for August and retired to the converted stable-
block, where councillors had to visit her on official business. The
vicar was persuaded to remonstrate with her. 'Do you think, Mrs
Anderson,' he began cautiously, 'that it is quite suitable for a
mayor to live in a stable?' 'Why not?' she answered, 'Your Lord
was *born* in a stable.' No more was heard about the matter. At the
beginning of her term of office she firmly sent the mayoral robes
to the dry cleaners. 'But', she told her brother Sam and his wife,
'even though cleaned, I cannot wear that hat!' She ordered from
her milliner a tricorne in black velvet, which she wore to the
royal garden party for mayors at Buckingham Palace. 'You look
very charming, Mrs Anderson, but I am not quite sure if I like
the hat,' said Edward VII with the freedom of old acquaintance.
'I'm sorry, Sir, but *my* people do,' said the mayor, quite unabashed.

It was the last time she saw King Edward before his death.
When the news of it reached Aldeburgh, she determined to do what
no other woman had done before, and proclaim his successor.
She described her tactics to Skelton's cousin Adelaide Anderson.

[1] Borough of Aldeburgh, Committee Minutes, Nov. 1908–Nov. 1910,
passim.

I took good care not to raise any question. The Lord Chamberlain's missive reached me at six-thirty on Monday morning. Happily I was already up and dressed, so I jotted down the various bodies who ought to be asked, went to the deputy Mayor [who received her astounded at his bedroom window], declined all offers of help, gave my orders, wrote eighteen or twenty notes of invitation and had all organized by eight-thirty and out of reach of discussion!

She led the procession up Church Hill, preceded by the mace-bearers, and followed by the Corporation, the volunteers, the lifeboat crew and the Boy Scouts, a little old woman in robes and black velvet bonnet, with a mayoral chain and an unfurled umbrella. Bravely she stepped out in her stout laced boots to play her part and uphold the dignity of her office. Four hundred people assembled for her to read the proclamation and, to her satisfaction, 'the furthest off heard every word'.[1]

Elizabeth Garrett Anderson's election to a second term of office had not gone uncontested. One section of the Borough Council resented this elderly lady's modernist tendencies. Moreover she took a dangerous line on the vexed question of Votes for Women. Elizabeth had been a lifelong supporter of the constitutional movement for women's suffrage, headed by her sister Millicent Fawcett. In 1908, feeling that progress was too slow, she began to show an interest in the new, militant movement, and joined the Women's Social and Political Union. Despite the protests of several councillors, she invited Emmeline Pankhurst to stay. Elizabeth had always felt warmly towards younger women and Mrs Pankhurst, by common consent, was a spellbinder. Elizabeth yielded to the charm of that slender figure, the transparent pallor, the violet eyes and marvellous speaking voice. While Aldeburgh looked on in horror, a women's suffrage meeting was organized from Alde House.

[1] Elizabeth Garrett Anderson to Adelaide Anderson, 11 May 1910. Anderson family papers.

All this was remembered on 9 November 1909, mayor-making day in the sixteenth-century moot hall at Aldeburgh. A councillor arose and demanded the election of Mrs Garrett Anderson's deputy in her place. The deputy, embarrassed and uncomfortable, 'deprecated his nomination and requested the members of the Council not to vote for him'.[1] Of the fourteen councillors present, nine voted for Elizabeth Garrett Anderson, and she accordingly took her place at the head of the long table on which lay the silver maces marked with Queen Elizabeth's cypher. Suddenly the objecting councillor stood up again. Mrs Anderson *must* be made to understand that during her year in office she should not invite Mrs Pankhurst or anyone of that sort to her house. Members of the public, who remembered Newson Garrett's rages, stirred in anticipation on their benches. Elizabeth, veteran of many committees, never showed her scathing calm to better effect. Glancing at the agenda, she merely remarked, 'Gentlemen, our first business is the election of aldermen', and the improper interruption was ignored.[2] It was not forgotten. Votes for Women agitated the whole kingdom and anyone supporting the militants did so at her peril. On 27 May 1910 Elizabeth Garrett Anderson stood for election to the aldermanic bench, but a hotel-keeper was elected in her place by a large majority. Furthermore, to the intense disappointment of Ford Anderson and other relatives, she received no royal or official recognition for a life of outstanding public service. They went on hoping, but still 'Royalty gave no sign'.

It was nothing new for Elizabeth Garrett Anderson to make personal sacrifices for a cause and she did not appear to regret it. She was not willing to desert the women's movement while she still had health and strength, and in her widowhood she had grown to need the companionship of younger women. To entertain friends she bought for the summers a small house in the Scottish Highlands, at Newtonmore, which she named Alde Cottage. Here Mrs Pankhurst arrived by the car in which she

[1] Borough of Aldeburgh, *Council Minutes*, 9 Nov. 1909.
[2] Anderson, L. G., op. cit. p. 273.

travelled like a nomad from meeting to meeting, still drafting propaganda even when jacked up for a wheel change. She was driven by Britain's first *chauffeuse* in navy-blue serge skirt, military tunic and peaked cap. Colin Anderson, Elizabeth's grandson, then aged about five, was offered as a treat a ride beside this figure of the new womanhood. He refused in some alarm and spent the rest of the day in bed, disgraced.[1]

To the militant suffrage movement, Elizabeth Garrett Anderson, the first woman doctor and the only woman mayor, was a valuable acquisition. Its newspaper *Votes for Women* published an account of her life as one on whom members of the Women's Social and Political Union 'look with love and reverence and with whom they feel privileged to work'.[2] The affection was sincere, but considering her years they worked her very hard. She opened a W.S.P.U. Exhibition at the Prince's Skating Rink, Knightsbridge, a vast, many-girdered hall containing for the occasion an 'Anti-Suffrage Waxworks' and a model prison cell. Speaking to a crowded hall, she said she wanted to give them three reasons why she was a suffragette. First, it was unjust that women who paid taxes should be denied the elementary privilege of having a voice in the selection of their Parliamentary representative. Secondly, she felt very strongly that there was a broader reason, namely that in the present state of things one half of humanity was left out. Until the masculine and feminine parts of mankind would help each other and have each other's interests at heart humanity would remain imperfect. Thirdly, she was a suffragette because of the industrial interests of women. 'A wave of sentimentality is sweeping the country, nominally in the interests of women,' she said. 'Many people think it kind to deprive them of employment; they seem to imagine all women would be so much better sitting on sofas.' If poor women were to do that, she asked, who would feed them and their children? She ended with a personal avowal. 'I am often asked, am I really in favour of militant methods. I

[1] Personal information, Sir Colin Anderson.
[2] *Votes for Women*, 22 April 1910.

always answer quite frankly, "Yes, I am".' Among shouts of 'Bravo!' she moved off to empty her purse and fill her shopping basket at the stalls.[1]

In March 1909 Elizabeth was invited to address a militant meeting convened by a woman doctor at Sheffield. The thought of the journey was daunting, but she was determined to do her best. 'I am a thorough-going suffragist,' she wrote, 'but I am also, alas, an old woman . . . and never a good traveller. If I can be quiet and not have to talk or behave prettily, I shall probably be fit for my job at 8 p.m. but not otherwise.' She went, presided at the meeting, refusing to wear a gown since 'men never do for the purpose', and thoroughly enjoyed seeing so many medical women all doing well.[2] In the same month she travelled to Manchester to address a meeting, and later to Glasgow to open the W.S.P.U.'s Scottish Suffrage Exhibition.

These public appearances were exhausting for a woman of her age, but they were not dangerous. The situation altered when Elizabeth Garrett Anderson felt she must obey Mrs Pankhurst's printed summons 'Help the Suffragettes to RUSH the House of Commons'. She had already marched beside Millicent and Emily Davies in a peaceful procession 13,000 strong, but on a Tuesday evening, 18 October 1908, she prepared to join a raid on Parliament and the inevitable scuffle with police. Millicent Fawcett, who knew the risks her sister would run, was appalled. On the morning of the raid, Lady Frances Balfour found her walking up and down her room at Gower Street in real agitation. 'Elizabeth is over seventy and not fit to be arrested,' she said. 'I dread what may happen.' Without saying a word Lady Frances went straight to the Home Secretary and secured a written promise that Mrs Garrett Anderson should not be arrested. The raid took place; the police repulsed it. Women were torn from the railings of the Abbey and thrust between crowds of spectators and a

[1] *Votes for Women*, 21 May 1909.
[2] Elizabeth Garrett Anderson to Dr Helen Wilson, 29 Jan., 1 Feb., 25 March 1909. Fawcett Library.

massive force of police. The centre of the battle swayed to and fro; the suffragettes fought back, giving as good as they got. The police had what were discreetly called 'special instructions' and in all the shouting and confusion Elizabeth was untouched. Alan Garrett Anderson, having failed to persuade her to fall out, walked beside his mother along the last stretch of Whitehall. He observed that she was mystified and indeed rather put out at not having been molested in some way by the police. If she had known the reason she would have been furious.[1]

For the next three years Elizabeth Garrett Anderson was a conspicuous and popular figure at militant demonstrations. When she was unable to be present she sent a message. 'For more than forty years we have been asking for the recognition of women as citizens. The road has been long and often rough. But the women in our ranks have had faith, courage and self devotion. No great cause has in the end ever failed while these have endured.'

In the summer of 1910 it seemed, briefly, that the vote might even be won by peaceful means. An all-party committee of M.P.s was formed to draft a Conciliation Bill to enfranchise 'every woman possessed of a household qualification or of a ten pound occupation qualification', which might weather its passage through the House of Commons. Hopes were high. Four days after the Bill was introduced the W.S.P.U. staged a vast procession through the streets of London. Elizabeth led the 'Regiment of Portias', a detachment of eight hundred learned or professional ladies. It was observed that though a squad of male supporters shambled behind in an apologetic fashion, the elderly Portias swung along briskly with military precision.[2]

The Conciliation Bill was torpedoed in the House of Commons by the opposition of Winston Churchill who claimed, with some justice, that it was undemocratic. When Parliament met again in November 1910 the Prime Minister announced that there would be an immediate General Election, with no time to reconsider the

[1] Strachey, R., *Millicent Garrett Fawcett*, p. 219.
[2] Fulford, R., *Votes for Women*, p. 224.

Bill. The news of this shipwreck of all the women's hopes broke on the dank and cheerless afternoon of 10 November, 'Black Friday' in the mythology of the suffragette movement. While Asquith was still making his announcement in the House, Mrs Pankhurst led a deputation asking him to withdraw his veto on the Conciliation Bill before Parliament dissolved. To accompany her she chose the most popular figure she could command, Elizabeth Garrett Anderson. Elizabeth was seventy-four. Because of the cold she wore a fur bonnet tied with ribbons under the chin, and a seal-skin jacket with sable border, remarkably like the engagement present Skelton had given her forty years before. Her plain old face was engraved by character and determination. She was a reminder of the great days of Victorian feminism, wise, dignified and appealing. The police met her with respect and courtesy and a pair of constables escorted her, with Mrs Pankhurst, to the House of Commons.[1] This goodwill did not extend to the women who followed, advancing with banners in parties of twelve. According to Sylvia Pankhurst, who was watching from a taxi, the police snatched their flags, tore them to shreds, smashed the sticks, struck the women with fists and knees, knocked them down, kicked them, dragged them up, carried them a few paces and flung them into the crowd of sightseers. For six hours this continued. A hundred and fifteen people were arrested.[2]

Millicent Fawcett, now President of the National Union of Constitutional Suffrage Societies, disapproved strongly of all militant tactics. 'I never can feel', she said, 'that setting fire to houses and churches and letter-boxes and destroying valuable pictures really helps to convince people that women ought to be enfranchised.' Nor was militancy really in accord with Elizabeth's lifework, which had been to show that trained women were capable of first-class professional work. She had been drawn into the W.S.P.U. by her sympathy with young people and her love for Louie, who became a passionate suffragette. Elizabeth was grow-

[1] ibid. p. 230.
[2] Pankhurst, S., *The Suffragette Movement*, p. 243.

ing old, and her head no longer ruled her heart with the firmness of younger days. The intellectual cut and thrust of discussion, which she had always loved, sometimes degenerated into argument. 'You are the only person who can attack me without quarrelling,' she said rather pathetically to a friend of whom she was particularly fond. To disagree with Millicent was a grief to her, but they had disagreed before and it was the family tradition to be independent. Each had to judge for herself.

In December 1911 Elizabeth decided that she could no longer support the militant suffragettes. The reason was not old age or failing courage but her insistence on using her own judgment. The W.S.P.U. was disciplined like an army; unquestioning obedience was demanded of every recruit. At this time Mrs Pankhurst was on a lecture tour in America and day-to-day policy was dictated by her daughter Christabel. The year had seen a six months' truce to militancy in hopes of the Conciliation Bill. The Liberal government now proposed instead a Male Franchise Bill, which might be amended by a free vote in the House of Commons to include women. To Elizabeth, as to Millicent Fawcett, this seemed worth having. Christabel Pankhurst and the leaders of the W.S.P.U. thought otherwise. They wanted the justice of their demands admitted by a Bill solely concerned with votes for women. In a general Franchise Bill the principle would be adulterated. 'War is declared on women,' announced Christabel Pankhurst. At a huge, excited meeting in the Albert Hall, she denounced the offer as a trick. Soon hundreds of women all over London were smashing windows.

Elizabeth protested to Christabel Pankhurst but was ignored. Millicent wrote making her attitude plain.

I personally feel that the attitude of the W.S.P.U. about the prospect of W.S. next session is a very big blunder, and we shall lose no opportunity of disowning it and making people understand that we condemn it. It is horrid to do it, but I feel we have no choice. . . . I hope we shan't drift apart over this, but I believe the chances of this misfortune (which would be a very great one to me) are less if we are quite frank with one another.

To this letter Elizabeth replied the next day. As Ford Anderson had said, she was honest enough to admit a mistake.

Dearest Milly, – I am quite with you about the W.S.P.U. I think they are quite wrong. I wrote to Miss Pankhurst before (no, I think it was the day after) the demonstration, but she took no notice. I have now told her I can go no more with them. It is dreadfully sad to have to be divided but I cannot help it. I was meaning to write to you yesterday. I had waited several days in case C.P. answered.[1]

Her Indian summer of ardent feminism was over. The following year, in June 1912, Asquith's Franchise and Registration Bill came before the House. Elizabeth signed a protest which deeply deplored the 'provocative and bellicose' attitude of the W.S.P.U. when offered some measure at least of enfranchisement. 'There is, in our judgment, one thing only that can now imperil our position and that is the renewal of militancy.'[2] Militant tactics, by a fatal necessity, grew more and more sensational – slashed pictures, burnt letters, window smashing, bombs, finally suicide. They attracted publicity among the sensation-seekers, but did little to convert a reasoned public opinion. Louisa Garrett Anderson remained a militant. She lectured for the W.S.P.U., helped to organize a medical petition against forcible feeding and was imprisoned for a short time in 1912. Elizabeth thought her daughter mistaken, but could not influence her; it was at least a comfort to be reunited with Millicent until old age swallowed up all their divisions.

Death continued to narrow the circle of her friends. Elizabeth Blackwell died in 1910, exactly fifty years after she had noticed the 'bright, intelligent young lady' whose interest was aroused by her

[1] Strachey, R., *Millicent Garrett Fawcett*, pp. 220–1.
[2] *Votes for Women*, July 1912.

345

lecture on medicine as a profession for women. Joshua Plaskitt, once Apothecary to the Middlesex Hospital, died in 1912. As a very old man he still remembered with gladness the years when Miss Garrett had been his apprentice.[1] In the same year Sophia Jex-Blake died peacefully sitting in her chair. Mr Westlake, treasurer of the New Hospital for many years, died. 'I hope he did not suffer at the end?' wrote Elizabeth to the widow. 'By God's mercy, I think conscious suffering at the end is rare.'[2] She wrote as her last published work in August 1910 an obituary notice of Skelton's sister Mary Marshall, M.D., which summed up her ideal of all a woman doctor should be. 'She was immensely kind to everyone who came into her circle and to her patients above all. She was rich in good judgment and good taste. In dealings with her fellow practitioners she was absolutely loyal, just and considerate.'[3]

At seventy-five Elizabeth Garrett Anderson seemed as healthy and vigorous as she had ever been. During 1912, however, she noticed disquieting symptoms. One day, looking for a letter, she found herself standing blankly before her bureau; she had forgotten what she wanted there. 'Hardening of the arteries,' she said to her sister-in-law's young companion who was in the room with her. 'It means, of course, softening of the brain.' That summer she went as usual to Newtonmore, where the view over the distant mountains and the crystalline air were an unfailing delight to her. At the beginning of July she fell ill, but was soon well enough to potter about over her tulip bulbs and walk on the moor. To Alan, who had written in some anxiety, she replied:

Nothing is worth taking much to heart except sin or incurable folly in ourselves or those we love. I have had a long and very happy and successful life. It would be very poor and wretched

[1] New Hospital for Women *Annual Report*, 1913.
[2] Elizabeth Garrett Anderson to Mrs Westlake, 15 April 1913. Elizabeth Garrett Anderson Hospital.
[3] *British Medical Journal*, 20 Aug. 1910.
[4] Personal information, the late Miss Rhoda Power.

if I could not take what comes as to its ending with a heart full of thankfulness for all my great blessings.[1]

She returned to Aldeburgh and took up her old activities. She gave a thousand pounds each to the building fund of the School and of Girton College, and drawing the cheques pleased her greatly. She even went to London to take the chair at the opening of the winter session of the School of Medicine. She announced a great improvement in the housekeeping, 'in which as women we all take a very great interest. It is, I think, most important that the students' meals should be good and substantial and cheap.' She was loudly applauded.[2]

The next year passed quietly. She was pleased when the hospital opened a country House of Recovery at Barnet, where patients could enjoy quiet and country air. She had lived long enough to see the School established, the Hospital growing and women doctors welcomed by colleagues and patients alike. Walking hand in hand with her grandson she confided in him: 'Colin, I have had a very happy life.' In July 1914 she fell ill again. Everyone spoke of care, of recovery, but she was seventy-eight and a doctor.

It is not breakfast in bed, or having someone sitting in the room or driving with me, that can check the downward tendencies of old age once they begin [she told her son]. I wish it could. I would dearly love to think I might have a few more years of mental activity . . . the only thing to do is to arrange to be as little of a worry to everyone else as I can.[3]

Her brief, businesslike will was already made. She left small bequests to her old servants, an annuity to Josephine who was not well off, and another to poor Newson Dunnell, who did not live

---

[1] Elizabeth Garrett Anderson to Alan Garrett Anderson, 10 July 1912 Anderson family papers.

[2] *The Times*, 16 Oct. 1912.

[3] Elizabeth Garrett Anderson to Alan Garrett Anderson, 24 July 1914. Anderson family papers.

to inherit it. Otherwise she left Alde House and its gardens to Alan, and the cottage in Scotland with its contents to Louisa, who had loved her father so dearly. She told them both 'not to waste money on me' since her condition was incurable.

A month later war broke out, but already Elizabeth Garrett Anderson was finding the present hard to grasp or understand. On 14 September 1914 she was brought to London to see her daughter leave with the first unit of medical women for service in France. Leaning on the arm of Mr Pollock, chairman of the New Hospital, she made her way slowly along the platform at Victoria. The long train was being loaded with equipment, tons of lint and cotton wool, cases of instruments, crates of drugs and chloroform all marked *Women's Hospital Corps.* Young women doctors in the uniform of the corps answered confidently to their roll call. She was puzzled. 'Aren't they splendid?' she said to Mr Pollock wistfully. 'If only I were a little younger, how I should love to be going with them!' 'Mrs Anderson,' said Pollock emphatically, 'it is thanks to your life work that these women are able to go on such an enterprise.' She looked at him wonderingly. What had she done? She could no longer remember. At last she said simply, 'So many helped me.'[1]

It was true. Her mother had given her a happy childhood and health of body and mind. Her father had handed on as a birthright the confidence that man can master circumstance. Whatever doors money could unlock were opened to her. Distinguished men of science had given their time to teach her. She had been fortunate in friends and colleagues from the earliest until the last; Emily Davies, caustic and loyal, Barbara Bodichon, the brilliant Mary Scharlieb, Sophia Jex-Blake, so difficult to work with yet so worthy of respect. The staff of Hospital and School had served her faithfully; the students had warmed her with their youthful admiration. Skelton Anderson's love and wisdom had enriched her working days. Yet all these together had not been

[1] Pollock, A. G., MS. draft for a speech, 30 June 1925, Elizabeth Garrett Anderson Hospital.

enough. Something more was needed, and had been found, the mysterious alchemy of character which transformed a Suffolk girl into one of the most successful revolutionaries of the Victorian age.

She was taken home to Aldeburgh. The next three years were a tragedy, pitiful to watch. She complained, 'I have such a tired, *fading* brain', yet she lived on. The oaken constitution which had been her stronghold became her prison. Business and money affairs confused her, her own mistakes and muddles vexed her spirit. 'Lay down your cares and accept help' well-meaning relations urged. She could not do it. She had taken heavy responsibility and delighted in it. To be helpless spelt boredom and humiliation. She had healed others all her working life, but no one could heal her. On good days her old philosophy reasserted itself, and on one of these, 7 April 1915, after a specialist had visited her, she wrote to Louisa,

> I have delayed passing on to you the news of my probable fate, g.p. or some variant of that. I shd. have been thankful for keeping to my brains to the end, but it is not for me or another to dictate how the end shall come. I have had a very happy life and I am content that the end shall be chosen by the Almighty.

The effort of will which drove her pen over the page exhausted her. 'You must not grieve over much, my dear one. . . .' After a few lines the writing wavers and breaks off.[1]

Gradually she sank into acceptance and forgetfulness. Her niece Gladys came to keep house. Martha, her old parlourmaid, and three devoted nurses cared for her. Toddy, old and grizzled but still ready to fly at any other dog, walked stiffly beside her wheel-chair. Letters fell unopened from her lap, though to the last to hear from her children gave her pleasure. Louisa served as chief surgeon to the military hospital at Endell Street, staffed by

[1] Elizabeth Garrett Anderson to Louisa Garrett Anderson, 7 April 1915. Anderson family papers.

women only. Alan, a Controller of the Navy, was created K.B.E. in the last year of his mother's life. He lent her portrait by Sargent to the New Hospital and it hung over the platform at a meeting to celebrate the fiftieth anniversary of her dispensary in Seymour Place. She was no longer aware of it, nor of the coming triumph of the Women's Suffrage movement, nor of Europe's tragedy.

By 1917 the war was at a critical stage. 'Ten dear young men' of the Garrett family had died in the fighting. Half the households in the country were in mourning. Women and children had to wait for hours in the wet and cold hoping for groceries or meat or bread. A pioneer of fifty years ago had no place in the present struggle for survival. On 17 December 1917, almost unnoticed by a world she had forgotten, Elizabeth Garrett Anderson died.

By her life she convinced a reluctant society that a woman could qualify for an exacting profession, and in it win the trust of her colleagues. No one could pretend that the early women doctors, so earnest and hard-working, were always popular with the men, but their conscientious devotion raised the tone of the profession, just as their presence ended for ever the brutalizing obscenities of the old medical education. In all this, Elizabeth Garrett Anderson faithfully played her part. She had brought the warmth of an entirely feminine temperament to serve the demands of a masculine discipline. As long as strength lasted she tried to serve the calling of medicine and the women's cause. Death blotted out the tragedy of her last years, leaving her achievement radiant and intact. 'I rejoice', wrote a friend, 'to think of her free at last.'

Middlesex Hospital Medical School Committee Minutes Vol. III, 13 June 1861

Mr Shaw in the Chair, Dr Thompson, Mr Heisch, Dr Murchison, Dr Cobbold, Mr Flower, Dr Greenlow, Mr Moore, Mr de Morgan, Mr Taylor, Mr Henry, Mr Sibley, Mr Nunn.

The following memorial from the Students was read and ordered to be entered in the Minutes:–

To the Lecturers of the Middlesex Hospital Medical College. Gentlemen –

We the undersigned students of your School respectfully solicit your attention to the following Memorial in reference to the admission of female students to the classes of the College:–

We consider 1st that the promiscuous assemblage of the sexes in the same class is a dangerous innovation likely to lead to results of an unpleasant character.

2nd That as in cases where the study of any other science is pursued by both sexes a separate class is formed for each (e.g. the government classes for the study of the fine arts) so must such provision be made for females before they can study the science of surgery or medicine with such advantages as are due to the importance of the subject.

3rd That the lecturers are likely (although unconsciously) to feel some restraint through the presence of females in giving that explicit and forcible enunciation of some facts which is necessary for their comprehension by the student.

4th That the presence of young females as passive spectators in the operating theatre is an outrage on our natural instincts and feelings and calculated to destroy those sentiments of respect and admiration with which the opposite sex is regarded by all right-minded men, such feelings being a mark of civilization and refinement.

Further we beg to state that the presence of a female student in the Middlesex School has become a byword and a reproach amongst similar institutions in this metropolis and that its members are subjects to taunts of a nature calculated to undermine those feelings of pride and satisfaction which ought to possess every student in reference to the School with which he is connected.

In approaching this subject we feel we have undertaken a task at once delicate and disagreeable; we have strictly avoided all allusion to the capabilities of women and the privileges of the sexes but have endeavoured to state our opinion with all respect to the feelings and sex of the person most concerned. In memorialising our Lecturers on the subject we entirely repudiate any idea of dictating or suggesting any course of conduct, yet we respectfully hope that a knowledge of the feelings which exist among the students may be of some service in guiding them in their future deliberations on this unfortunate matter.

Dated June 7th 1861. Signed James S. Turner. Chairman
4 members of committee &
38 other students

The following letter from Miss Garrett and given to the Secretary to be communicated to the Lecturers was read and ordered to be entered on the Minutes.

'Suggestions relative to the endowment of a medical scholarship for the use of women in connexion with the Medical School of the Middlesex Hospital:–

£2,000 to be invested in the Funds or in land and the interest to be paid annually to the Treasurer of the School for the perpetual education of one woman student. Candidates for the scholarship must not be less than 24 years of age. [*Elizabeth Garrett was just* 25].

Every candidate will be required to show a first class certificate for Latin and a second class certificate for Greek and Mathematics, the certificates to be those of the Queen's College, London.

Every candidate will be required to spend at least six months in the Hospital for preparatory study before she can be elected. For the opportunities of instruction she will there enjoy she will be expected to give £10 to the funds of the Hospital. [*Elizabeth Garrett had just fulfilled both these qualifications.*]

Any other woman conforming in all respects to the regulations laid down for the guidance of the candidate for the Scholarship will be admitted as a student to all classes and examinations upon paying the fees required from men students.'

It was resolved – that it is inadvisable to admit Ladies to any of the lectures delivered in this College.

Resolved – that the Students be informed that this memorial has been the means of bringing before the Lecturers a subject which would have occupied their attention previous to the next Session, and that although the Lecturers are unable to agree with much of the reasoning in the memorial they have come to the conclusion that for several reasons it will be inexpedient to admit Ladies to the Lectures in future sessions. This motion was carried by a majority of 7 to 1. [*The names of the voters are not given and it is therefore impossible to be certain who the one opponent of the resolution was. The most probable candidates – though for differing reasons – were the Dean and Mr Heisch.*]

The Secretary was directed to send a letter to Miss Garrett expressive of the Lecturers regret at their being obliged to come to the foregoing resolution. [*This paragraph has been squeezed in as an addition at the foot of the page in the Minute Book.*]

Apothecaries' Hall

[Entries in registers, showing lectures and clinical instruction completed by Elizabeth Garrett, with names of lecturers and place of work.]

FIRST YEAR

Classes	Date	Lecturer
Chemistry	Oct. 1861	Redwood Taylor (Middlesex Hospital)
Anatomy and Physiology	Nov. 1862	George Day (Prof. in the Univ. of St Andrew's)
Dissections	Oct. 1863 –Mar. 1864	Mr Little (demonstrator London Hospital)
Botany	May 1861	Bentley
Materia Medica & Therapeutics	May 1861	Dr. Thompson (Middlesex Hospital)
Practical Chemistry	May 1861	Heisch (Middlesex Hospital)

SECOND YEAR

Classes	Date	Lecturer
Anatomy	Oct. 1863 –Mar. 1864	Adams (London Hospital)
Anatomical Demonstrations & Dissections	Mar. 1864	L. S. Little (London Hospital)
Principles and Practice of Medicine	April 1865	Goodfellow (Middlesex–a complete course)

Appendix II

Clinical Medical Practice	Oct. 1860 to Mar. 1861	Middlesex Hospital
Midwifery & Diseases of Women & Children	July 1863	Keiller (Edinburgh)
Forensic Medicine & Toxicology	Aug. 1865	Harley (University College)
Clinical Medical Practice	1 Oct. 1861 –31 Mar. 1861 and April–Sept. 1861	Middlesex Hospital

THIRD YEAR

Classes	Date	Lecturer
Principles and Practice of Medicine		see above
Clinical Medical Lectures		Goodfellow
Morbid Anatomy & Clinical Medical Practice	April 1865	L. J. Little (London Hospital)
Practical Midwifery	9 July 1864	55 cases certified by Mr Heckford (London Hospital)
Vaccination	9 July 1864	Heckford (London Hospital)
Morbid Anatomy and Clinical Practice	1 Oct. 1863 –31 Mar. 1864	London Dispensary Spital Fields

[*Copy of Candidates' Entry Book, 31 March 1864*]

10. M̶r̶.*iss* Elizabeth Garrett

Daughter s̶o̶n̶ of Newson and Louisa Garrett

Born June 9 1836

355

Appendix II

An Apprentice to Mr. Joshua Plaskitt
  25 Chapel St., Belgrave Sq:
Apothecary for five years *Indenture dated* October 1st 1860
Testimonial of Moral Character Joshua Plaskitt Sept. 27
First Examination by Dr. Ward *and* approved.

  [*then follows résumé of lecturers as in large register with entry added*]
Attendance on Cases 100

  [*a marginal note records*]
Arts Exam^n. Apoth^s Hall 27th Septr 1862

  [*Copy of Candidates' Entry Book, 28 Sept. 1865*]
M$_r$.^{iss} Elizabeth Garrett
See March 31 1864 no. 10 *and* approved
2 *Examination by* Mr. Wheeler *and* approved.

APPENDIX III

Royal College of Physicians

[*Elizabeth Garrett to the Secretary Royal College of Physicians, 5 April 1864. Library of the Royal College of Physicians*]
Sir,

I wish to present myself as a candidate for the License of the College of Physicians. I have been registered as a medical student at the Apothecaries Hall, where I have also passed the preliminary examination in Arts and the first professional examination for the License.

I have at present been engaged in medical study for three years and a half (including nearly two years hospital or dispensary practise) and I can produce all necessary certificates of study from recognized teachers in acknowledged schools of medicine.

I trust you will pardon me if I mention, in addition to these details, my special reasons as a woman for desiring to become a candidate for the License of the College. In endeavouring to open the profession of medicine to women I have wished above all things *not* to assist in lowering the standard either of preliminary or professional education; and since it is proved that they cannot legally be excluded from the License of the Apothecaries Hall, and that they will in this way be able to become registered practitioners, I believe that in the interests of the public and for the honour of the profession women should be subject to the severest tests open to men. It is no longer possible to exclude women from the profession; it is only possible to confine them to one and that a comparatively easy mode of entrance.

I have the honour to remain
Sir,
Your obedient servant,
Elizabeth Garrett.

357

The Paris M.D. Examination

[Translations of Extracts from Chapter XII]

p. 190 (*a*) 'Miss Garrett,' expostulated the examiner, 'do you not know about the great men of your country?'
'But, Sir,' she replied undismayed, 'we have so many!'

p. 190 (*b*) ... severe disability of migraine proper, 'an acute pain in the head, which can be felt from time to time ... almost always accompanied by vertigo, nausea, and vomiting'.

p. 190 (*c*) 'Migraine,' she observes, 'is a genuine neurosis, and not merely the result of a disturbed digestion.'

p. 191 (*d*) ... the principal lesion is the result of malnutrition of the nervous tissues. The immediate consequence is an over-rapid discharge of the electrical impulses, which are inherent in the molecules of the nervous system.

p. 191 (*e*) It is inadvisable to attempt treatment of any sort during the attack. The efforts of friends to persuade the patient to eat, or to take some form of stimulant or remedy only increase his suffering. Generally speaking the patient needs only air, and to be alone in a darkened room in peace and quiet. Any movement is sheer torture, be it nothing but the sound of footsteps or the ticking of a watch. . . . Large quantities of very hot tea are to be recommended, whether it acts as an emetic or purge, or whether the heat has a sedative effect on the nerves of the Stomach, and of the Duodenum.

Appendix IV

Final Viva Voce Examination

[*Questions answered by Elizabeth Garrett. Translated from Collection de Thèses de l'Ecole de Medicine de Paris, Tome V, pp. 31–2.*]

Normal Anatomy and Histology
Concerning the joints of the head.

Physiology
Concerning the secretion of tears and the lachrymal ducts through which they pass to reach the exterior.

Physics
Hygrometry – the effects of the humidity of the air – variations in the level of humidity.

Chemistry
Concerning the oxygen compounds of arsenic and antimony – their preparation and their properties.

Natural History
General characteristics of the fish – classification of the species – concerning the electric fish and the venomous fish – concerning the oil obtainable from fish liver.

External Pathology
Concerning the treatment of dislocations, complicated by bone fractures.

Internal Pathology
Concerning secondary Pneumonia.

General Pathology
Concerning the influence of age on the course of different diseases.

Pathological Anatomical Abnormalities
An anatomical study of Thrombosis.

Surgical Medicine
Concerning the catheterization of the Eustachian Tube.

Pharmacology

Concerning the ether employed in the preparation of ethereal tinctures. How are these prepared? Name those most frequently used. What are the principal substances found in plants which dissolve in ether?

Therapeutics

Concerning the permissible doses of medicine in the treatment of different illnesses, according to the differing age and physical condition of the individual.

Hygiene

Concerning the effects of the varying density and rarefaction of the air on the organism.

Forensic Medicine

What are the methods employed in taking impressions of prints made by feet, or other objects, in mud, snow, etc.

Gynaecology

Concerning extra-uterine pregnancy.

Surgical Practice

[Summary of gynaecological cases treated by Elizabeth Garrett Anderson as sole surgeon at the New Hospital for Women in an average year. Reprinted from the Annual Report 1876.]

Name of Disease	Cured	Relieved	Incurable	Died
Pelvic cellulitis	3			
Ovarian tumour		1		
Ovaritis	1	4		
Menorrhagia		3		
Dysmenorrhoea		5		
Amenorrhoea		2		
Metritis	2	9		1
Subinvolutio uteri		2		
Anteversion		1		
Anteflexion		1		
Retroversion	2			
Retroflexion		2		
Procedentia		2		
Fibroid of uterus	1	4	1	
Fibroid with polypus	1	1		
Fibroma	1			
Suppurating ovarian cyst			1	
Hypertrophy of cervix		1		
Vaginal catarrh	1			
Vaginitis	1	1		
Fistula	3			
Recto-vaginal fistula		1		
Cystitis		1		
Renal disease		2		
Renal cyst		2		

Name of Disease	Cured	Relieved	Incurable	Died
Cancer of rectum		2		
Carcinoma of uterus		7		
Chlorosis	3	7		
Hysteria	3	7		
Hysterical paraplegia		2		
Hysterical coxalgia		1		
Sarcoma of breast		1		
Double mammary cancer				1
Vulvar abscess	1			
Urethral haemorrhoids	2	3		
Condylomata	1			
Umbilical hernia		2		

Readmissions 4
Total gynaecological cases 112

[*These figures cover in-patients only. Out-patients in the same year totalled 7,946 visits, of which no detailed analysis is available.*]

The Building of the New Hospital for Women

The idea of a new building in the Euston Road had great advantages. It would almost double the number of beds for clinical teaching, and reduce the waiting lists of patients. Patients too weak to walk far in all weathers could travel by train to Kings Cross and St Pancras, or by Metropolitan railway or horse bus to the Euston Road. Students could walk from the School in a few minutes. Near at hand to the north were settlements of poor and crowded dwellings. Somerstown was full of tenements, every door open, every window broken, every passage-way full of ragged children. Agar town, huddling under the arches of the Great Northern Railway, was a collection of shanties in muddy yards. The new hospital, accessible to the world, would never lack needy patients on its own back doorstep. The difficulty of the building plan was that it would cost at least £20,000 as well as the annual ground rent of £272. The idea of any public assistance or government grant was unthinkable. Elizabeth Garrett Anderson prepared to raise the sum on her own initiative. Five people, including Elizabeth and Skelton themselves, gave £1,000. Up and down the country volunteers held drawing-room meetings and filled collecting cards. Church collections, Jewish charities, dissenting chapels and Anglo-Catholic convents subscribed according to their means. Elizabeth had cast her net wide. In two years she raised over £21,000. Thereafter her energies were devoted to endowing the existing beds by yearly subscriptions and bequests and adding a maternity ward, a cancer ward, Finsen light and X-ray departments, as money became available.

The Building of the London School of Medicine for Women[1]

The Dean drew on a fund of experience gained in the rebuilding of the New Hospital. She took a long lease from the ground landlords, the Foundling Hospital, and incorporated the School under the Companies Act to free the trustees from personal responsibility. On her advice J. M. Brydon was again engaged as architect. The estimated building time was three to four years and the cost 'certainly not less than £20,000', of which £12,000 was already in the building fund. A letter to *The Times* produced an immediate £1,750, but there was no money to spare. It was necessary to raise a mortgage of £8,000 and there were very heavy expenses to pay. The Dean allowed herself a reasoned optimism. 'The School will be able,' she said, 'taking one year with another, with economy and with the help of occasional wind-falls in the way of legacies and donations to pay its way.' She herself gave sums up to a hundred pounds each year.

[1] Now the Royal Free Hospital Medical School.

SOURCES

I. Manuscript and Privately Printed

Letters of Elizabeth Garrett Anderson in:
the Anderson family papers
the Fawcett Library
the Elizabeth Garrett Anderson Hospital
the Royal Free Hospital School of Medicine
the Wellcome Historical Medical Library
the Library of the Royal College of Physicians

Reports and Minutes of:
the Society of Apothecaries
the Faculty of Medicine of Paris
the Middlesex Hospital
the London Hospital
Queen Elizabeth Hospital for Children
St Mary's Dispensary
the New Hospital for Women
the Royal Free Hospital School of Medicine
the Royal College of Surgeons of England
the School Board for London
Aldeburgh Borough Council

M.S. notes by:
J. Ford Anderson, M.D., *A Pioneer*
Sir A. G. Anderson, *The Garretts of Suffolk*
Louisa Aldrich Blake, Mrs Garrett Anderson's lectures on
Medicine at the London School of Medicine for Women, 1889

II. Publications by Elizabeth Garrett Anderson

'Volunteer Hospital Nursing', *Macmillan's Magazine*, April 1867.

'An Enquiry into the nature of the C.D. Acts', *Pall Mall Gazette*, 25 Jan. 1870.

'Sur la Migraine', École de Medicine de Paris: Thèses, 1870.

Autobiographical note, *Hampstead and Highgate Express*, 29 Oct. 1870.

'Clot in Heart and Cerebral Embolism' *British Medical Journal*, 14 Dec. 1872.

'Wholesome Houses', letter to *The Times*, 21 Jan. 1873.

'Medical Education of Women', letter to *The Times*, 5 Aug. 1873.

'Education of Girls', *Fortnightly Review*, May 1874.

Progress in Medicine, H. K. Lewis, 1877. Inaugural lecture.

'Conjoint Board Examinations', letter to *The Times*, 5 May 1878.

The Students' Pocket Book. Macmillan, 1878.

'Educational Pressure', letter to *The Times*, 15 April 1880.

'Examinations for Girls', letter to *The Times*, 17 Feb. 1881.

'Medical Women for India', letter to *The Times*, 31 Oct. 1881.

'Women's Franchise', letter to *The Times*, 31 May 1884.

'Educational Pressure', letter to *The Times*, 19 Aug. 1884.

'Medical Education of Women', letter to *The Times*, 26 Jan. 1889.

'Medical Women at Oxford', letter to *The Times*, 15 Nov. 1890.

'Clinical Teaching at Edinburgh', *The Scotsman*, 2 March 1891.

'History of a Movement', *Fortnightly Review*, March 1893.

'Appeal for London School of Medicine for Women and New Hospital for Women', letter to *The Times*, 11 Dec. 1896.

'Midwives Registration Bill', letter to *The Times*, 30 April 1898.

'Vaccination', 2 letters to *The Times*, 31 Jan., 1 Feb. 1899.

'History of Vaccination', *Edinburgh Review*, April 1899.

'Ethics of Vivisection', *Edinburgh Review*, July 1899.

'Medical Education of Women', letter to *The Times*, 24 Nov. 1900.

'Women Doctors at Pekin', letter to *The Times*, 26 April 1901.

Sources

'Vaccination', 3 letters to *The Times*, Oct.–Nov. 1901.

'Imperial Vaccination League', 3 letters to *The Times*, Feb.–
Sept., 1903.

'The Progress of Medicine since 1803', *Edinburgh Review*, Jan.
1903.

Contributions to *Encyclopaedia Medica*, Green & Sons, 15 vols.

'Medical Women in General Hospitals', letter to *The Times*,
17 Oct. 1903.

'Smallpox Hospitals', 2 letters to *The Times*, 12 and 26 Jan. 1904.

'Factory Girls' Country Holiday Fund', letter to *The Times*,
30 Aug. 1905.

'Unmarried Daughters', letter to *The Times*, 29 Nov. 1909.

'Women Suffrage Deputation', letter to *The Times*, 22 Nov. 1910.

Mary Marshall, M.D., Obituary, *British Medical Journal*, 20 Aug.
1910.

III. Newspapers and Periodicals, 1863–1912

The British Medical Journal
The Lancet
The Times
The Scotsman
The Pall Mall Gazette
The Standard
Macmillan's Magazine
The Fortnightly Review
The Edinburgh Review
Punch
All the Year Round
The Englishwoman's Journal
The Queen
The Gentlewoman
Votes for Women
The Hampstead and Highgate Express
The East Anglian Daily Times

IV. Printed

ALDBURGHAM, ALISON *A Punch History of Manners and Modes.* Hutchinson, 1961.

ANDERSON, LOUISA GARRETT *Elizabeth Garrett Anderson.* Faber, 1939.

BANKS, J. & O. *Feminism and Family Planning in Victorian England.* Liverpool University Press, 1964.

BARNARDO, MRS, and MARCHANT J. *Memoirs of Dr Barnardo.* Hodder & Stoughton, 1907.

BELL, E. MOBERLY *Storming the Citadel.* Constable, 1953. *Josephine Butler.* Constable, 1963.

BIBBY, CYRIL *T. H. Huxley.* Watts & Co., 1959.

BLACKWELL, ELIZABETH *Pioneer Work in Opening the Medical Profession to Women.* Dent, Everyman, 1914. *Essays Medical and Sociological,* 2 vols. E. Bell, 1902.

BROADBENT, M. E., ed. *The Life of Sir William Broadbent told in his own letters.* John Murray, 1909.

BROWN, FORD K. *Fathers of the Victorians.* Cambridge University Press, 1961.

BURTON, HESTER *Barbara Bodichon.* John Murray, 1949.

BUTLER, A. S. G. *Portrait of Josephine Butler.* Faber, 1954.

BUTLER, JOSEPHINE *Personal Reminiscences of a Great Crusade,* 2nd edn. Horace Marshall, 1898.

CASTIGLIONE, A. *A History of Medicine,* 2nd edn. Alfred A. Knopf. 1947.

CHANCELLOR, E. BERESFORD *Life in Regency and Early Victorian Times.* Batsford, 1926.

CLODD, EDWARD (pub. anon.) *A Guide to Aldeburgh.* J. Buck, Aldeburgh, 1861.

CLODD, H. P. *Aldeburgh, the History of an Ancient Borough.* Norman Adlard & Co., 1959.

CRABBE, GEORGE *The Poetical Works* (ed. Ward, A. W.), 2 vols. Cambridge University Press, 1905.

DURUY, VICTOR *Notes et Souvenirs*. Paris Hachette, 1882.

Encyclopaedia Medica, 15 vols. W. Green & Sons, 1899–1910.

FAWCETT, M. G. *What I Remember*. T. Fisher Unwin, 1924.

FONTANGES, H. *Les Femmes Docteurs*. Alliance Co-operative du Livre, 1901.

FRAZER, W. M. *English Public Health, 1834–1939*. Baillière, Tindall & Cox, 1950.

FULFORD, ROGER *Votes for Women*. Faber, 1957.

GEDDES, AUCKLAND CAMPBELL, LORD *The Forging of a Family*. Faber, 1952.

GLYNNE-GRYLLS, R. *Queen's College 1848–1948*. Routledge, 1948.

GORDON, H. L. *Sir James Young Simpson*. Masters of Medicine series.

HECKFORD, SARAH (foreword) *Voluntaries for an East London Hospital*. David Stott, 1887.

HOLLINGSHEAD, JOHN *Ragged London*. Smith Elder, 1861.

HUNTLEY, E. A. *The Study and Practise of Medicine by Women*. Lewes Farncombe & Co., 1886.

HUXLEY, LEONARD *Life and Letters of Thomas Henry Huxley*. Macmillan, 1900.

LIPINSKA, M. *Histoire des Femmes Medicins*. Paris: Jacques, 1900.

McGREGOR, O. R. *The Social Position of Women in England, 1850–1914*. (Reprinted from *The British Journal of Sociology*, March 1955.)

McKENZIE, K. A. *Edith Simcox and George Eliot*. Oxford University Press, 1960.

MARTINDALE, LOUISA *The Woman Doctor*. Mills & Boon, 1922.

A Woman Surgeon. Gollancz, 1951.

MEAD, K. C. H. *Women in Medicine*. Haddam Press, 1938.

MITCHISON, NAOMI (contributor) *Revaluations – Studies in Biography*. Oxford University Press, 1931.

MOORE, N. *History of St Bartholomew's Hospital.* Arthur Pearson, 1918.

MORRIS, E. W. *The History of the London Hospital.* Arnold, 1910.

MURRAY, FLORA *Women as Army Surgeons.* Hodder, 1920.

NEWMAN, CHARLES *The Evolution of Medical Education in the Nineteenth Century.* Oxford University Press, 1957.

OKEY, THOMAS *A Basketful of Memories.* J. M. Dent, 1930.

PAGET, STEPHEN *Memoirs and Letters of Sir James Paget, F.R.S.* Longmans, 1901.

PANKHURST, SYLVIA *The Suffragette Movement.* Longmans, Green, 1931.

POWER, D'ARCY *British Medical Societies.* Medical Press and Circular, 1939.

PRATT, EDWIN A. *Pioneer Women in Victoria's Reign,* Newnes, 1897.

RIVINGTON, WALTER *The Medical Profession,* 1st edn 1879, 2nd edn 1887. Baillière, Tindall & Cox.

ROSE, MILLICENT *The East End of London.* Cresset Press, 1951.

ROSS, ISHBEL *Child of Destiny.* Gollancz, 1950.

RUSSELL, BERTRAND and PATRICIA (ed.) *The Amberley Papers,* 2 vols. Hogarth Press, 1937.

SANDWITH, FRIEDA *Surgeon Compassionate – the Life of William Marsden.* Peter Davies, 1960.

SAUNDERS, HILARY ST GEORGE *The Middlesex Hospital.* Max Parrish, 1947.

SCHARLIEB, MARY *Reminiscences.* Williams & Norgate, 1924.

SCOTT, J. H. *A Short History of Spitalfields.* Privately printed, 1894.

SIMPSON, JAMES YOUNG *Obstetric Memoirs,* 2 vols. A. & C. Black, 1855.

SPRIGGE, S. SQUIRE *Life and Times of Thomas Wakley.* Longmans, 1897.

STEPHEN, BARBARA *Emily Davies and Girton College,* Constable, 1927.

STEPHEN, LESLIE *Henry Fawcett.* Smith Elder, 1886.

STRACHEY, R. *Millicent Garrett Fawcett.* John Murray, 1931. *The Cause.* Bell & Sons, 1928.

SUTHERLAND-ORR, MRS *The Life and Letters of Robert Browning.* Smith Elder. 1891.

THOMSON, H. CAMPBELL *The Middlesex Hospital Medical School.* John Murray, 1935.

THORNE, ISABEL *The Foundation and Development of the London School of Medicine for Women.* Privately printed, 1905.

TODD, MARGARET *The Life of Sophia Jex-Blake.* Macmillan, 1918.

TREVES, SIR F. *The Elephant Man and Other Essays,* Cassell, 1923.

VARIOUS HANDS *Ideas and Beliefs of the Victorians.* Sylvan Press, 1949.

VAUGHAN, PAUL *Doctors Commons – a history of the British Medical Association.* Heinemann, 1959.

WAUCHOPE, G. M. *The Story of a Woman Physician.* N. Wright & Sons, Bristol, 1963.

WHITE, W. HALE *Great Doctors of the Nineteenth Century.* Edward Arnold & Co., 1935.

Index

EGA throughout stands for Elizabeth Garrett Anderson.
N refers to footnote.
Main references only are listed for Aldeburgh, medicine, surgery, and Elizabeth Garrett Anderson.
Illustrations, and footnotes citing sources of information, are not included in the index.

Index

378

379

Index

Index